KU-775-670

Brief contents

Research Methods for Nursing and Healthcare

PEARSON EDUCATION

NURSING&HEALTH

FIRST FOR HEALTH

We work with leading authors to develop the strongest educational materials in nursing, bringing cutting-edge thinking and best learning practice to a global market.

Under a range of well-known imprints, including Pearson Education, we craft high-quality print and electronic publications that help readers to understand and apply their content, whether studying or at work.

To find out more about the complete range of our publishing, please visit us on the World Wide Web at: **www.pearsoned.co.uk.**

Research Methods for Nursing and Healthcare

John Maltby
University of Leicester

Glenn A. Williams
Nottingham Trent University

Julie McGarry
University of Nottingham

Liz Day
Sheffield Hallam University

Harlow, England • London • New York • Boston • San Francisco • Toronto
Sydney • Tokyo • Singapore • Hong Kong • Seoul • Taipei • New Delhi
Cape Town • Madrid • Mexico City • Amsterdam • Munich • Paris • Milan

Pearson Education Limited

Edinburgh Gate
Harlow
Essex CM20 2JE
England

and Associated Companies throughout the world

Visit us on the World Wide Web at:
www.pearsoned.co.uk

First published 2010

ISBN: 978-0-273-71850-5

British Library Cataloguing-in-Publication Data
A catalogue record for this book is available from the British Library

Library of Congress Cataloging-in-Publication Data
Research methods for nursing and healthcare / John Maltby . . . [et al.].
    p. ; cm.
 Includes bibliographical references and index.
 ISBN 978-0-273-71850-5
1. Nursing–Research. I. Maltby, John, 1969-
 [DNLM: 1. Nursing Research–methods. WY 20.5 R43215 2010]
 RT81.5.R464 2010
 610.73072–dc22

                                        2009049015

10 9 8 7 6 5 4 3 2 1
13 12 11 10

Typeset in *9.5 /13 pt Interstate Light* by *73*
Printed in Great Britain by Henry Ling Ltd, at the Dorset Press, Dorchester, Dorset

The publisher's policy is to use paper manufactured from sustainable forests.

Contents

Contents

Preface

We all use research skills constantly in our everyday lives. Sometimes research skills are used to describe the different numbers in our lives. We know how much of our income we spend on different things, for example, approximately how much on rent/mortgage payments, food and clothes. You would also be able to estimate what percentage of your income you spend on these things. We know roughly, on average, how much a week we spend. We know the average house prices on the street where we live. We could also find out from looking at the house prices which house in our neighbourhood is the most expensive and which is the cheapest. You also know how people generally feel about living in your neighbourhood, how people view your community and to what extent you live in a close-knit community. You use research skills to gain knowledge and to be able to assess these things.

Research skills in nursing are very similar. Nurses need to know about which sorts of drugs and treatments work and the best way to administer them, which patients have suffered the most side effects with a certain drug, which patients have had the least side effects and to what extent they have felt these side effects. Nurses have to know about which percentage of patients with a leg ulcer recover the quickest with a certain treatment so that they can implement practice that is evidence-based. Nurses should know about the likelihood that patients with a specific cancer can survive with early treatment by using facts and figures of survival rates and also differences in approaches to treatment. Nurses also need to understand service users' and carers' perspectives and experiences of health and health care. In the nursing profession, many of the things that affect your work have been guided by research skills.

The aim of this book is to provide an introduction to research methods and analysis tools using a simplistic approach to give you a basic working understanding of research methods and analysis skills in a real-world health setting. There is a multitude of research methods available to researchers and in this book we will present research methods, analysis and decisions in research to you in a user-friendly, approachable and practice-based way. This will help you address issues underpinning more advanced thinking and research problems in research. This progression will help you create a knowledge and skills base for yourself, giving you confidence, knowledge and skills that will be invaluable throughout your nursing career.

Acknowledgements

Our appreciation goes to the whole editorial and production team at Pearson Education that have been involved in producing this book: David Harrison (Acquisition Editor); Georgina Clark-Mazo (Senior Editor); Sophie Playle (Editorial Assistant); Kay Holman (Production Controller); and Colin Reed (Text Designer).

We would also like to thank the reviewers. We would like to especially thank them for devoting their valuable time, incredible patience and superb guidance.

John Maltby
Glenn A. Williams
Julie McGarry
Liz Day

Publisher's acknowledgements

We are grateful to the following for permission to reproduce copyright material:

Figures
Figure 7.1 adapted from *Experiential Learning: Experience as a Source of Learning and Development*, Prentice Hall, NJ (Kolb, D.A.) p.21 copyright © 1984, adapted with the permission of Pearson Education, Inc., Upper Saddle River, NJ.; Figure 7.3 after *Becoming Critical*, Falmer Press, Lewes (Carr, W. and Kemmis, S. 1986), copyright © Taylor & Francis Books, 1986; Figure 12.2 adapted from 'General Medical Practitioners need to be aware of the theories on which our work depend', *Annals of Family Medicine*, 4(5), pp. 450–4, July/August 2006 (P. Thomas, FRCGP, MD), copyright © Annals of Family Medicine.

Screenshots
Screenshot 4.1 Output from a search on Google for 'What information is out there on older people and their quality of life in community settings?', www.google.co.uk, copyright © Google; Screenshot 4.2 A typical screen dump from Google Scholar with a search of 'What information is out there on older people and their quality of life in community settings?', www.google.co.uk, copyright © Google; Screenshot 4.3a 'The disability paradox: high quality of life against all odds', *Social Science & Medicine*, 48 (8), pp. 977–88 (Albrecht, G.L. and Devlieger, P. J. 1999), Elsevier, copyright © 1999 Elsevier Science Ltd, all rights reserved; Screenshot 4.3c 'Measuring health status in older patients. The SF-36 in practice' by Parker, S.G., Peet, S.M., Jagger, M.F., Farhan and Castleden, C.M., *Age and Ageing*, copyright © 1998 Oxford University Press and granted with permission of Oxford University Press and Professor Stuart G. Parker; Screenshots 4.10, 4.11, 4.12, 4.13 from ISI Web of Knowledge from Thomson Reuters, granted with permission.

Tables
Table 6.2 from *Qualitative Research Practice: A Guide for Social Science Students and Researchers*, Sage, London (Ritchie, J. and Lewis, J. 2003), reproduced by permission

Text

Chapter 1

An introduction to research methods

KEY THEMES

Research process • Theory • Research • Quantitative research • Qualitative research • Variables • Evidence-based practice

LEARNING OUTCOMES

At the end of this chapter you will be able to:

- Outline the research process

- Understand the nature of variables and how to identify them in research papers

- Outline the distinction between theory and research and see how the two are intrinsically linked

- Understand that there is a distinction between quantitative and qualitative research

- Understand what is meant by variables and how they are important to the research process

- Appreciate how theory, research and the research process fit into ideas of evidence-based practice and implementation.

Introduction

You engage in research every day. Don't believe us? Well take for example the scenario that you get up slightly late and you are wondering whether you should skip breakfast this morning. You know that if you skip breakfast in the morning that it is possibly bad for you, but you know that you will be ok. That is, you have researched it. You know from reading health articles that there is evidence that people who skip breakfast are less able to concentrate during the day. However, you know that you have missed breakfast on a number of occasions and are quite able to skip breakfast regularly without any noticeable effect on your concentration. Therefore the whole issue of whether you can skip breakfast or not, you have researched. You have collected evidence from magazines and your own experiences and you analysed this research and decided that on balance you can skip breakfast this morning. This, basically, is what research is. It is the process of collecting evidence that allows you to make decisions regarding certain questions.

And there is a lot of it. Research is going on all the time. You are surrounded by research. Research is going on every minute of the day, and it is informing all sorts of things, including the type of food that is available to you in your local supermarket, the type of television that is scheduled for you to watch in the evening, what the current interest rates are and what clothes are fashionable. For the large majority of aspects of life out there, research will have been involved. Your local supermarket will have researched what types of food are bought regularly by people in your area, and this will inform what is available. Television researchers will have found out what types of programmes are more popular in the evening and this will inform the schedules. Those determining interest rates will have researched whether prices of a range of commodities will have gone up.

Of course in your profession there is also a lot of research going on. Medical researchers investigate what are the best types of drug. Surgeons will have determined what the best operating procedures are. Your hospital will have researched what is the best type of care to provide to individuals on head injury wards. You yourself will have researched the best way that you can help a patient on a ward who is in distress. The role of research in your profession is crucial, from the types of drugs you administer to the level of care you provide.

As a nurse you will use research in your practice: in your work you must carry out evidence-based practice, that is, nursing involves making decisions in your work on patient characteristics and situations but also on the available evidence. Research informs that available evidence and therefore you need to be able to search out, understand and use research to support your practice. For example the National Institute for Health and Clinical Excellence (NICE), an independent organisation responsible for providing national guidance on promoting good health and preventing and treating ill health, emphasises the importance of evidence-based practice and proper implementation of research by suggesting in their guidelines that all practitioners use the best available evidence for the appropriate treatment and care of people.

The aim of this book is to break down the research process for you and show you how it applies not only to your academic thinking but your everyday practice, so you can carry out evidence-based practice. There are many different types of research out there and we will slowly and deliberately take you through many of these aspects so you can build up your confidence and repertoire of research methods.

1.1 The research process

Formally the research process looks something like Figure 1.1. Generally all research projects will follow a certain order of stage and in Figure 1.1 we have outlined each of these stages. In the first column we outline these stages in everyday language. In the second column, each corresponding row gives more formal titles to each stage.

Therefore all research processes start with an assessment of what is known about a particular topic (1), going on to some sort of determination of something that we need to know more about with regard to that topic (2). The next stage of the research process is to devise a way to look at that something we need to know about and then after looking at it (3). Then after looking at the topic, we determine what we have

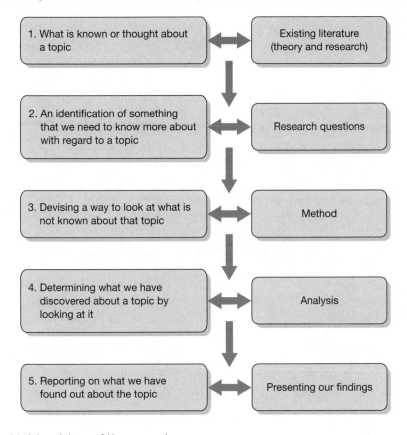

Figure 1.1 A breakdown of the research process.

discovered about a topic (4). We then present to others on what we have found out about the topic (5). To then present this in more research-based language:

- All research processes start with an assessment of what is known or thought about a particular topic (1), = **existing literature** (theory and research, i.e. books and journal articles on the topic).
- Going on to some sort of determination of something that we need to know more about with regard to that topic (2) = **research question.**
- The next stage of the research process is to devise a way to look at that something we need to know about and then after looking at it (3) = **method.**
- Then after looking at the topic, we determine what we have discovered about a topic (4) = **analysis.**
- We then report to others on what we have found out about the topic (5) = **presenting our findings.**

Let us illustrate with an example you are likely to come across in your sample. Say for example a new disease is discovered that attacks the liver. We will first visit the existing literature, i.e. what theory and research exists. Within this **literature** we discover there is good and bad news. The bad news is that we find out that there is no cure for this disease. However, the good news is that the **literature** suggests that the development of a drug will combat the disease, as similar drugs have been used with similar diseases and have cured such a disease. We will then have a **research question,** will developing a compound of these drugs help us combat the disease? We will have to develop a **method** for seeing whether it will work, i.e. we will have to trial the drug among patients. We will have to perform an **analysis** of the effects of the drug on those patients will inform us whether the drug can successfully combat the disease. Let us imagine that the drug is successful (it is too early in the chapter to bring bad news). We would then **present our findings** (by talking about them, written reports or discussion) back to the medical community reporting on the success of the new drug.

A further point is that what you will find in the research process usually forms a circle of activity (see Figure 1.2), with the presentation of findings feeding into the

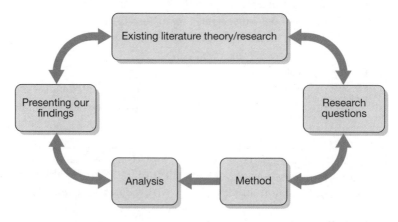

Figure 1.2 The research process cycle.

literature and researchers thinking up further research questions, methods and analysis to carry out leading to more and more presentations of findings. Nonetheless the chapters in this book are broken down into the first cycle of stages, and we will use the next sections to introduce you to each of these stages (literature, research questions, method, analysis and reporting your findings), before you go on to study them in detail in the different chapters. Though you will see that it is sometimes useful to pair these process together.

1.2 Variables

In the last section we introduced you to the research process. One central key aspect to the research process is the variable. The **variable** is the most crucial part of research. If we were to describe the research process as a moving car, then we would call the 'variable' the engine of the car, the mechanism that drives the car (research) so that it can move forward.

How do you view the world? Do you view it as made up of good and evil, of right- or left-wing political thought, or of those who are rich and those who are poor? Or do you view the world in terms of your profession, those who care for others, and those who are cared for? Or those who are well or those who are ill? In this section we are going to introduce you to another way of viewing the world . . . that is, by seeing the world as made up of variables.

IMAGINE THAT . . .
You are a leg ulcer specialist nurse and are trying to decide on the most effective methods for treating your patients' leg ulcers – do you use a short-stretch bandage or a medium-stretch one? How would you assess the effectiveness of the dressing? Through its (1) comfort, (2) ability to alleviate pain or (3) effect on how quickly the leg ulcer heals? All three ways of looking at the effectiveness of a type of dressing can be labelled 'variables' as they can vary for different groups of patients and depending on how severe the leg ulcer is (another variable). We will be identifying more variables in this chapter as the notion of having variables to analyse is the cornerstone of any statistics that you will be doing in your studies and your nursing career.

The idea of *variables* is central to statistics. In this chapter we are going to tell you what variables are and get you working with them. You use variables every day in your life (the time you get up in the morning, the amount of money you spend on different things during the day), and the notion that many things are variables in your life is a key aspect of statistics. What we will show you in this chapter is how variables can be understood and defined in our lives, which will then give you a powerful basis for understanding some of our later points about research methods and statistics.

Variables are quite simply things that vary. We are surrounded by variables, for example different types of events or objects, our feelings and attitudes and other people's feelings and attitudes. Instances of these could be the different times that people get up in the morning, the different types of breakfast they might have (if any), the way that people feel about work, the number of hours they spend watching television at night and the time they go to bed. These examples are slightly flippant, but valid. As researchers we tend to be interested in those variables related to our discipline. An economist would be interested in interest rates, unemployment figures and levels of supply and demand. However, as nurses, you will be most interested in how well patients recover after becoming ill, the different types of illness they face, and the treatment options available to them.

In this section you will explore how to identify variables and then how to do so within academic titles and text.

Identifying variables

One important skill that researchers must have is to be able to identify accurately the variables which exist in an area of research. We are going to spend a little time looking at how to develop the skill of identifying variables. Read the article by James Meikle in Box 1.1.

BOX 1.1 TASK

Scientists warn of 30 per cent rise in human BSE

Government scientists yesterday warned of a sharply accelerating trend in the incidence of human BSE after studying the pattern of the disease so far.

They said the number of reported cases may in fact be rising at between 20 per cent and 30 per cent a year despite the apparently varied annual death rates over the past five years.

The prediction came as it was revealed that the death toll from the incurable condition officially known as vCJD had risen by a further 2 in the past fortnight to a total of 69, and 14 so far this year.

The scientists said that there was now a 'statistically significant rising trend' in the number of victims since the first casualties first displayed signs of the disease in 1994, although it was still too early to forecast the ultimate number of deaths caused by vCJD.

This year's toll is already equal to that for the whole of last year when the number dropped. A further seven people still alive are thought to be suffering from the condition. The scientists have come to their conclusion about the progress of the disease after analyses of monthly figures, including studying the dates at which friends, relatives or doctors first noted symptoms.

The period between this and eventual death has varied between 7 and 38 months, with an average of 14 months, although the incubation period before symptoms become evident is believed to be several years longer.

Stephen Churchill was the first known death from the disease in May 1995, although it was not formally identified or officially linked to the eating of beef in the late 1980s until March 1996. Three people died in 1995, 10 in 1996, 10 in 1997, 18 in 1998 and 14 last year.

Members of the government's spongiform encephalopathy advisory committee took the unusual step of publishing the figure immediately after their meeting in London yesterday because of the recent interest in a cluster of five cases around Queniborough in Leicestershire. These included three victims dying within a few of months in 1998, a fourth

▶

who died in May and another patient, still alive, who is thought to be suffering from the same disease.

The scientists said this was 'unlikely to have occurred by chance but this cannot be completely ruled out' and they would be closely informed about local investigations. The Department of Health last night said it could not elaborate on the significance of the new analysis until ministers and officials had considered the scientists' new advice.

The figures came amid reports that sheep imported by the US from Europe were showing signs of a disease, which could be linked to BSE in cattle. Government scientists are to hold talks with their US counterparts after the US agriculture department ordered the destruction of three flocks of sheep, which were in quarantine in the state of Vermont.

Source: James Meikle, 'Scientists warn of 30 per cent rise in human BSE: What's wrong with our food?', *The Guardian*, 18 July 2000. © The Guardian Newspapers Limited, 2000, reproduced with permission.

You will see from this article that there are many variables in which government scientists are interested. At one level it may seem that scientists are interested only in the levels of vCJD, and in how many people have died of vCJD. However, there are other variables that can be identified within this article:

- the year in which people died (to consider trends in the disease);

- changes in the frequency of vCJD, by looking at changes from one year to the next;

- the time period between which 'friends, relatives or doctors first noted the symptoms' and eventual death, which varies from 7 to 38 months;

- whether people have died of vCJD or another related disease;

- where the vCJD case occurred. Here there is an emphasis on Queniborough in Leicestershire.

We can see, therefore, that even within a fairly straightforward area of research, many variables emerge during the course of an investigation.

A useful thinking skill that you can develop is to be able to identify what possible variables are contained within a research area. Read the next article by Kirsty Scott, which appeared in the same issue of *The Guardian* (Box 1.2). Try to identify, and list in the box, as many variables as you can see emerging from this report. You should be able to name several.

Identifying variables within academic titles and text

What is particularly interesting about the example in Box 1.2 is that the report begins to speculate about some of the causes of lung cancer. The researchers suggest that a number of different variables have contributed to lung disease. These include whether workers have worked excessive hours, the number of times they may have worked excessive hours, and whether protective equipment is worn.

Also, being able to identify how variables relate to other variables is central to any research. All researchers are interested in asking, and trying to answer, research

BOX 1.2 TASK

Miners' long hours blamed as lung disease returns

Miners at a Scottish colliery are suffering from a serious lung disease that health experts thought had been virtually eradicated.

Routine tests have found that nine miners at the Longannet colliery in Fife have developed pneumoconiosis, or black lung, which is caused by inhaling coal dust. A further 11 have abnormalities in the lungs, an early stage of the condition. The condition, which can lead to debilitating and sometimes fatal respiratory disease, was thought to have almost disappeared with the introduction of new safety and screening measures in the mid-1970s.

Last year a compensation scheme was agreed for miners affected by the disease after the biggest ever personal injury action in the UK. A Health and Safety Executive report on the Longannet findings is expected to blame excessive working hours and a failure to use protective equipment properly.

Dan Mitchell, HSE chief inspector of mines, said it was unusual to have found such an outbreak. 'But certainly in recent years the number of workers in mines attending for X-ray has been falling,' he said. 'It's not as good as it used to be and we only know about the prevalence of disease from the people who are X-rayed.'

The re-emergence of the disease has also surprised medical authorities at the Scottish pulmonary vascular unit at the Western Infirmary in Glasgow. 'I am really quite surprised because we have known about this condition for years and screening measures have been in place for years,' said the unit head, Andrew Peacock. 'We know what causes it. We expect old cases from the past but new cases coming along now does surprise me.'

Under regulations introduced in 1975 miners are only supposed to work 7-hour shifts, but many work overtime. They are also expected to have lung X-rays every five years, but at Longannet only around 70 per cent of men took part on the last occasion.

Representatives from the National Union of Mineworkers met HSE officials yesterday to discuss the situation. Peter Neilsen, vice-president of the NUM in Scotland, said: 'We thought that disease had disappeared. As a union we are concerned and it is our intention to take stock of the situation.'

The Scottish Coal Deep Mine Company, which runs Longannet, issued a statement saying that health of employees was of the utmost concern. More than 82,000 claims for compensation have been filed since the miners won their health case against the government and the nationalised coal industry. They claimed it had been known for decades that dust produced in the coal mining process could cause diseases like emphysema and chronic bronchitis and that not enough was done to protect them.

Source: Kirsty Scott, 'Miners' long hours blamed as lung disease returns', *The Guardian*, 18 July 2000. © The Guardian Newspapers Limited, 2000, reproduced with permission.

Now list as many variables as you can find in the above article.

....

....

....

....

....

questions about the relationships between variables. Some researchers will refer to research questions in different ways as hypotheses, aims or objectives, but basically these are terms used to answer a question about research. Therefore, a research question a nurse might ask is whether smoking (Variable 1: whether a person smokes) is a cause of heart disease (Variable 2: whether a person develops heart disease).

So far, we have used examples where researchers may be seeking to establish connections between variables. However, it is also worth noting that researchers are sometimes equally interested in *not* finding relationships between variables. For example, a research nurse would be interested in ensuring that a new drug does not have any major side effects.

Using the captions from the newspaper articles in Box 1.3, try to identify the variables and what possible links the journalists and researchers are trying to identify and establish.

BOX 1.3 TASK

Try identifying variables from these headlines from a variety of nursing publications.

Adult branch nursing articles

'Cold comfort: the impact of poverty on older people's health'
Nursing Standard (2004) 19(5): 1

'Pain-free heart attacks raise risk of death'
Nursing Times (2004) 100(33): 6

Learning disability branch nursing articles

'The impact of nurse education on staff attributions in relation to challenging behaviour'
Learning Disability Practice (2004) 7(5): 16

'Choice-making for people with a learning disability'
Learning Disability Practice (1998) 1(3): 22

Mental health branch nursing articles

'Half of mental health service users back concept of compulsory home treatment'
Nursing Times (2004) 100(41): 5

'The role of lithium clinics in the treatment of bipolar disorder'
Nursing Times (2004) 100(27): 42

Child branch nursing articles

'Sedentary kids more likely to get ME'
Nursing Times (2004) 100(41): 9

....

'How nurse intervention is tackling child obesity'
Nursing Times (2004) 100(31): 26

....

Repeat the exercise with some academic journal titles (Box 1.4).

BOX 1.4 TASK

Try identifying variables from these journal article titles.

'Symptoms of anxiety and depression among mothers of pre-school children: effect of chronic strain related to children and child care-taking'
(Naerde, 2000)

....

'Characteristics of severely mentally ill patients in and out of contact with community mental health services'
(Barr, 2000)

....

'Gender and treatment differences in knowledge, health beliefs, and metabolic control in Mexican Americans with type B diabetes'
(Brown *et al.*, 2000)

....

So now you should be thinking of many things as variables. This is an important research skill to learn, so let us do a little exercise to finish. In your nursing practice, you will need to handle different ways of measuring things, ranging from assessing a patient's health needs to seeing how well a treatment has worked. In Box 1.5, write down

BOX 1.5 TASK

Energiser table

Things measured in nursing practice	Unit of measure
1. Size of leg ulcer	In cm^2
2. Patient's pain	From 1 to 5 (1 = low pain to 5 = extremely severe pain)
3. Severity of person's learning disability	From 'mild' to 'moderate' to 'severe'

▶

4. ....

5. ....

6. ....

7. ....

8. ....

9. ....

10. ....

in the space provided the things that you may need to measure in your everyday practice. Also, write down in the second column how you measure these things. Three examples have been provided to give you some ideas.

1.3 Looking more closely at aspects of the research process

Now you have seen the important aspects of the research process there are two important distinctions in the research cycle that we want to bring to your attention:

- The distinction between theory and research
- The distinction in research between qualitative and quantitative research

The distinction between theory and research

The literature on any topic you are likely to study is likely to be huge. The first way that you can break down any literature is by **theory** and **research**. You may have used the term theory, before, in sentences such as 'it's only a theory' as if to say 'it's only an opinion' or 'it's just pure speculation'. In the nursing literature (and indeed many literature), a theory does not mean opinion or speculation. A theory means a framework for describing a set of phenomena.

To use a rather simple example, let's imagine there are two wards in a hospital, Ward A and Ward B. Both wards deal with similar sorts of patients, female patients over the age of 65 who have had some minor surgery. You regularly work on Ward A with a team of four that you have worked with over the last 18 months, however they require some cover on Ward B because there have been a lot of illnesses and time off among staff on that ward. So you have taken some shifts on Ward B. You've only worked a few shifts on Ward B, but despite dealing with similar patients you've noticed a number of differences between the two wards. What you've discovered is that in contrast to Ward A, there seems to be a high level of non-concordance, for example

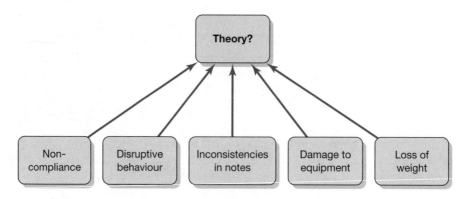

Figure 1.3 Creating a theory.

treatments and medication not administered as prescribed and patient complaints. You've found a lot of inconsistencies in the notes of patients, that there is damage to equipment and among many of the patients there is a tendency to lose weight.

You might wonder why this is happening. Clearly something is happening on Ward B that marks it out from Ward A, despite dealing with a very similar ward of patients. A good theory would be something that sought to explain this set of phenomena; i.e. non-compliance, disruptive behaviour, inconsistencies in notes, damage to equipment, loss of weight). In the box in Figure 1.3 write down your theory which might explain the following phenomena.

We would argue that it is not just to do with the type of patients admitted to Ward B. It would be unusual if a series of patients with these potential problems ended up on a particular ward, while those who did not have these potential problems ended up on another. We would suggest therefore that it may be something to do with the environment, and one possible theory (and we emphasise theory) here is that it is to do with high levels of staff turnover on Ward B while Ward A seems to have relatively low levels of staff turnover, with the same four people working on the same ward for 18 months.

However, we never know whether a theory has any support or not, regardless of how likely or reasonable it is that the theory might explain a phenomena. For example you may have come up with another theory which might equally explain the set of phenomena describe above. However, there is a way you can find out whether there is any support for your theory, and this is where research can help.

To see if you could find some support for your theory you could try to find evidence by carrying out **research** in other hospitals and examine whether wards in other hospitals show a similar pattern, i.e. do patients in wards with high staff turnover show higher levels of patient complaints than patients in wards with a low staff turnover? The research part of the process would be to identify wards where there had been a lot of absence through illness and time off among staff and identify wards where this was much less common. Then you would find a way of assessing non-concordance and complaints, inconsistencies in notes, damage to equipment and loss of weight among these wards.

When you had finished this research, if you found a similar pattern of behaviour in other hospitals to the first hospital, this finding would provide further support for your theory. If you didn't find a similar pattern, and there were similar behavioural patterns across wards with high and low staff turnover, then you did not find support for your theory.

This is the main point about theory and research. They are intrinsically linked. Theory informs research, and research informs theory. All theories, particularly scientific ones, are always provisional and always subject to modification or to be challenged, when considered in the context of research findings. For example, in the light of finding similar behavioural patterns across both wards with high and low staff turnover you might reject your theory or modify your idea in some way.

The distinction between quantitative and qualitative research

One of the main themes of this book is the distinction that is made between quantitative and qualitative research. All through this book we will illustrating the different aspects of these two different types of research, but we're just going to spend a little time here outlining their characteristics.

Put simply quantitative research is based around numbers. You remember maths at school, no doubt with fondness. It involved numbers, but it also emphasised other things. Quantitative research does so in much the same way: it uses numbers, measurement, quantities and patterns and it seeks to quantify information. On the other hand, qualitative research aims to provide an in-depth understanding and seeks to explore the reasons behind any phenomena. Therefore it is concerned with meaning, particularly the meaning people attach to their actions and their beliefs.

To illustrate this, we are going to give you a simple example, by asking you a question, and we would like an honest and full answer. We're going to use your answer to illustrate some of the points we are going to make in this chapter. Don't worry, there are no right or wrong answers, so we are not going to analyse it (there is no key at the end of this chapter saying if you put this you are mostly this . . .) but we need you to answer it as honestly and as fully as you can.

In the box below, answer the question 'How do you know that *you* (as in you the person reading this book) are a good person?' Try to write as many things as possible.

Now you, and other people, will have written different answers to this question. They will be many and varied, but we can use some of the possible answers to this question to illustrate the distinction between quantitative and qualitative research.

Some people might have written down answers such as:

I give money to charity.

I do volunteer work.

I am kind to people.

These answers lend themselves to the quantitative side of research because we can do things with these questions that lend themselves to ideas of quantity, measurement and numbers. For example, we can quantify how much money people give to charity, or how often they give to charity. We can quantify how often people do volunteer work or what type of volunteer work they do. We can quantify how kind people are to others or in what ways they are kind. The point is that we can quantify these questions in terms of understanding 'what it is to be good'. That is, we can research the idea in a quantitative way by measuring how often or how much people engage in certain acts.

Imagine someone had written in response to the question above:

I have a kind and caring nature, and believe that we should help people whenever possible. This is important because it helps society as a whole, because kind acts can be passed on from one person to another. I had a difficult childhood and I wouldn't want people to suffer in the same way.

This comment is much more difficult to quantify. It would be really hard to measure this, in the same way that we can easily attach numbers to how much people give to charity. Nonetheless it does provide us with a very powerful example of what it is to be good. That is because it lends itself much more readily to the qualitative tradition by providing an in-depth understanding of a question, and seeks to explore reasons behind any phenomena.

This is perhaps a good starting approach: you should employ research methods when first considering quantitative and qualitative research. That is, these research distinctions allow us to approach questions and problems in research in different ways that can be used largely to complement each other. A good way of remembering this distinction is that quantitative research is primarily concerned with the *What*, *Where*, and *When* of research and qualitative research is concerned with the *How* and *Why* of research (see Figure 1.4).

Please note we have presented a rather simplistic interpretation of the differences between quantitative and qualitative research as there are debates about this distinction. However, we have done this to get you started in the area and the way we have presented these two research traditions is an excellent starting point. We will expand your view and appreciation of the differences and similarities between the research traditions over the course of this book.

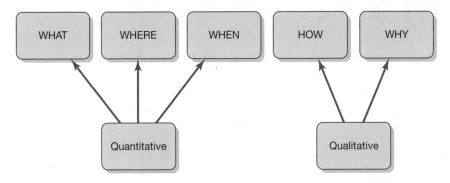

Figure 1.4 The what, where, when, how and why of research.

1.4 The research process, theory and research: quantitative and qualitative aspects: analysing variables – the basis of the book

The reason we have highlighted the research process, theory and research and quantitative and qualitative aspects to research is that these themes continue through the rest of the book. Again and again throughout this book you will be revisiting these distinctions and ideas. Therefore, in this last section we are going to set out the rest of the book so you can not only plan your study but will also be aware about how the book is telling you about each of the main aspects of the research at each stage. We have presented an overview of this in Figure 1.5.

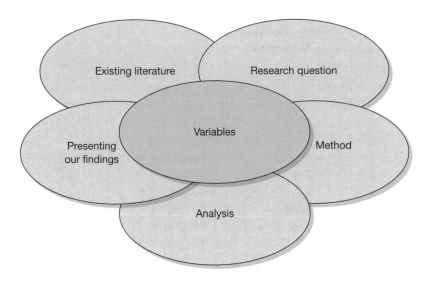

Figure 1.5(a) An overview of the development of core themes of the book.

	The Research Process					Theory and research		Quantitative and qualitative	
	Existing literature	Research questions	Method	Analysis	Presenting findings	Theory	Research	Quantitative	Qualitative
Chapter 2 Quantitative methodologies and research designs			✓			✓	✓	✓	
Chapter 3 Qualitative research methodologies and methods			✓			✓	✓		✓
Chapter 4 Reading the literature and generating research ideas	✓	✓				✓	✓	✓	✓
Chapter 5 Setting up your study: methods in data collection	✓	✓	✓					✓	✓
Chapter 6 Qualitative analysis: a step-by-step guide				✓			✓		✓
Chapter 7 Blending qualitative and quantitative methods: action research				✓				✓	✓
Chapter 8 Quantitative analysis: using descriptive statistics				✓			✓	✓	
Chapter 9 Interpreting inferential statistics in quantitative research				✓		✓	✓	✓	
Chapter 10 Critical appraisal of quantitative and qualitative research				✓	✓	✓	✓	✓	✓
Chapter 11 Presenting your work to others	✓	✓	✓	✓	✓	✓	✓	✓	✓
Chapter 12 Advanced thinking in research methods and practice: from novice to expert nurse researcher	✓	✓	✓	✓	✓	✓	✓	✓	✓
Chapter 13 Going forward: a step-by-step guide from research idea to ethics application	✓	✓	✓	✓	✓	✓	✓	✓	✓

Figure 1.5(b) Continued

As you can see from Figure 1.5, we start looking at some of the thinking and theory that underpin research methods. In Chapters 2 (Quantitative methodologies and research designs) and 3 (Qualitative research methodologies and methods) we look at different research designs and methods but draw a distinction between how quantitative and qualitative dimensions of research impacts on different research methods. These chapters will inform a decision-making process and demonstrate the theoretical emphasis when planning research designs and the general research approaches that one can take in selecting a research method. In these chapters we will detail the types of method that are available to you such as experiments, clinical trials, surveys, interviews, focus groups and case studies, and the type of research designs that underpin these methods.

In Chapter 4, Reading the literature and generating research ideas, we will be concentrating on the literature and research question aspects of the research process, emphasising theory and research. First we will provide a systematic approach to finding and appraising relevant literature for any topic. In this chapter we will include information about how to identify good literature sources and use them effectively. We will then visit research ideas, identifying avenues for generating research ideas and how to identify important research questions.

In Chapter 5, Setting up your study: methods in data collection, we will get you started in actually carrying out research. As you can see from Figure 1.5, this research concentrates on the 'methods' side of the research process and is based around the idea of things to consider before collecting data. This chapter will also detail the different considerations that need to be made before and when collecting your data depending on the type of methodology chosen.

Chapters 6, Qualitative analysis: a step-by-step guide, 7, Blending qualitative and quantitative methods: action research, 8, Quantitative analysis: using descriptive statistics and 9, Interpreting inferential statistics in quantitative research, deal with the analysis side of research and are again split, largely, between quantitative and qualitative analysis techniques. In these chapters we will introduce you to a number of qualitative analysis techniques such as conversational analysis, discourse analysis, grounded theory, interpretative phenomenological analysis and content analysis, and quantitative analysis techniques such as descriptive and inferential statistical tests.

Chapters 10 and 11 are designed to get you thinking properly and accurately about your research and the possible contributions that it can make in terms of two aspects of the research process, analysis and presenting your findings. Chapter 10, Critical appraisal of quantitative and qualitative research, is concerned with critical appraisals of your research using both quantitative and qualitative approaches and will contain techniques and strategies for making sure you get the best out of your research analysis. Chapter 11, Presenting your work to others, is concerned with presenting your research, whether it be in oral or written form. Therefore this chapter contains sections on being an effective speaker and presenter, deciding on your message and using feedback effectively.

Chapters 12 and 13, Advanced thinking in research methods and practice: from novice to expert nurse researcher and Going forward: a step-by-step guide from research idea to ethics application, bring together all aspects of the research process in the context of considering theory and research, as well as quantitative and qualitative aspects of the research process. In Chapter 12 we will raise some is-sues that you may immediately find of benefit when taking your research forward, but may not have encountered in the first instance during the book. Chapter 13 is designed to get you to experience parts of the next stages in research that you are likely to experience so you are able to move on confidently to more independent research work.

1.5 Evidence-based practice

All of this knowledge feeds into the approach adopted in nursing today of evidence-based practice. The need for knowledge in research has become increasingly crucial in the practice of nursing in modern-day medicine. Previously, nursing emphasised the medical model, that is, health problems were diagnosed and treated medically. However, today this type of practice has evolved into another model, **evidence-based practice**.

Within nursing evidence-based practice (EBP) is an approach where all people involved in the profession use the best, most appropriate, most suitable methods to treat patients. The approach is a framework for you to work within and it is re-ferred to continually throughout health care. As a nurse evidence-based practice will help you make sense of knowledge derived from research and use it as a basis for making decisions. Evidence-based practice emphasises that nursing care today is complex, treatments are uncertain, patients are different, nothing always works 100 per cent, no provision of care is always effective, and patients react differently to different types of care. EBP is designed to highlight these issues, and ensure that your judgement is based on a number of sources. That your treatment of any patient is based on the integration of a number of sources about the patient which includes:

- Patient reports (i.e. what the patient tells you) and information from relatives, carers and views from other health professionals, your observations about the patient, and
- Research-based evidence.

It is this last section of this list, research-based evidence, that this book con-tributes to. It is important for the modern-day nurse to bring research-based evi-dence to their everyday practice: evidence-based practice relies on you as a nurse reviewing information and collecting data, rather than just relying on the rules of the profession or single observation of patients. The rest of the book will teach you all about different aspects of research so you can identify, understand and use research evidence in your practice.

Self-assessment exercise

At the end of each chapter we are going to give you a quick task to do. You will have done a number of tasks throughout the chapter to test your learning but here we're going to give you a task to help you in your research career. For this chapter your task is to do the following:

● Register with *Nursing Times*. The journal details nursing practice, clinical research, and NHS and health care news with nurse specialist pages. It can be found online at **http://www.nursingtimes.net/**.

● Throughout this book you will asked to look up research. At this stage, you should find out what online library resources including databases and e-journals you have access to.

Summary

You have now been introduced to some of the main ideas that will be detailed throughout this book. You know the main aspects of the research process; literature, research questions, method, analysis and presenting your findings. You know how variables are important to research, and you should also be able to outline the distinction between theory and research and appreciate how the two are intrinsically linked. You should now appreciate that there is a distinction between quantitative and qualitative research. Finally, you should now know how the development of your research knowledge will aid you in your evidence-based practice.

In the next two chapters we are going to tell you about all the different methodology and research designs that are available to you in your nursing research. In these chapters we want to give you a background to what methodologies and research designs are out there for you to use. There are many of them, and all of them can be used to answer a research question, but they split down into two main areas; quantitative and qualitative. We will cover quantitative research methodologies and designs in Chapter 2, and qualitative research methodologies and designs in Chapter 3.

Chapter 2

Quantitative methodologies and research designs

KEY THEMES

Quantitative methodologies • Quantitative designs • Positivism •
Experimental • Quasi-experimental • Survey designs • Clinical trials •
Randomised controlled trials • Case-control design • Cohort studies •
Cross-sectional surveys • Longitudinal surveys

LEARNING OUTCOMES

At the end of this chapter you will be able to:

● Describe how quantitative methodology results from the philosophy of
  positivism, and that certain assumptions are being made about the way the
  world can be measured in a scientific and objective way

● Appreciate that positivism underpins three major groups of quantitative
  research designs in nursing research: experimental, quasi-experimental and
  survey designs

● Understand that the methodologies and research designs covered in this
  chapter, and the next chapter, all help to inform evidence-based practice in
  nursing.

Introduction

In this chapter, we are going to learn more about research that involves the measurement of health and health care in a **quantitative** way, which means information is collected in quantities. The common theme to virtually all quantitative research is that it involves the handling of numerical information (information involving numbers) and quantitative research is best known for its use of numerical information. Numbers can provide insights into many aspects of health and health care. It can inform you how common a disease is at any given time among the population (i.e. prevalence, the percentage of the population who have a disease comprises numerical information), the risks of contracting a disease (the odds of catching a disease comprises numerical information) and can tell you a lot about whether one method of treating an illness is better or worse than another mode of treatment by comparing the number of symptoms of people following each mode of treatment (the number of symptoms comprises numerical information). Therefore quantitative research and the use of numbers can be used to inform effective evidence-based practice. Let us look at a typical example of why quantitative methods are so important . . .

IMAGINE THAT . . .
You are a hospital trustee of a new hospital, Saint Research Methods hospital. Your job as a trustee is to find out all about our hospital. In each area of the hospital you will find a little bit more about research methods, so by the end of your tour you will be fully versed with all aspects of research methods. You may think of it as a simple hospital visit, or try to think of it as the nursing equivalent of a visit to Willy Wonka's chocolate factory – only with research instead of chocolate as the main product!

So welcome! Sir, Madam. Welcome to Saint Research Methods hospital. This hospital was built in recognition of all the nursing research stuff that goes on in the world and today we are going to show our different departments. We have broken your visit to the hospital up into two areas that comprise the west and east wings of the hospital (see Figure 2.1). We have split up the hospital into two areas, an area that is concerned with quantitative research methods and an area that is concerned with qualitative research methods.

In the west wing is the area concerned with quantitative research methods that contain two related areas:

- Quantitative methodology
- Quantitative research methods.

In the east wing is the area concerned with qualitative research methods that represent two related areas:

- Qualitative methodology
- Qualitative research methods

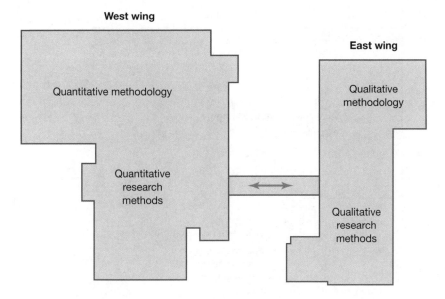

Figure 2.1 Map of Saint Research Methods Hospital.

We are first going to visit the west wing with our quantitative methodology and quantitative research methods in this chapter and follow up with qualitative methodology and qualitative research methods in Chapter 3. Figure 2.2 shows what is available in our high prestige west wing.

In the west wing there is activity relating to quantitative aspects of research in two areas of activity. The first area is concerned with quantitative methodology and here you will find out about:

- The theory that lies behind all quantitative research designs, which is known as positivism.

The second area is to do with research designs. There are a number of different research designs that can be put into three groups:

- There are experimental research designs which involve different types of clinical trials and randomised controlled trials
- There are quasi-experimental research designs that involve case-control and cohort research designs
- There are survey research designs that involve cross-sectional and longitudinal research designs.

It is this wing of the hospital we are going to visit first in Saint Research Methods Hospital; the department that deals with quantitative methodology.

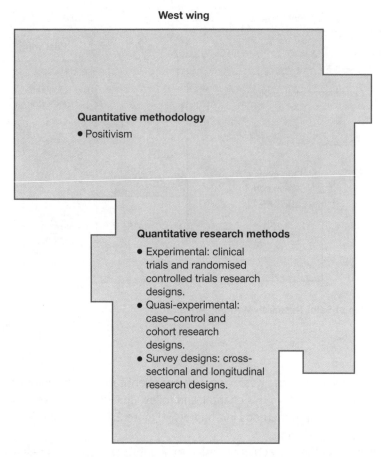

West wing

Quantitative methodology

- Positivism

Quantitative research methods

- Experimental: clinical trials and randomised controlled trials research designs.
- Quasi-experimental: case–control and cohort research designs.
- Survey designs: cross-sectional and longitudinal research designs.

Figure 2.2 The west wing of Saint Research Methods Hospital: quantitative methodology and research designs.

2.1 Quantitative methodology

The word methodology is a very specific term. It refers to the general outline, or approach, of a number of methods (which are more specific approaches), rules and procedures that allow the systematic investigation of a particular discipline or profession (e.g. nursing). Therefore, a methodology can be a number of concepts or ideas; it can provide an overview of an area which allows the comparison of different approaches within the area. Most of all it is an overall rationale, a philosophy, that guides practice in that area.

The philosophy that underlies quantitative methodology is positivism. Positivism was developed by a French nineteenth-century sociologist called August Comte. Comte saw all societies as going through three stages following a universal rule; theological, metaphysical and scientific. The first stage, theological, reflects society's view of the truth about the world relying on belief in God and the word of formal religion. Therefore, in this stage the knowledge of what we know about the world is based on religious teachings and belief.

The second stage is metaphysical, and this emphasises what is called logical rationalism. The second phase is concerned with the nature of philosophy and deals with knowledge that concerns philosophical thinking. The knowledge and awareness of humanity in this stage would have concerned discussion on determinism and free will, mind and matter, ideas of space and time and identity and change.

The third stage is what Comte emphasised as the scientific stage (or positivism) and the emphasis that all knowledge is scientific, that everything can be explained through science and all things are observable and measurable. Therefore, this approach emphasises that many things can be explained if we look for laws and principles. You will recognise this approach because it underpins much of your practice. The administration of drugs to patients to help them combat disease is based on the scientific approach rather than the metaphysical or the theological approach. You will also recognise this approach from your time at school in subjects such as physics, chemistry and biology where you did experiments use the scientific approach.

It is the scientific/positivist approach that underpins much of the quantitative approach. Quantitative research is very much concerned with the systematic and scientific investigation of phenomena and the relationship of particular phenomena to other phenomena. Therefore, the objective of quantitative research is to use observations, numerical analysis, hypotheses and measurement to understand the world. Some of these terms – measurement, hypotheses, etc. – may be new to you, so let us give you a general introduction to some of these ideas.

Hypotheses

Simply put, **hypotheses** are suggested explanations for phenomena or a suggestion of the possible relationship between different phenomena. You make hypotheses all the time.

In quantitative research methods, researchers are usually looking to test hypotheses. At a simple level, researchers may have an idea and they want to see if that idea has any worth. Usually, researchers will be trying to test hypotheses based on things that the discipline may have previously observed, or trying to advance scientific theories. Every time someone introduces a new drug, their general hypothesis is that it will make people taking the drug 'better', given that previous drugs have made people better.

Hypotheses take many forms. Sometimes they will be designed to suggest that one thing causes another. So for example, a new drug might be expected to cause greater recovery rates in individuals. However, sometimes a **hypothesis** might just say there is a relationship between two variables. Therefore, we expect one thing to be related to another thing, inflation related to higher living costs, eating chocolate to be related to gains in weight, and use of a new drug to be related to better health.

Another distinction made in research methods is between the '**alternative hypothesis**' and '**null hypothesis**'. Alternative hypotheses are the sort of hypotheses outlined above and will suggest that something will occur between the variables being studied. The two hypotheses above of causation and relationship are examples of hypotheses (e.g. 'a certain drug will lead to people getting better'). However, we sometimes identify the null hypothesis. This is a statement that runs contrary to the alternative hypothesis and suggests that one variable won't cause an effect on the other, or that there won't be a relationship between the two variables. That is, we have to consider that a certain drug will not lead people to get better. How and why these different hypotheses operate will be discussed later in the book. What is important to note now is that in quantitative research methods, the ideas of testing a hypothesis, be it to say something will happen, or that it won't happen, is important in research.

Measurement and statistics

When you can measure what you are speaking about, and express it in numbers, you know something about it; but when you cannot express it in numbers, your knowledge is of a meagre and unsatisfactory kind; it may be the beginning of knowledge, but you have scarcely in your thoughts advanced to the state of science.

Lord Kelvin (in a lecture to the Institute of Civil Engineers)

This is a well-used quote and illustrates the nature of measurement very well. Lord Kelvin is saying that when you are interested in a particular phenomenon, to gain a real and fruitful understanding, you need to somehow measure it with numbers. Not surprisingly, a major aspect underlying quantitative research methods is the idea that everything is quantifiable and therefore measurable. Formally, measurement means the estimation regarding the properties of any variable. For example, this might be height or your weight. In nursing, it might be a patient's temperature, average waiting times in Accident and Emergency, or length of remission. There are many different ways of measuring things in quantitative research methods. Some of these are based on categorising things (i.e. putting people into different wards in a hospital, for example, surgical or medical ward) or assigning numbers to things (temperature, the amount of a drug a person needs, the number of hours an average nurse does during the week). Measurement allows you to be precise, and to some extent accurate, about things in nursing. What dire straits might we be in if we had to guess at how much of a drug designed to lower blood pressure we had to administer to a patient and we were unable to list its side effects or assess the possible improvement to a patient's blood pressure.

One important thing to note here is that measurement often leads to lending numerical values to phenomena. This is something we will explore in greater depth in this book, but the important thing to remember here is that quantitative researchers are very interested in describing phenomena in numerical terms.

So, if we go back to the Saint Research Methods Hospital that we introduced you to at the beginning of the chapter, you will find the staff in the quantitative methods wards talking about their research in terms of possible hypotheses and measurement. For example Charge Nurse Williams in Room 222 has hypothesised that if his patients drink five cups of green tea per day, this will reduce their risk of heart problems. Next door, in Room 223, Sister Day is testing out a new drug Dayloxophine, and has hypothesised that administering 200mg of the new drug daily to patients suffering from headaches will reduce the amount of pain they feel by 60 per cent. Equally, this wing's administrator, Mr Maltby, is looking at ways to reduce hospital waiting times. Here, he has hypothesised that hiring three more doctors will halve patients' waiting times for receiving elective surgery within an acceptable six-month period. It is in all these situations that our team are generating hypotheses that they can test in order to have a positive effect on the hospital, and are assessing their results by numbers.

So, now we have introduced you to positivism, hypotheses and measurement, let us take you to the next part of the west wing of Saint Research Methods Hospital, and introduce you to some specific research designs that are used in quantitative research methods that are influenced by the ideas of positivism, hypotheses and measurement.

2.2 Quantitative research designs

From the positivist methodology a number of quantitative research designs emerge. In this section we are going to show you three quantitative designs that are commonly used in the hospital:

● Experimental design

● Quasi-experimental design

● Survey design.

2.3 Experimental design: clinical trials and randomised controlled trials

The first set of quantitative research designs is known as experimental designs. You will remember experiments at school, in chemistry or physics, where you tested out scientific ideas (i.e. chemical reactions, the movement of objects) under controlled conditions (in a laboratory, using test tubes) to examine particular phenomena. Our first set of quantitative research designs very much follow in this tradition, and they are clinical trials and randomised controlled trials.

Clinical trials

The use of **clinical trials** was first introduced around the year 1025, in *The Canon of Medicine* (or The Law of Medicine), which was a 14-volume medical encyclopaedia written in Arabic by the scientist and physician Avicenna. In this medical encyclopaedia Avicenna wrote guidelines for examining the effectiveness of new medical drugs which still underpin many modern-day clinical trials. He said clinical trials of a drug should ensure:

● There must be no strange or accidental influences on the drug being tested.

● The drug must be used on a simple disease, not a disease made up of separate parts or elements.

- The drug should be tested on two very different types of disease. Avicenna suggested this on the basis that a drug may cure one disease due to the unique qualities of the drug, but there may be other properties in the drug that may cure another disease.

- The quality of the drug must in some way correspond to the strength of disease. Avicenna was advocating that drug treatment must start with a weaker type of disease and then be used with diseases of gradually increasing strength.

- That the effects of the drug must be closely observed to ensure that any beneficial effects can be attributed to the drug and not the result of accidental causes.

- That the effects of the drug must have a constant effect, i.e. the drug should consistently help people improve, and among many people, or else it again could be attributed to an accidental effect.

- That experimentation with the drug must be done among humans, as testing among another species (i.e. animals) might not prove anything about the effect of the drug on a person. So for example, testing a drug on rats and observing an improvement does not necessarily mean we will see an improvement among humans.

THINGS TO CONSIDER

Intervention studies versus observational studies

Researchers conduct clinical trials in one of two different ways; intervention and observation. In an **intervention study**, researchers administer a medicine or another intervention to a group of participants and compare this group with another group of participants who are taking a **placebo** (i.e. an inactive pill, liquid or powder that has no treatment value); the researchers can then assess the effects of the intervention. For example an intervention study might involve the researcher administering a new drug to groups of patients.

The **observational study** is where researchers observe effects of a phenomenon. Here the researcher will simply observe the subjects and measure the outcomes, but at no point do they actually make an intervention (i.e. administer a treatment). Sometimes this is referred to as a natural experiment. One example of an observational study is the series of Nurses' Health studies. The Nurses' Health studies consist of two studies, the first established by Dr Frank Speizer in 1976, the second by Dr Walter Willett in 1989. These studies have been described as 'One of the most significant studies ever conducted on the health of women' by Donna Shalala, Former Secretary of the US Department of Health and Human Services. This observational study followed over 120,000 female nurses, initially aged 30 to 55, from 1976 to look for risk factors in cancer and cardiovascular disease. This also involved assessment of diets and exercise and analysing relationships with risk of sudden cardiac death or breast cancer survival.

However, the organisation and carrying out of clinical trials are much more developed today. Today, clinical trials are classified in different ways. The United States of

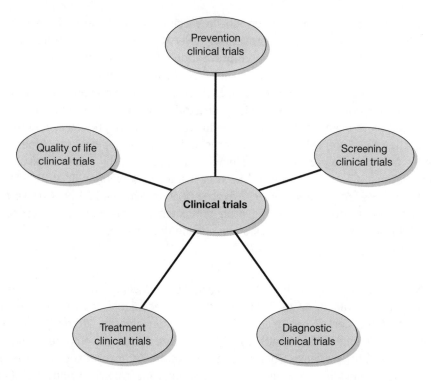

Figure 2.3 Different types of clinical trials.

America's National Institutes of Health, which is the primary organisation of the USA's government responsible for health-related research, has found a way of classifying clinical trials by their purpose. The National Institutes of Health suggest there are five different types of clinical trials (see also Figure 2.3):

- Prevention clinical trials
- Screening clinical trials
- Diagnostic clinical trials
- Treatment clinical trials
- Quality of life clinical trials.

To illustrate these different types of trials we are going to use some examples of the treatment of cancer, and specific examples described by the National Cancer Institute (National Cancer Institute, 2008) which forms part of the USA's National Institutes of Health.

Prevention trials

In **prevention trials** there are research methods for looking for better techniques to prevent disease. You may take a lot of preventative measures in your life to guard against disease. Eating five portions of fruit and vegetables a day, taking vitamins, taking regular exercise, having your rubella vaccine as a child, are all preventative methods that are undertaken to prevent or lower the chances of contracting a disease in the future. In nursing research prevention trials are a research method that looks at the way of preventing disease. This might be to prevent the disease occurring among individuals who don't have the disease, or it may be to prevent the disease occurring among individuals who may be prone to the disease. These measures could prevent a disease from recurring among individuals who have previously had the disease or they could prevent the chance of the individual developing a new type of disease. An example of a prevention trial in nursing research is the research carried out by the National Cancer Institute on the Breast Cancer Prevention Trial (BCPT). Between April 1992 and September 1997 over 13,000 women aged 35 or over were recruited to test whether taking the drug tamoxifen can prevent breast cancer in women who are at an increased risk of developing the disease.

Screening trials

Screening trials are research methods designed to develop and assess screening tools to detect certain diseases. Therefore, they are techniques designed to see if it is possible to detect certain health conditions before they emerge. Often this is done to see whether finding certain health conditions before symptoms emerge would help the treatment of the disease. Therefore, at the National Cancer Institute in the USA they use screening trials to study ways of detecting cancer before symptoms of cancer display themselves in the individual. These could lead to the development of screening tests. The sort of tests that emerge from screening trials might be:

- *Imaging tests*: these are screening tests that use X-rays, radioactive particles, sound waves or magnetic fields whose information can be analysed after passing through tissues of the body and that produce pictures of areas inside the body. In cancer a mammography (X-ray study of the breast) can be used to screen for cancer even though there are no symptoms of the disease.

- *Laboratory tests*: these are screening tests that check body fluids, such as blood or urine, and tissues. These tests would be used to see whether the results of whatever is being checked for in the individual falls inside the normal ranges expected. Also tests may be compared to previous tests for the individuals, so changes can be checked for.

- *Genetic tests*: these are screening tests that look for inherited genetic markers that may have a link to some cancers. For example, genetic make-up has been linked with bowel/womb cancer and breast/ovarian cancer. Within these screening tests, not only is the individual's genetic make-up examined, but deoxyribonucleic acid (DNA) (a person's genetic code) from family members is also analysed by collecting samples of blood or saliva. This allows a series of screening tests, including a mutation search, which sees whether there is a changed gene (mutation) that might run in your family that is linked to cancer. Then a genetic test screening will be used to see if the individual has inherited this mutation of the gene that is linked to cancer.

Diagnostic trials

Diagnostic trials are research methods that surround developing tools that can be used for recognising or detecting a particular disease. When a certain disease or health problem is suspected, diagnostic tests can be used to diagnose the underlying disease or problem. For example, in detecting lung cancer, imaging technologies such as magnetic resonance imaging (MRI) or computed tomography (CT) provide re- searchers with information on changes in the anatomy of the individual, but recently, researchers using diagnostic trials have found that positron emission tomography (PET) imaging, which uses biochemical processes, may be able to detect lung cancer before anatomic changes occur (Ung *et al.*, 2007). The purpose of diagnostic and screening trials are often the same, i.e. to detect the health problem or condition early. Therefore, you will often find these two terms being used together, because a screen test can also be a diagnostic test.

Treatment trials

Treatment trials are research methods that are used to test new drugs or new com- binations of drugs, new treatments, or new types of surgery. For example in the treat- ment of cancer, there are always treatment trials being carried out, in terms of a new drug to treat cancer, new approaches to surgery and new types of radiation treat- ment. These treatment trials involve comparing differences before and after treat- ment has been received to see if the spread of the disease has been halted. A typical treatment trial design can be seen in Figure 2.4.

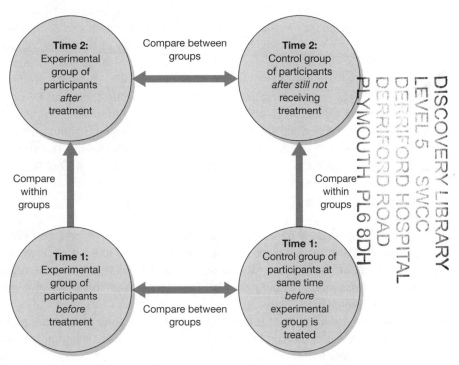

Figure 2.4 A treatment trial design.

Quality of life trials

Quality of life trials are a research method for exploring ways to improve the quality of life for individuals with an illness. Therefore, in the exploration and treatment of cancer, quality of life trials would look at ways of helping individuals who were suffering from the effects of cancer, such as nausea, problems with sleeping, or depression. If you look back over Avicenna's original criteria you will see that there is an emphasis on closely controlling the conditions of the experiment while observing, testing and exploring other elements in terms of beneficial effects. This emphasis still underlies the way that many of the different clinical trials are carried out today. In the next section we are going to concentrate on a particular feature of clinical trials, called randomised controlled trials, a method in clinical trials that helps researchers establish confidence in the findings and the effectiveness of the clinical trial.

Randomised controlled trials

Randomised controlled trials (RCTs) are the most commonly used in nursing and medicine across all the types of clinical trials described above. Randomised controlled trials are research designs that are considered to be of a high-quality standard, as it can provide researchers with some of the strongest evidence that the treatment, or intervention, has had the expected effect on treatment outcomes.

One of the major threats to any nurse researcher is the issue of bias. Bias exists in our everyday life: sometimes it happens naturally, sometimes it happens deliberately. Certain newspapers have a bias toward certain political thought, some we might consider more closely aligned to right-wing thought, and some more closely aligned to left-wing thought. You are biased in terms of what type of clothes you wear, whether you would prefer to take a friend or a stranger out for dinner, unless of course that stranger was Brad Pitt or Angelina Jolie. Therefore, we have certain biases towards certain strangers. We show bias in our choice of TV programmes we watch. We would like to watch a programme that interests us rather than bores us. Bias is an exciting part of our life. It helps us understand about ourselves (shopping or the library?). However, when it comes to establishing the truth, bias can sometimes distort that. Take for example our politicians. All politicians claim to act in our best interests, but we know that sometimes politicians are biased and may try to spin the 'facts'. Therefore, we can never be certain of what the 'truth' of the matter is.

This is also an issue when it comes to research methods. In research it is important that we establish the truth (or as close to it as we can). For example, if we are trialling a new drug, we want to know that if people get better when using the drug, it is the drug that is actually helping people. Therefore, researchers are always guarding against potential bias.

The main aspect of RCTs is the idea of controlling against potential bias to establish confidence in the result. You can read more about RCTs, and how to implement them, in Chapter 5.

THINGS TO CONSIDER

The four phases of new treatments

When a new treatment or drug is being introduced clinical trials using that treatment (i.e. drug) are often classified into four phases. The drug-development process can take many years, so that everyone involved in making and administering the treatment can be as sure as possible of its effectiveness and any potential problems, and that it can then be approved by the national regulatory authority. Though there are many issues surrounding these four phases, in very simple terms they are:

- **Phase 1 trials** are the earliest trials in the process. These would establish whether the trial treatment is actually safe or whether it has any harmful side effects. Examples of phase 1 trials might be to see how the body copes with the treatment or to see which is the best level of dose of the drug or treatment to use. If the treatment is considered safe enough, then the testing will move onto Phase 2.

- **Phase 2 trials** will comprise studies that look at how well a treatment works. Therefore, studies in Phase 2 will look at the effectiveness of the treatment, which aspects of the disease does the treatment work well for, how possible side effects can be managed. If these trials provide evidence to suggest the treatment is positive then researchers will move onto Phase 3.

- **Phase 3 trials** will comprise studies that test the new treatment against existing standard treatments, or the best available treatments. For example, Phase 3 studies will compare the new drug against an existing drug. If the new drug seems to provide evidence of its effectiveness, particularly over other treatments, it is at this stage that it will be granted a licence by the national regulatory authority.

- **Phase 4 trials** are research studies carried out after the new treatment has been licensed by the national regulatory authority. Researchers will carry out further studies about the drug as they collect information about its effectiveness and side effects among the general population. It is at this stage, over a longer period of time, researchers will be able to assess the long-term risks and benefits of the treatment.

EXERCISE 2.1

Below are two trials that are undergoing in our research methods hospital. Decide whether each is a prevention, a screening, a diagnostic, a treatment or a quality of life trial.

- A trial to measure the effect of a new cancer drug upon anxiety and depression.
- A trial designed to see whether taking the drug Foscrar-O can prevent prostate cancer.

2.4 Quasi-experimental research designs: case-control and cohort research designs

In the next section we are going to introduce you to **quasi-experimental** designs. Although experimental randomised controlled trials are recognised as a high-quality standard for quantitative research by attempting to minimise bias and only focusing on the impact of one intervention, sometimes in research it is not always possible to give placebos to a control group or carry out randomised experiments. For example, if researchers want to look at the growth or development of the disease within a particular community or population particularly over a period of 20 to 40 years (e.g. the development of lung cancer) a randomised controlled trial would not be the best approach to take. Here, quasi-experimental designs (quasi meaning resembling) may be more appropriate. Quasi-experimental designs 'resemble' experimental designs, but they differ from experimental designs in one important aspect, quasi-experimental designs lack the random assignment to treatment groups and presence of placebos that you are likely to see in experimental design, e.g. RCTs. In this section we are going to introduce you to two quasi-experimental research designs, case-control designs and cohort designs, and show you how they can be important research designs to researchers.

Case-control designs

Case-control designs are research designs that researchers use to identify or study the possible variables that may contribute to various health factors. For example, if a researcher was looking at the possible influences on the development of heart disease, they would compare the life of a group of patients who have heart disease with a group of patients who do not. Therefore, in case-control designs, researchers **look back** over individual's clinical, medical and lifestyle history and compare people who have the disease with those who do not. An example of a case-control design can be seen in Figure 2.5.

One of the most famous case-control designs was carried out by Richard Doll and Austin Bradford Hill in the 1950s. Today it is generally accepted that tobacco smoking is a major cause of all lung cancer mortality in the Western world. However, in 1950 no-one knew the extent of the health problems associated with smoking. In a research study Doll and Hill (1950) looked at the various factors by surveying patients in 20 London hospitals. These authors were able to determine that when comparing lung cancer patients with non-lung cancer patients smoking was the only variable that was strongly related to lung cancer, as the disease was rare in non-smokers. This study by Doll and Hill also showed that smoking was linked to heart attacks and emphysema (disease of the lungs evidenced by an abnormal increase in the size of the air spaces, resulting in difficult breathing and increased susceptibility to infection). Most notably this research study was the basis for the first health reports and concerns regarding the possible dangers of tobacco.

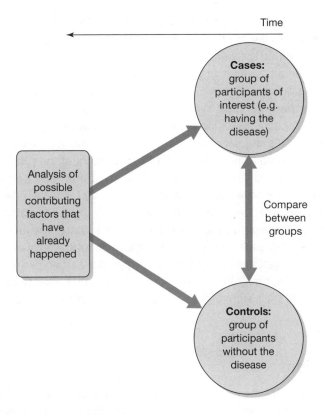

Figure 2.5 A case-control research design.

A recent example of case-control study is by Norwegian researchers (Jacobson *et al.*, 2008). Here, the researchers were interested in incidence and the risk of formation of a thrombus within the veins (venous thromboembolism) in pregnancy and in the four-week period following childbirth. The researchers looked at a number of variables from 613,232 pregnancies from between 1990 to 2003 in Norway, and compared those individuals who had developed thrombus within the veins with those who had not. They compared these two groups on a number of antenatal (before childbirth) and postnatal (subsequent to childbirth) factors. The antenatal factors included assisted reproduction (e.g., *in vitro* fertilisation [IVF]), gestational diabetes, whether the age of the mother was older than 35 years, whether the mother had had multiple pregnancies, and primi-parity (whether this was a first pregnancy). The postnatal factors included whether the mother had received a Caesarean section, pre-eclampsia (a type of blood poisoning associated with pregnancy, characterised by hypertension and fluid retention), assisted reproduction, abruptio placenta (refers to separation of the normally located placenta after the twentieth week), and placenta previa (a complication that occurs in the second and third trimesters of pregnancy). From comparing these two groups on these different antenatal and postnatal factors, Jacobson *et al.* (2008)

found that assisted reproduction and gestational diabetes were significant antenatal risk factors and Caesarean section and pre-eclampsia were strong postnatal risk factors for thrombus within the veins.

One of the main advantages of case-control studies is that they is relatively simpler, cheaper and quicker than many clinical trial designs. For example, in the study above the researchers will have simply collected the data and then carried out the analysis, with no random allocation of people into groups or controlling for the influence of potentially biasing variables. However, these advantages from case-control studies are not as strong as RCTs with regard to the extent of the conclusions you can draw. For example, with a case-control study, you can't draw exact effects of certain variables, because they have not been closely controlled for. If the researchers found out, among patients with lung cancer that they had smoked, while among those who hadn't got lung cancer that they hadn't smoked, this indicates the influence of smoking. However, what it doesn't do is tell you too much about the level of risk or the incidence of smoking. Often, case-control studies suggest a certain pattern of disease or certain risk factors that may then lead to other studies that need to be conducted to look more exactly at the nature of the relationships. One of this type of study is cohort designs.

Cohort designs

A **cohort** study ('cohort' means a group of people) is a study that examines a common characteristic among a sample of individuals. This characteristic might be the year they were born, or the area in which they live, or something that has happened to a group (e.g. a breakout of a disease in a residential area) or whether they are given a particular treatment or drug. The crucial feature to remember about cohort studies is that researchers **look forwards** and focus on a group of people who are tracked **over a period of time** and their health/illness patterns are tracked simultaneously, along with factors that might contribute to the cohort's health or illness. An example of a **cohort study design** can be seen in Figure 2.6.

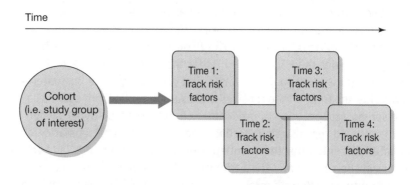

Figure 2.6 A cohort study research design.

Let us return to our example of smoking and lung cancer. In a cohort study the researchers would recruit a sample of smokers and non-smokers. They would follow this cohort for a period of time to see whether smoking or the degree of smoking leads to the development of lung cancer. One important aspect of this research would be that the groups would be matched. In many quantitative research designs you see that the groups are 'matched'. Researchers then match these samples on a number of criteria. Matching samples in research is where you ensure that the samples of participants are as alike as possible, therefore a researcher may try to match a sample based on a number of variables, i.e., sex, age, employment status, area of residence. A researcher in a study on smoking and health would make sure that if there was a 23-year-old, unemployed male who was a father of two who lived in a city in the smoking sample, the researcher would get another 23-year-old, unemployed male who was a father of two who lived in the city who didn't smoke to be in the non-smoking sample. Matching is done in research so that researchers can be sure that when they find a difference between the two groups (i.e. development of lung cancer) they can strongly suggest it is the result of differences between the two groups in terms of smoking, rather than the result of another variable, i.e. sex, age, employment status, how many children you have. Like many quantitative research designs, matching is a process designed to reduce possible error, control for other variables and establish confidence in your results.

A cohort study is a research design that is used to try to confirm or negate the proposed existence between certain variables and a disease. So for example, following the case–control study by Richard Doll and Austin Bradford Hill in the 1950s, with the possible link between smoking and lung cancer, one avenue for researchers would have been to carry out a cohort study of smokers to try to confirm or refute the findings. Imagine for example that they found evidence to support the link between smoking and lung cancer, researchers could also overcome one of the disadvantages with a case–control study and draw a conclusion about the amount of risk that smoking poses. For example, at the end of our smoking and lung cancer cohort design researchers would have information about the extent of risk **over time**. They would have statistics that would tell them that, within a defined time point, 6 in 10 people in the smoking group had gone on to develop lung cancer, whereas only 1 in 10 people in the non-smoking group had developed lung cancer during the same time, giving us some idea of the extent of the risk.

Other advantages of the cohort study are that it is longitudinal in nature, which means that researchers follow a sample of individuals over time by collecting data at regular intervals to examine the onset and extent of the influences of certain variables on disease (for example, does lung cancer first emerge after 5 years, 10 years, or 20 years of smoking regularly?). However, cohort studies do have issues to consider. They are time-consuming and individuals may drop out of the study.

Therefore, in contrast to case–control designs, where researchers look back over individuals' clinical, medical and lifestyle history and compare people who have the disease versus those who do not, cohort designs look at things that are likely, or expected, to happen; these studies are carried out over time and look for factors to see how a disease has been acquired.

THINGS TO CONSIDER

An example of a cohort study – the Framingham Heart Study

The Framingham Heart Study (based in Massachusetts, USA) is a cohort study looking at cardiovascular disease (CVD), the leading cause of death and serious illness in the United States. Cardiovascular disease refers to diseases that affect the heart or blood vessels (arteries and veins). The Framingham Heart Study started in 1948 and has informed medical research and knowledge on the effects of things such as diet, exercise, high blood pressure, high blood cholesterol, smoking and the use of medicine on heart disease. Significant findings include cigarette smoking being found to increase the risk of heart disease (1960), physical activity found to reduce the risk of heart disease (1967), high blood pressure found to increase the risk of stroke (1970) and a link between hypertension (elevation of the blood pressure) and heart failure (1996).

The study comprises three cohorts:

- *Original cohort*: this is an original cohort of 5,209 men and women aged between 30 and 62 years from the town of Framingham, Massachusetts. The study has involved participants undertaking medical history and lifestyle interviews, physical examinations and laboratory tests every two years from 1948, with the data then being used to understand the development of CVD. Participants were examined again every two years to establish a detailed medical life history.

- *Offspring cohort*: this is the next generation of participants and comprises 5,124 of the original participants' adult children and their spouses. This cohort underwent similar physical examinations and lifestyle interviews every two years.

- *Generation III cohort*: this is the next generation of participants and this cohort comprises around 4,095 grandchildren of the original cohort.

For more details on the Framingham Heart Study go to http://www.framinghamheartstudy.org/.

2.5 Survey designs: cross-sectional and longitudinal

The final quantitative research design we are going to highlight here is **survey** research designs. This is when researchers administer a survey to a number of people to find out about general attitudes, opinions, or certain behaviours. One of the features of surveys is that they can additionally be made up of a number of questions about a number of things. While clinical trials or cohort studies look for information relating to a particular disease, or testing of a drug that looks to get information on peoples' lifestyles (how much they smoke), or health (i.e. have they developed a certain disease), what you will see sometimes in surveys are a lot more questions about attitudes or behaviours that may be used to answer a number of different research ideas. So, typically, a survey may ask a respondent about their health behaviours, their attitudes to local health services, their relationships and all sorts of topics. Different surveys are designed to get different information. We are going to go over the development of survey questions in a later chapter, however, be aware that in surveys

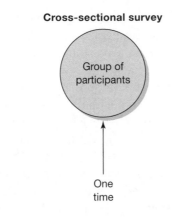

Cross-sectional survey

Group of participants

One time

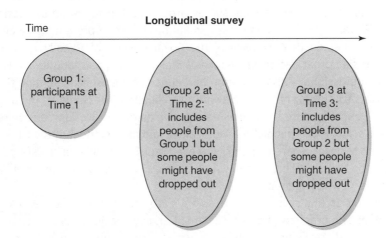

Longitudinal survey

Time

Group 1: participants at Time 1

Group 2 at Time 2: includes people from Group 1 but some people might have dropped out

Group 3 at Time 3: includes people from Group 2 but some people might have dropped out

Figure 2.7 Cross-sectional versus longitudinal survey research designs.

you might be asking many different questions about various aspects of individuals' lives (i.e. their opinions, their hopes, their feelings as well as getting information about health behaviours or medical records). The best example of a survey is the National Census. In the United Kingdom, the Census is a survey of all people and households in the country and the questions are designed to provide the government with essential information about society. Surveys can occur at a single point in time (i.e. cross-sectional designs) or over a number of different time-points (i.e. longitudinal designs). A comparison between cross-sectional and longitudinal survey designs can be seen in Figure 2.7.

Cross-sectional survey research designs

Cross-sectional surveys are research designs that provide the researcher with a picture of what might be occurring in a sample or population of people at a particular time. The important thing to remember about cross-sectional designs is that it's like taking a snapshot with a camera. You are looking at a group of people at only one moment in time. All of the information that you get from these people will be 'frozen' in time. If you want to see if people's experiences of health and illness have changed over time, then it might be best to use a longitudinal survey design, which we will tell you more about later on in this chapter.

Surveys can be used for a number of reasons. Examples of cross-sectional surveys would include a researcher trying to gain an assessment or understanding of the prevalence of a disease, or the researcher may look for information on general attitudes towards a number of things in society (e.g. drinking, smoking) or the engagement in a number of behaviours (e.g. smoking, visits to the doctor). Cross-sectional surveys can also be used to explore links between variables. For example, a researcher might use a survey to see whether there is a connection between poor diet and being overweight, or to examine the relationship between the amount an individual smokes and drinks and the number of times an individual is absent from work.

An example of a cross-sectional survey arose in 2006 following discussions between the Royal College of Nursing (a nursing organisation promoting excellence in practice and shaping health policies), the Royal College of Paediatrics and Child Health (a nursing organisation which takes a major role in postgraduate medical education and professional standards) and the Council of Deans (representing the views of university facilities for nursing, midwifery and health professionals). Together, they organised a questionnaire to establish a national picture of workforce requirements for children's and young people's services, and examine the effect of the NHS deficits on children's services. Therefore, they surveyed registered and non-registered nurses working in the NHS in children's and young people's services on a number of issues in their practice to investigate just that.

You will tend to find cross-sectional surveys are used in three main areas of nursing; **attitudes and practices**, **need assessment** and **evaluation**. A cross-sectional survey looking at attitudes and practices are used across nursing research to engage current attitudes and practices within the profession. So for example, Eller, Kleber and Wang (2003) used a survey of 746 health professionals (including 538 nurses) to assess general practice-based **knowledge and attitudes** about research among the profession. In this survey they found that current knowledge and practices about the research was high, so the authors felt they could make recommendations about the usefulness and development of multidisciplinary teams. The use of surveys to help nurses gain an understanding of **needs** in an area is also a common feature in nursing research. Often in community nursing, surveys will be used to assess the needs of certain populations, particularly those who are potentially vulnerable (i.e. old people; disabled people), so practitioners and service providers working in the area can develop policy and strategies for meeting that need. Finally, surveys can be used to **evaluate** an area's practice and outcomes within nursing. For example, Limb (2004) carried out an evaluation survey of limb reconstruction, a procedure used in orthopaedics following surgical intervention, with the application of the new limb requiring extensive rehabilitation. In Limb's (2004) survey of 60 patients who underwent these procedures, the researcher was able to evaluate the patients' recovery in terms of the patients' self-concept and physical, social and personal well-being.

Longitudinal survey research designs

In contrast to cross-sectional surveys are **longitudinal survey** designs in which the same surveys are observed repeatedly over a period of time. There are two main types of longitudinal research designs – cohort/panel surveys and those that look for trends.

The first longitudinal survey design is a cohort/panel survey design. We've already mentioned what a cohort design is. This is a research design that follows the same sample (cohort) over a period of time, and therefore a cohort survey design is a research design where the same survey is administered to a cohort over a period of time. A common example of a cohort survey design is a panel survey. A panel survey is one that takes samples of certain populations and presents the same survey (or similar surveys) to respondents over a period of time.

An example of a panel survey in nursing takes place in the USA and is known as The National Nursing Home Survey. These surveys are a continuing series of national sample surveys that are conducted in over a thousand nursing homes throughout the USA that were first carried out between 1973 and 1974, and have been repeated regularly since then (1977, 1985, 1995, 1997, 1999 and 2004). In the survey, questions are asked about the nursing homes, their staff and their residents. Data for the surveys are gathered from service providers or administrators of the nursing home and from family members. Consequently, reports are made regarding each survey so that, over time, results can be compared. So for example, Gabrel and Jones (2000) reported on the 1995 survey, and Jones (2002) reports the following findings from the 1999 survey. Here, researchers can view findings from the two surveys to see how nursing homes have changed over time. Figure 2.8 shows some of the findings from the two surveys.

Here you can appreciate from these two simple facts that people concerned with nursing homes, be it through government or health provision, would see from the survey there had been a growth in residents received nursing home care (from 1.5 million to 1.6 million) and that there had been a rise in how many of these residents were 65 and over (from nearly 90 per cent to 90 per cent). Therefore, someone concerned with nursing policy for care of the older person would use the information to help them plan resources strategically, i.e. you would be aware that there was an increasing demand to provide for those needing care. Typically, these type of surveys deal with a lot of information. For example the 1999 survey (Jones, 2002) told nursing researchers information such as:

- 72 per cent of current residents were female,
- 57 per cent of current residents were widowed.

1995 survey (Gabrel and Jones, 2000)	1999 survey (Jones, 2002)
About 1.5 million residents were receiving care during 1995	About 1.6 million current residents received nursing home care during 1999
Nearly 90 per cent of the residents were aged 65 years and over	90 per cent of current residents were aged 65 years or over

Figure 2.8 Comparing panel survey data collected in 1995 and 1999.

- Nearly half (46 per cent) of current residents were admitted to the nursing home from a hospital.

- The average length of time since admission for current residents was 892 days.

- Most nursing home discharges were female (62 per cent). The main reasons for most discharges were admission to a hospital (29 per cent) and death (24 per cent).

- The average length of stay for a discharge was 272 days.

All this information allows researchers in later years to compare findings from one panel survey to another.

The other type of longitudinal survey research design is trend analysis. This is similar to a cohort study, but where a cohort study may look at a number of variables at fairly regular intervals that may be over a number of years, trend analysis is a research design that aims to collect information on specific variables to identify a particular pattern or trend in data over time, but at much shorter and more regular intervals. The most obvious example of trend analysis that you will come across is housing prices. Here, building societies collect information monthly across the country regarding one variable, housing prices. This allows people to look for trends in house prices in the housing market. Typically though, the important thing about trend analysis is that it is used to make forecasts about the future. By monitoring house prices, commentators are able to say from data collected whether they expect house prices to continue to increase, or note that they are beginning to slow down in their increase and, therefore, might predict that in the long term there may be a market crash. You will see trend analysis used in all types of things in everyday life, particularly the stock market, and it will be used by the Bank of England in terms of deciding interest rates (i.e. if the Bank of England believes there is a trend for inflation in the country, they will increase interest rates to curb inflation).

In nursing, trend analysis survey designs are used to do similar things; i.e. forecast future events. For example, Xu and Kwak (2007) used trend analysis to help them understand trends and implications for the nursing profession of using internationally educated nurses in the US workforce, given that there is a nursing shortage in the USA and employers were targeting their employment efforts towards internationally educated nurses. What Xu and Kwak (2007) were able to show was that, when compared to US-educated nurses, internationally educated nurses were younger but more clinically experienced as nurses, and better prepared educationally; the internationally trained nurses had worked more hours in both primary and secondary nursing positions and they were primarily employed in urban hospitals as staff nurses in direct care roles. This type of information would have led policy makers to decide in the nursing profession that in the future there may not be a problem in recruiting more and more internationally educated nurses into the US workforce. Xu and Kwak (2007) also forecast that recruiting these nurses would relieve the US nurse shortage and make important contributions to the care of Americans, particularly older Americans, and those cared for in inner-city hospitals.

There is one major thing to note in regards to quasi-experimental cohort research designs and the longitudinal surveys mentioned in this section. A distinction between a quasi-experimental cohort research design and the longitudinal surveys mentioned here is that while the quasi-experimental cohort research design looks at the same population over a period of time, longitudinal surveys may look at the same population on each occasion but that population may change. For example, in the panel survey in nursing homes mentioned earlier, the survey would be conducted in as many nursing homes as possible; therefore, it is possible that certain nursing homes might be included in the second survey that weren't included in the first. Similarly, with trend analysis it may be that when looking at trends in nurse employment, you would be looking at different individuals each time, because nurses are entering and leaving the nursing profession all the time, and therefore, at each data collection point, the sample will contain many different people. In theory, if the time gap between two data collection points was substantial it might be a completely different sample, which could occur if the trend analysis was looking at attributes of nurses entering their first year of their qualification (as this would change yearly).

Self-assessment exercise

Identifying different types of quantitative studies: which is which?

These abstracts are from real-life research studies that have been carried out. After reading each abstract, have a go at trying to identify what type of study has been conducted and give a reason for your answer. Choose from the following:

- Randomised controlled trial (RCT)
- Cohort study
- Case-control study
- Cross-sectional study

Study 1

The aim of this study was to describe the incidence and prognosis of wheezing illness from birth to age 33 and the relation of incidence to perinatal, medical, social, environmental, and lifestyle factors.

Reference: Strachan, D.P., *et al.* (1996) Incidence and prognosis of asthma and wheezing illness from early childhood to age 33 in a national British cohort. *British Medical Journal, 312*, 1195-1199.

Subjects: 18,559 people born on 3-9 March 1958. 5801 (31 per cent) contributed information at ages 7, 11, 16, 23, and 33 years. Attrition bias was evaluated using information on 14,571 (79 per cent) subjects.

Main outcome measure: History of asthma, wheezy bronchitis, or wheezing obtained from interview with subjects' parents at ages 7, 11, and 16 and reported at interview by subjects at ages 23 and 33.

Results: The cumulative incidence of wheezing illness was 18 per cent by age 7, 24 per cent by age 16, and 43 per cent by age 33. Incidence during childhood was strongly and independently associated with pneumonia, hay fever and eczema. There were weaker independent

▶

associations with male sex, third trimester antepartum haemorrhage, whooping cough, recurrent abdominal pain and migraine. Incidence from age 17 to 33 was associated strongly with active cigarette smoking and a history of hay fever. There were weaker independent associations with female sex, maternal albuminuria during pregnancy and histories of eczema and migraine. Maternal smoking during pregnancy was weakly and inconsistently related to childhood wheezing but was a stronger and significant independent predictor of incidence after age 16. Among 880 subjects who developed asthma or wheezy bronchitis from birth to age 7, 50 per cent had attacks in the previous year at age 7, 18 per cent at 11, 10 per cent at 16, 10 per cent at 23 and 27 per cent at 33. Relapse at 33 after prolonged remission of childhood wheezing was more common among current smokers and atopic subjects.

What type of study is this? _____

Study 2

The aim of this study was to compare the clinical effectiveness of general practitioner care versus two general practice-based psychological therapies for depressed patients.

Reference: Ward, E. *et al.* (2000) Randomised controlled trial of non-directive counselling, cognitive-behaviour therapy, and usual general practitioner care for patients with depression. I: Clinical effectiveness. *British Medical Journal, 321*, 1383-1388.

Results: 197 patients were randomly assigned to treatment, 137 chose their treatment, and 130 were randomised only between the two psychological therapies. All groups improved significantly over time. At four months, patients randomised to non-directive counselling or cognitive-behaviour therapy improved more in terms of the Beck depression inventory (mean [SD] scores 12.9 [9.3] and 14.3 [10.8] respectively) than those randomised to usual general practitioner care (18.3 [12.4]). However, there was no significant difference between the two therapies. There were no significant differences between the three treatment groups at 12 months (Beck depression scores 11.8 [9.6], 11.4 [10.8], and 12.1 [10.3] for non-directive counselling, cognitive-behaviour therapy, and general practitioner care).

Conclusions: Psychological therapy was a more effective treatment for depression than usual general practitioner care in the short term, but after one year there was no difference in outcome.

What type of study is this? _____

Study 3

The aim of this study was to assess the impact of a social marketing programme for distributing nets treated with insecticide on malarial parasitaemia and anaemia in very young children in an area of high malaria transmission.

Reference: Abdulla, S., *et al.* (2001) Impact on malaria morbidity of a programme supplying insecticide treated nets in children aged under 2 years in Tanzania: community cross-sectional study. *British Medical Journal, 322*, 270-273.

Design: Data were collected at the beginning of the social marketing campaign (1997) and the subsequent two years. Net ownership and other risk and confounding factors were assessed with a questionnaire. Blood samples were taken from the children to assess prevalence of parasitaemia and haemoglobin levels.

Setting: 18 villages in the Kilombero and Ulanga districts of south-western Tanzania.

Participants: A random sample of children aged under 2 years.

Main outcome measures: The presence of any parasitaemia in the peripheral blood sample and the presence of anaemia (classified as a haemoglobin level of <80 g/L).

Results: Ownership of nets increased rapidly (treated or not treated nets: from 58 to 83 per cent; treated nets: from 10 to 61 per cent). The mean haemoglobin level rose from 80 g/L to 89 g/L in the study children in the successive surveys. Overall, the prevalence of anaemia in the study population decreased from 49 to 26 per cent in the two years studied. Treated nets had a protective efficacy of 62 per cent (95 per cent confidence interval 38 to 77 per cent) on the prevalence of parasitaemia and of 63 per cent (27 to 82 per cent) on anaemia.

Conclusions: These results show that nets treated with insecticide have a substantial impact on morbidity when distributed in a public health setting.

What type of study is this? _____

Study 4

The aim of this study was to investigate the association between consumption of green tea and various serum markers in a Japanese population, with special reference to preventive effects of green tea against cardiovascular disease and disorders of the liver.

Reference: Imai, K. and Nakachi, K. (1995) Cross-sectional study of effects of drinking green tea on cardiovascular and liver diseases. *British Medical Journal, 310,* 693-696.

Setting: Yoshimi, Japan.

Subjects: 1371 men aged over 40 years resident in Yoshimi and surveyed on their living habits including daily consumption of green tea. Their peripheral blood samples were subjected to several biochemical assays.

Results: Increased consumption of green tea was associated with decreased serum concentrations of total cholesterol (P for trend < 0.001) and triglyceride (P for trend = 0.02) and an increased proportion of high-density lipoprotein cholesterol together with a decreased proportion of low and very-low lipoprotein cholesterols (P for trend = 0.02), which resulted in a decreased atherogenic index (P for trend = 0.02). Moreover, increased consumption of green tea, especially more than 10 cups a day, was related to decreased concentrations of hepatological markers in serum, aspartate aminotransferase (P for trend = 0.06), alanine transferase (P for trend = 0.07), and ferritin (P for trend = 0.02).

Conclusion: The inverse association between consumption of green tea and various serum markers shows that green tea may act protectively against cardiovascular disease and disorders of the liver.

What type of study is this? _____

Study 5

This study was aimed at investigating the association between keeping birds and the risk of lung cancer in Sweden.

Reference: Modigh, C., *et al* (1996) Pet birds and risk of lung cancer in Sweden: a case-control study. *British Medical Journal, 313*, 1236–1238.

Design: Study based on cases of lung cancer and community controls. Interviews were performed by two nurses specially trained for this project.

Setting: Three major referral hospitals located in south-west Sweden.

Subjects: All patients aged 75 and under with newly diagnosed lung cancer and of Scandinavian birth who lived in one of 26 municipalities in Gothenburg and Bohus county or Alvsborg county. Potential control subjects matched on county of residence, sex and closest date of birth were selected from population registries. In the context of a larger study, information on pet birds was obtained from 380 patients with lung cancer (252 men) and 696 controls (433 men).

Main outcome measures: Odds ratios for lung cancer in relation to whether or not pet birds were kept and the duration of keeping pet birds.

Results: The adjusted odds ratio for ever versus never exposed to pet birds at home was 0.94 (95 per cent confidence interval 0.64 to 1.39) for men and 1.10 (0.64 to 1.90) for women. There was no evidence of a trend for increased risk of lung cancer with duration of bird ownership.

Conclusion: Bird keeping does not seem to confer any excess risk of lung cancer to Swedish men or women.

What type of study is this? _____

Summary

So far, we have introduced you to a range of research designs in our west wing of Saint Research Methods Hospital. With the description of positivism as a philosophy for informing and guiding research practice, we've introduced you to:

- experimental designs through clinical trials, and in particular, randomised controlled trials,
- quasi-experimental designs such as case-control and cohort studies, and
- survey research designs which comprise cross-sectional and longitudinal studies.

Now, in the next chapter we're going to take you to our east wing, where qualitative methodology and qualitative research methods are being used.

Chapter 3

Qualitative research methodologies and methods

KEY THEMES

Qualitative methodology • Qualitative research methods • Phenomenology • Ethnomethodology • Symbolic interactionism • Grounded theory • Constructivism • Interviews • Case studies • Focus groups • Participant observation • Ethnography • Action research • Fourth generation evaluation

LEARNING OUTCOMES

At the end of this chapter you will be able to:

- Recognise that phenomenology, ethnomethodology, symbolic interactionism, grounded theory and constructivism guide the use of qualitative research methods in nursing research with data collection, analysis and interpretation

- Appreciate that the use of qualitative research methods involves deploying a range of tools, including interviews, case studies, focus groups, participant observation, ethnography and action research.

Introduction

In this chapter, we are going to learn more about research that involves the measurement of health and health care in a qualitative way, which means the in-depth, rich experiences of participants are unearthed through a range of philosophical approaches and methods. To tap into the deeper experiences of these participants, this will often require a great deal of time and effort and revisiting the data you collect on many occasions. Just as if you were immersing yourself into a swimming pool, **qualitative** approaches usually need you to 'immerse' yourself in the worlds of your participants and understand the world from their perspective. You will often need to be 'knee-deep' in plenty of transcripts from interviews you have conducted or in observations that you have made and recorded in your observation diary. Let us introduce you to what qualitative research is all about in nursing research . . .

IMAGINE THAT . . .

You are that very same cardiac nurse from the Introduction in the previous chapter. You have got the most trustworthy statistics about smoking as posing a major risk to heart health and you regularly give this information to your patients. However, you have found that many of the patients do not give much credence to the statistics that you quote to them. They say to you that you don't know what it's like to be a smoker and they also mutter to you that they don't like the double standards of some of the health professionals who advise giving up smoking and yet these health professionals don't stick to their own advice when it comes to smoking. Something tells you that you may have missed out on the all-important 'human' dimension. These patients are human beings who are interacting with others around them; they are not passive recipients of advice and they may use role models who have smoked for many years and still not become ill from it. These patients are not worried about statistics. Instead, you perhaps need to focus on these patients' lifestyles, how they see themselves and their health and how others might influence what they do. You'll need to use qualitative research to get insights into these areas . . .

3.1 Qualitative methodology and research designs

Figure 3.1 shows you the work that is available in our high-quality east wing. In this wing we have activities relating to many aspects of qualitative research. The first area is concerned with qualitative methodologies, and here we will cover things you need to consider with the overall philosophies and assumptions that are made when doing qualitative research. To develop on from these philosophies, there is the second area in the east wing, known as qualitative research methods, which is a part of the hospital to do with the tools that are used when undertaking qualitative research. So let us show you around and tell you about the work in the first area in the east wing.

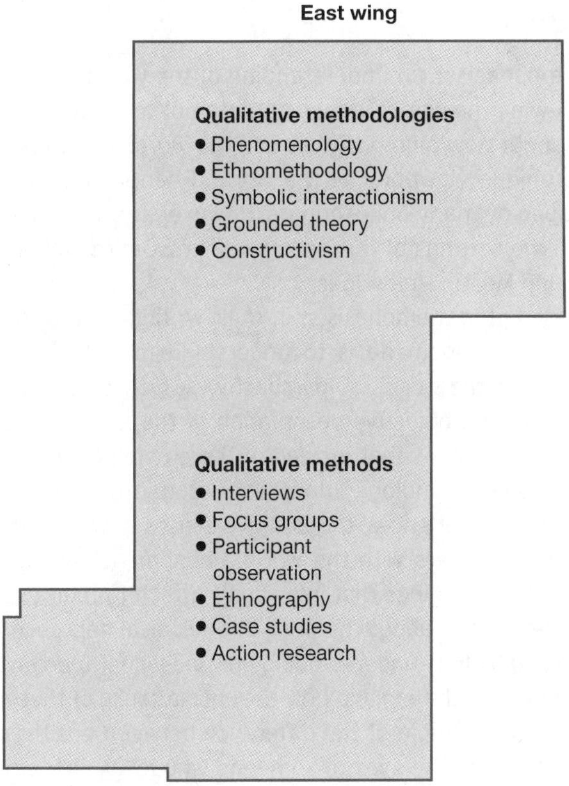

East wing

Qualitative methodologies
- Phenomenology
- Ethnomethodology
- Symbolic interactionism
- Grounded theory
- Constructivism

Qualitative methods
- Interviews
- Focus groups
- Participant observation
- Ethnography
- Case studies
- Action research

Figure 3.1 The east wing of Saint Research Methods Hospital.

3.2 Qualitative methodologies

Unlike quantitative methodologies, whose research designs are underpinned by the philosophy of positivism, qualitative methodologies have a number of philosophies that underpin the research that is done using this approach. In this section we're going to outline the more typical and popular qualitative methodologies. We're not going to cover all qualitative methodologies that exist, but we will rather give you a 'taster' of the major ones so that you get a feel for the main ideas underlying this area of research. In this section, we will introduce you to:

- Phenomenology
- Ethnomethodology
- Symbolic interactionism
- Grounded theory
- Constructivism.

Phenomenology

Phenomenology emphasises an understanding of the world from the view of the individual who is viewing the world; it does not attempt to come to a consensus and an objective 'truth' about how all individuals see the world but it instead gives priority to each person's unique viewpoint of the world. Phenomenology has been written about and developed by many philosophers. However, for our purposes we are going to concentrate on the writings of three philosophers, Georg Wilhelm Friedrich Hegel, Edmund Husserl and Martin Heidegger.

What all of these authors emphasised in their writings is that the key importance of understanding any phenomena is to understand from the first-person point of view. This differs from the positivist perspective, which emphasises that only true knowledge comes through objective observation of the area of interest. By contrast, **phenomenology** acknowledges that instead of there being only one 'truth', there can be many 'truths'. In phenomenology, knowledge results from uncovering each individual's perceptions, their experiences, the intuitive senses of what they are thinking and feeling in different encounters with the world. Phenomenology also attaches importance to measuring the meanings that individuals attach to their experiences. Overall, the main thing to remember about the phenomenological approach is that the key to knowledge is obtained by fully understanding how individuals *perceive* the phenomena (i.e. the experiences) around them and how they *make sense* of these phenomena.

Let us give a simple example of the difference between positivism and phenomenology. Let us see through the eyes of someone who loves shopping. A positivist researcher would emphasise the person's love of shopping via how much they spend, how much time they spend shopping, how many shops they visit. That is, they observe the person's behaviour and measure their love of shopping. However, a phenomenologist would emphasise the love of shopping through the person's 'eyes', i.e. their personal experience of shopping. They would want to know how they feel as they enter the shops, what feelings they experience as they cast their eyes over a product they want but wonder whether they can afford it, how excited they feel when they've bought something they really love and they rush home to try it out.

When researching health and health care, phenomenological research can be used to explore and understand how people cope with chronic illness. It could analyse how these people see their illness as an integral part of who they are and their relationships with others. For example, does a person with type 1 diabetes see the diabetes as being a vital part of who they are? Do they feel that they are meeting with 'kindred spirits' when meeting other people who also have type 1 diabetes? Or do they reject the 'diabetic' label and see the disease as only a small part of themselves? Many of these questions were asked by Watts, O'Hara and Trigg (in press) who explored the phenomenologies (i.e. experiences) of people with type 1 diabetes.

Ethnomethodology

Ethnomethodology was developed by Harold Garfinkel in the 1960s. It emphasises that people make sense of the world and are active agents in it; they communicate the way they understand the world to others and construct a **social world** from those shared understandings. To remember what ethnomethodology is all about, think about the phrase 'ethnic' (as in 'ethnic group') as a clue to the perspective that is taken when using this approach. With ethnomethodology, we are looking at a collective group of people, with their unique practices in doing things; through careful observation of their rites and rituals, ethnomethodology can show you how practices and procedures in a given group were developed and how certain ways of doing things are reinforced so that newcomers to this shared social world will be able to re-enact such practices. Nursing research based on ethnomethodological perspectives would be to treat the area to be researched as if someone is an outsider and studying a totally new tribe in an undiscovered world. The questions to be answered in health care research would be directed at learning more about this 'tribe'; for example, many nursing students have probably adopted this approach when first starting up on a new clinical placement. They would be looking for the formal, but also the unspoken informal, rules in the placement. How do fellow nurses treat each other and how do they interact with other health professionals, the administrators and the patients? Which administrator is the most influential if you want to get appointments changed? What jargon should you be using to showing that you are one of the health care team?

This approach can be contrasted with the positivist philosophy underpinning doing quantitative research with its emphasis on objective measurements. Instead, ethnomethodology emphasises the importance of context. Nurse researchers who used this approach would ask questions like 'what is going on in the social context within which nurses are building a rapport with their patients? Do the nurses portray themselves as "experts" when it comes to the rights and wrongs of providing health care or do the nurses see the patients as "co-experts" of their own health and well-being?' The ethnomethodological perspective would also be enquiring with questions like, 'What do people usually do around here and how do they justify these habits?' As you can see, ethnomethodology works from the premise of learning more about the spoken and also the unwritten rules, the rites of passage that newcomers need to undertake, and the network of activities and interrelationships between people within a vibrant, ecosystem-like entity.

Symbolic interactionism

Symbolic interactionism was developed from the work of George Herbert Mead, though the term was introduced by a student of Mead, Herbert Blumer. Symbolic interactionism, like ethnomethodology, is an area of philosophy emphasising that people are products of the social world: it also emphasises that people are creative and have purpose within the social world. Let us unpack what symbolic interactionism is all about by dissecting its label - researchers using this approach are interested in the 'symbols' in our worlds and the 'symbolism' that certain objects and environments can assume. For instance, what might you be feeling and thinking when you see a fellow nurse in their uniform? Are you looking for any signs of rank or status to see who might be in charge? Is that person wearing a name badge to signify this status? What might be the importance of nurses introducing themselves to patients by their first name as opposed to their job title, rank or surname? How might the patients see these nurses as a result of being introduced on a more informal level? This is another crucial aspect to symbolic interactionism, namely that we **interact** with the objects that we're presented with. Some patients might feel more relaxed and communicated to as an equal if treated by a nurse who introduced themselves just by their forename. On the other hand, some patients might see such an approach as being too informal or disrespectful. As you can see from this example, the interactionist part of this research methodology shows that we are not passive recipients of information – we are continually responding to it.

In essence, with symbolic interactionism, people don't just conform to the social world; they place their own meaning and interpretation of social events within the world and interact in relation to these meanings and interpretations. Blumer (1969) suggested three things in human behaviour that are illustrative of the dynamic processes of symbolic interactionism. The first is that those individuals attach meanings to things, and act towards those things based on the meaning they have attached to other things. The second is that the reasons people develop and attach meaning to things, and how they do so, come from their social interactions. The third is that meanings that people possess are developed and changed as the person moves through life and the interpretations the individual makes to different life events.

An example of symbolic interactionism as a research methodology in a health care context can be found in Kelly Smith Papa's (2008) blog (i.e. a weblog or diary on the Internet), which recounts the findings from her Masters thesis investigating how older people react to the symbolism that the environment of a nursing home might evoke. In her research, she was able to illustrate through interview data from nursing home residents how they saw some of the threatening features that meant a nursing home was very unlike a 'home' in the conventional sense. For instance, the nursing homes that Papa (2008) studied were replete with symbolism of death, illness and dependency. Indeed, the environment often had a cold and 'clinical' feel to it with the following miscellaneous items . . .

> Unfamiliar medical tools such as blood pressure cuffs, medication cart, a poster on cardiopulmonary resuscitation, reminder notices about proper hand hygiene techniques, large linen carts, and a strange-looking mechanical lift cluttered the hallways.

Papa (2008) makes a strong case for being continually aware of the messages that can be conveyed through environments, objects, language and the ways in which all of this is used in a care setting. As a health professional, are you helping to reinforce a sense of helplessness and dependency among patients through symbols that foster such feelings? Or are you tapping into how your patients see you, your health care team and the care environment? Do you call them 'patients' or are they 'service users' or 'clients'? Symbolic interactionism gets you to be mindful of the impact that various symbols can have on the recipients of your care; these symbols can often be used to repress, but they might also be used to empower or liberate.

Overall, symbolic interactionism is an approach that demonstrates how people make sense of their role in different social contexts, their identity, their own and others' behaviours and their interactions with others, based on the meanings they attach to things. This approach is a significant contrast from positivist approaches and the use of quantitative research methods in nursing, which tends to assume that everything means roughly the same thing to people and everything is simply measurable and quantifiable. Symbolic interactionism emphasises the idea that even the same phenomenon can have many different meanings for many different people and these dynamics need to be explored through a range of tools that analyse how symbols are interpreted, and used to powerful effect in our social lives. This methodology is closely related to the development of grounded theory, which we shall turn to in the next section.

Grounded theory

Though often a research method, **grounded theory** is also a perspective (i.e. methodology) that informs modern qualitative research. This approach was developed from the 1960s onwards by Anselm Strauss and Barney Glaser (e.g. Glaser, 1978). It is intended to be '*a systematic way to generate theoretical concepts and/or concepts that illuminate human behaviour and the social world*' (Tavakol *et al.*, 2006; p. 1).

In a similar way to symbolic interactionism, grounded theory is often used to analyse social systems and dynamics that become more prominent through careful scrutiny of how people interact with each other. The analyst who employs a grounded theory approach is usually focused on the cycles of negotiation and re-negotiation between people as they develop social norms, values and standards of conduct.

The main thrust of grounded theory is directed towards building theory from specific samples of data (i.e. it is **inductive**), rather than having any hypotheses or theories that are generated first and then tested with the collection of data (this would be called a **hypothetico-deductive** or **deductive** approach). As a result, the development of research questions with grounded theory is one where there are no hypotheses; the questions set are open-ended and broad, which allows for an in-depth investigation of the subject of interest. Research questions evolve in the course of the entire study as several iterations of data generation and analysis take place.

With sampling of study participants, research using grounded theory does not start with a predefined sample. Instead, the process is driven by the principle of 'theoretical sampling' (Glaser, 1978). This means that data should be collected with the express intention of generating theory. To get theory to emerge, progressive cycles of collecting, coding and analysing data need to be undertaken. Along the way, the theoretical sampling will help inform decisions on what data to collect and from whom. Scott (2003) used theoretical sampling and a range of data sources (i.e. government reports, observations of practice and 25 interviews) to develop a theory about how Australian registered nurses adopt different positions when negotiating different encounters in the nursing home environment with staff and residents. Scott (2003) called this theory 'situational positioning' and she showed how these nurses needed to 'position' themselves according to who is making a request for an action, what decisions were required, etc. This meant the registered nurses needed to negotiate their position along two dimensions of being more (or less) flexible or rigid and more (or less) yielding or confronting towards those persons making a demand on the nurses' time. The theory that developed from Scott's (2003) work has implications for how registered nurses in such a setting can manage the demands of their roles; such research can show us how the ideals of high-quality nursing care can be compromised by the practicalities of juggling multiple roles. Overall, grounded theory, in the instance of Scott's (2003) research, was able to show us that registered nurses' roles were ill-defined and not used very efficiently. As a result, such research can help inform us of more effective ways of managing health care staff resources.

When using grounded theory, data collection and analysis is typically about 'immersing oneself' (i.e. living, breathing and regularly thinking about!) in the subject matter and the social context of the study. Grounded theory would entail collecting data through interviews (usually unstructured as there needs to be minimal bias from the researcher's perspective), observation and analysis of documentary evidence (textual and/or graphical, such as posters, minutes of meetings, etc.). Data collection, coding and analysis would all be done in a similar time frame. This would allow the study to take different turns, or it could progress in a similar direction, depending on how the first cycle of activity progresses. Overall, the key thing to bear in mind with many of these qualitative methodologies is that there is an acknowledgement of the socially constructed nature of knowledge and various perspectives of what constitutes 'reality'. We will now turn to this process of how knowledge is constructed over time and how this informs qualitative research that uses this approach.

Constructivism

Constructivism is a theory that was developed by Jean Piaget, who emphasised that individual knowledge in internalised within each person. Piaget argued that much of the knowledge that we gather through our lives comes from our own experiences, and that this new knowledge is then placed in our consciousness with all our other knowledge. However, constructivism emphasises that our previous knowledge impacts on how we treat new knowledge and what that means to us. Constructivism suggests that we have a framework of understanding that we use to interpret most new knowledge within that framework. For example, if you are at work and there is a new patient in the ward and they seem upset, you may understand this new experience as being a normal reaction by patients who are new to wards because they are clearly anxious or upset about being in hospital. What is important to note is that your knowledge has fitted into a framework of previous knowledge. However, what it also means is that we may sometimes misinterpret new knowledge, or have misunderstandings about knowledge. It may be that the patient is in pain or upset about something else altogether. Of course new experiences may change your framework. If, for example, you found out later that the new patient was in pain, the next time you saw a new patient crying you might additionally check whether they were in pain, thus changing your framework about knowledge of why new patients might cry.

What constructivism emphasises is that we are constantly receiving (formally known in the theory as accommodating) and changing (formally known in the theory as reframing) our knowledge about the world due to our experiences and the experiences of others.

What constructivism has particularly taught us is about learning – that learning is a very active process, in which we are accommodating and reframing what we know all the time. In nursing research, the theory of constructivism is used to inform certain research methods because research can be seen as a learning process, therefore if it is treated as such there is a need to acknowledge that in research knowledge needs to be accommodated and reframed based on our and others' experience.

Overall, as you walk around the east wing of Saint Research Methods Hospital you will see research that uses some of the above methodologies to get deeper insights into patient experiences and 'how things are done around here'. For example, nursing sister Day is looking at how patients due to have elective surgery perceive and understand the nature of their operation; she is examining the meanings that these patients are attaching to the consequences of the surgery and the impact on the patients' feelings about themselves before, and after, surgery. Nurse consultant McGarry is talking to older patients about the different types of social support they receive, and to what extent they feel they have experienced a network of support that meets their varying needs. Research nurse Maltby is talking to patients who do not have English as a first language, via an interpreter; he is asking them about how they access appropriate health services in primary care and whether they perceive any barriers to fully accessing health care for themselves or for other family members.

So it is within this part of the hospital you will find the staff talking about their research in terms of qualitative terms of perception, social interactions, meaning and experience. Let us take you to the next part of the east wing, and introduce you to some specific common qualitative research methods that are based on qualitative methodologies.

3.3 Qualitative research methods

In this section we are going to discuss the following research methods that are typically used in qualitative research:

- Interviews
- Focus groups
- Participant observation
- Ethnography
- Case studies
- Action research.

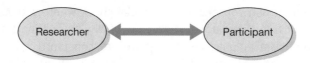

Figure 3.2 An interview research method.

Interviews

You will have come across the concept of the interview before. That is, an interview is one person asking another person questions and there is two-way communication in which the interviewee responds to the questions and further questions often arise as a result. For a typical illustration of an interview, have a look at Figure 3.2.

In nursing research, interviews are often used to get in-depth qualitative data. However, a distinction is made between different types of interview and centres on the difference between structured, semi-structured and unstructured interviews.

Structured interviews are designed to ensure that the interviewer covers the same specific areas with each interviewee. They would generally comprise of a list of questions all of which need to be asked and covered in a set order; the interviewer would normally not be allowed to ask additional questions. This would be done to ensure that the interviewer didn't influence the information given by the interviewee in any way. The interviewer might ask the interviewee to sometimes elaborate on something they have said, or clarify what they said, but the interviewer would not be able to ask a supplementary question or be permitted to give their own opinions on things.

In nursing practice you would tend to come across structured interviews in the assessment of patients. An example is the Edinburgh Postnatal Depression Scale (Cox *et al*., 1987) that health visitors sometimes use, in which a certain number of questions are asked about a mother's experiences after having given birth. Although the mother can elaborate on her responses, there is little in-depth, rich information that can be gleaned from this structured interview. The mother needs to give a rating for each question that is asked of her and a score is generated at the end of the interview session. Structured interviews could be used to gain information, give information or to motivate the patient/service user in some way.

Semi-structured interviews are a little bit like a natural conversation, in that the interviewer has a schedule of questions or topics that need to be covered, but there is less emphasis on these areas being covered in a set order or questions being asked in the same way. As a result, this approach seems to approximate more to a genuine interaction between interviewee and interviewer. The interviewer is looking at the content of the interviewee's responses and whether the interviewee is addressing the issues that are of interest or perhaps on the agenda for discussion later on in the interview schedule. The interviewer needs to be an active, responsive and flexible listener in relation to what the interviewee is saying.

In a similar way, unstructured interviews are more informal when compared to structured interviews and are also conversational in nature. There might be a few predetermined questions or topics for discussion but overall the interviewee is setting the agenda. The interviewer might be generally interested in a specific topic but there is sufficient flexibility for the interviewee to focus on a range of areas that the interviewer might not have anticipated beforehand. An unstructured interview might even be a lot more dominated by the interviewee doing most of the talking; it could result in a 'stream of consciousness' in which interviewees start to say almost everything on their minds unless there is some careful marshalling of the conversation to cover areas of mutual interest.

In nursing research, structured, semi-structured and unstructured interviews are used in many qualitative studies. An example of interviews used in research was published by Janice Brown and Julia Addington-Hall (2008). In this, research interviews were used to explore patients' experiences of living and coping with motor neurone disease. Motor neurone disease is a group of progressive neurological disorders that destroy the cells that control voluntary muscle activity such as speaking, walking and breathing and, therefore, many people who suffer from the disease experience the loss of mobility and the inability to communicate. From their interviews of 13 adults over an 18-month period, Brown and Addington-Hall were able to identify four major issues that were most prominent for a person with motor neurone disease. These were:

- Being able to live life as well as possible by keeping active and engaging fully in life.
- That motor neurone disease presents an insurmountable situation leaving the person feeling disempowered, unable to fight for life or against death.
- The person with motor neurone disease wanted to survive the disease.
- There were considerable feelings of loss and fear about what was going to happen to them.

Focus groups

In the last section we talked about interviews. A research design that is an extension of the interview is the focus group. A focus group is a qualitative research design in which a group of people are asked about their opinions and ideas on a particular topic. You may have heard of a focus group before. They are used extensively in marketing to discuss new products or to give feedback on services. Focus groups are also used in nursing research. Within a focus group a number of questions are put to the group and participants freely respond, often also interacting with each other, to the question. Figure 3.3 shows an example of what a focus group set-up might look like.

Focus groups are thought to present a more natural setting than interviews which are normally one-to-one, and can be quicker (due to there being a number of people) than gaining information on a one-to-one basis.

Focus groups can be set up in different ways. Sometimes the researcher won't run the focus group, but get what is known as a moderator to run the group while they observe the session. Sometimes the researcher might be in the room recording responses, or they might be behind a glass screen observing the focus group. In many cases the focus group session might be recorded (either video or audio) so that the opinions expressed can be accurately monitored. The reason for videoing such sessions

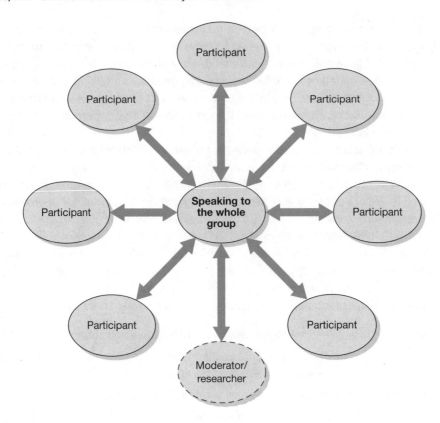

Figure 3.3 A focus group research method.

is that facial expressions, or expressions of mood, made by participants during the session might also be useful information to the observer. This type of information might help the researcher decide how strongly the group felt about something. For example, the idea of making patients pay for their time in hospital might be met with a sudden gasp and look of horror, rather than a collective shrug of shoulders.

There are different variations of focus groups, and the extent of the involvement of researchers in this process. For example, there is a **dual moderator focus group** in which one researcher ensures that the session runs well in terms of interactions between the participants, while another researcher ensures all the topics are covered. This contrasts with the **duelling moderator focus group** in which the researchers may take opposite sides of a debate. Indeed, one type of focus group research method is the **two-way focus group**, where one focus group watches another focus group and they themselves discuss the opinions of the other focus group.

There are some issues with focus groups. The most often cited problem is something called 'groupthink' (Janis, 1972). This is where people may tend to conform to the majority position or opinion, even though they don't really agree, because they feel they will be derided if they disagree with the group, or made foolish for expressing their own opinion. As a result, people might come up with extreme and radical proposals for action rather than taking a more careful approach if they were asked about things on their own. However, if a focus group is carefully facilitated by the moderator, it should be possible for the group setting to create original thought or generate ideas on a topic or phenomena that researchers wouldn't have found out about if they had just interviewed each of the participants on a one-to-one basis.

There are other issues that emerge with focus groups. For example, while in a one-to-one interview the researcher has greater control over the direction and the structure of the interview. However, with a focus group, keeping this sort of control over the discussion is much harder, and the group may wander off topic, or their reactions or opinions may be difficult to gauge.

An example of the use of focus groups in nursing research is presented by Willis and Wortley (2007). These authors were interested in finding out about attitudes towards influenza immunization among nurses. In the USA, the Advisory Committee on Immunization Practices suggests that all nurses are immunized against influenza to reduce the spread of influenza between workers and patients. However, Willis and Wortley wanted to find out why, despite these recommendations by the Advisory Committee, influenza immunization coverage of nurses is less than 50 per cent. These authors ran eight focus groups; four of which were nurses who had been vaccinated, and four of the groups contained nurses who had not been vaccinated. What Willis and Wortley were able to find out from these focus groups is that many nurses (whether they were vaccinated or unvaccinated) were concerned about influenza vaccine effectiveness and safety. They also found that unvaccinated nurses tended to be less aware of the Advisory Committee recommendations for vaccination.

Participant observation

In the last section we talked about the involvement of the researcher in the research process as part of the focus group. There is another research method in which the researcher 'immerses' themselves in the research process, which is known as participant observation. Figure 3.4 illustrates what the use of participant observation might look like.

Participant observation is a research method designed so that the researcher can get close to the research participants, and usually involves the researcher getting involved with the participants within their natural environment. The origins of this research method comes from sociology (the study of the origin, development, organisation and functioning of human society) and the work of sociologists in the study of different human societies. Some of the most famous work is Margaret Mead's work (e.g. Mead, 1928; 1930; 1935) looking at sexual practices among communities of South Pacific and South East Asian traditional cultures which sought to broaden traditional attitudes in the West towards sex in the 1960s.

In this work, the researcher goes into a particular community or **population** and lives within in that community by participating and observing that culture. In doing so they are able to develop accounts of the lives of that community and gain unique insights. Participant observation is often done over longer periods of time, sometimes a few months to many years. The reason for this is that the researcher, over longer time periods, will be able to get a detailed and more accurate picture of the community.

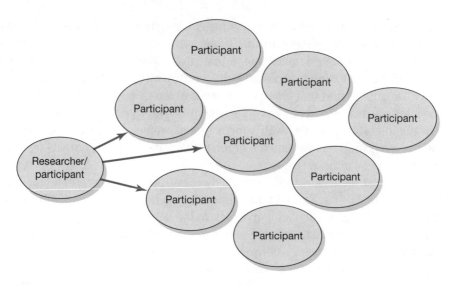

Figure 3.4 A participant observation research method.

There are three ways that the researcher might carry out a participant observation among a community.

- *Complete participant*: this is where the participant completely immerses themself in the community they are researching. Their participation in the community is not made known, and thus their true role will be hidden from the community. This is because the researcher may want to hide the research from participants. We've already talked in this chapter about how researchers might influence the research process, but participant observation is usually used when the researcher fears their presence might affect the participants or might affect the accuracy of the information. For example, if a researcher was investigating an extreme political party, they might join the party and pretend to be a member to do their research, not revealing anything about the research, because they may feel that individuals will moderate their views or actions if they knew a researcher was present.

- *Participant as observer*: in some situations it is not possible for the researcher to fully participate in a community. For example, if a researcher was investigating a drug community who took heroin, it would be ill-advised (in fact irresponsible) that they started taking heroin so they could undertake a participant observation. Here, the researcher tells the community they are studying what their role is and involves themselves in the everyday life of the community.

- *Observer as participant*: on this occasion, the researcher almost drops the whole idea of being a participant. They will visit the community, and may observe its practices over a period of time and will do in-depth interviews with many of the participants. However, they will tend to observe processes rather than participate in them. They will tend to do in-depth interviews with everyone in the community.

An example of how participant observation is used in nursing research was that carried out by McKnight (2006). One aspect of this study that the researcher was interested in was looking at how on-duty critical care nurses seek information about their practice in their job in terms of how to best treat their patients. McKnight carried out the information seeking behaviour of on-duty critical care nurses on a 20-bed critical care unit in a community hospital for 50 hours. McKnight found that the nurses' main information-gathering was centred on the patient, seeking information from people and records of the patient. McKnight found, however, that nurses tended not to use other information from research papers to inform their practice. She found that nurses felt taking time to read published information on duty was not only difficult, but perhaps also ethically wrong.

Ethnography

From participant observation comes **ethnography**. Ethnography is a research method used in nursing that has emerged from the qualitative methodology of ethnomethodology. It is used to present an overall picture of a population or sample that will use a number of methods to build up a picture, one of which could be participant observation. Figure 3.5 is an example of an ethnographic research method. As you can see,

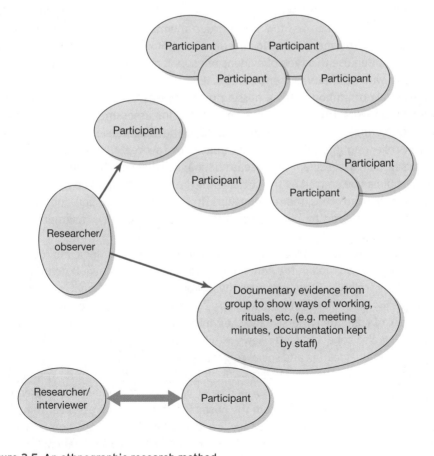

Figure 3.5 An ethnographic research method.

often ethnographers (i.e. those who do ethnography) might use more than one method to get insights about the social worlds of interest.

As with participant observation, the researchers will involve themselves with the population being studied over a period of time. They will not only rely on participant observation but use a number of further techniques to present an overall picture of that population. Therefore, an ethnographer will undertake a number of activities in an ethnographic study, including:

- Making direct observations of daily behaviour; this may include participant observation but can involve other methods of observation, such as unobtrusive observation.
- Conducting interviews and conversations with members of the groups that the researcher is interested in. This might range from minor conversations to in-depth interviews.
- Examining documentary evidence about how people in the group of interest do things through documented meetings, displaying signs showing what is or isn't acceptable behaviour, emails that are sent among group members, etc.

We've put ethnography in the qualitative research method chapter, however, the evidence collected in ethnography could include quantitative (i.e. number-based) research information, such as how often group members meet, which of the group members speak the most often in meetings, etc. However, effective ethnographic analysis will often use this type of evidence to supplement the data collected from in-depth observations, interviews and the like.

An example of ethnography in nursing research was carried out by Laurie Clabo (2008). In this work, the researcher examined nursing assessment of pain across two postoperative units in one teaching hospital in the USA between 2003 and 2004. Through collecting information from a number of sources, Clabo was able to show that nurses' pain assessment practice is not shaped solely by their education and experience but can be shaped by the social context of the unit on which practice occurs, suggesting that the ethos, the relationships that exist within the unit and the general understandings shared by people working in the unit influence how nurses assess pain among patients.

In the United Kingdom, McGarry (2009) has used an ethnographic approach to explore how nurses working in the community and older patients negotiated the boundaries of their relationships and how these boundaries can impact on the caring experience for these older patients. McGarry collected data via participant observation of the work of community nurses and their interactions with each other and with the patients. She also conducted interviews with the community nurses and older patients and found that the location and social context of care was pivotal to effective caring relationships; most importantly, McGarry was able to find that the taken-for-granted relationships between community nurses and older patients are significantly altered when the location of care has shifted from the hospital to the home. In essence, community nurses are often keenly aware that they are 'guests' in the patients' homes and that appropriate boundaries and methods of building a rapport between patient and nurse need to acknowledge the social context of delivering care.

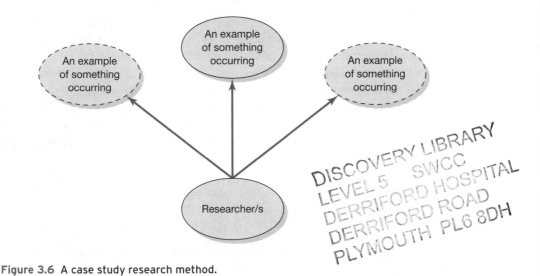

Figure 3.6 A case study research method.

Case studies

In nursing research a case study details a particular instance, or instances, that can be used to provide evidence or data for researchers. A graphic illustration of what goes on in using the case study can be seen in Figure 3.6.

For example, a nursing researcher wants to look at practices that occur in an accident and emergency department. To present a case study our researcher might, for example, visit one hospital and collect information about the practices that occur within that department over a week. Then, when the researcher has finished, they would present the information collected about the practice in that department as a case study.

The case study is a research method that investigates a phenomenon within a real-life context. A case study might be a single example or the combination of many examples, and it may include a range of different sources of evidence. In fact like ethnography, we've put case study in the qualitative research method section; however, the evidence for a case study might include qualitative and quantitative research information. A case study might seem like an ethnographic study at face value, but the important difference is ethnography seeks to describe a community or population to a full extent based around a social context, whereas a case study will look at an instance, or instances, to illustrate a particular problem(s) or issue(s).

An example of a nursing case study was carried out by Lauretta Luck, Debra Jackson and Kim Usher (2008) looking at violence in emergency departments. These authors picked up on the fact that the prevalence of violence in health sector situations, particularly in accident and emergency departments, is very high and nurses have an increased risk of being victims of such violence. Luck *et al.* were particularly concerned at looking at why violence incidents are under-reported by nurses. In this study Luck and her colleagues looked at the meanings that emergency department nurses place on individual acts of violence from patients, their family and friends and what impact these meanings have upon how they respond to such acts. They explored this in an Australian emergency department among 20 consenting registered nurses. Using a case study design, in which the researchers used a mixture of qualitative and quantitative research methods (participant observation, semi-structured interviews, numerical data including counts of the number of incidents of violence), Luck *et al.* found out three things that were common to nurses' assessments of violence in their workplace. They discovered that nurses don't interpret all violence in the same way, and don't simply report all violence; instead they take into account how much they feel the violence was personal towards them, what mitigating factors there were and the reason for the violence in the first place. Therefore, the meanings that nurses ascribe to the violence contributed to the under-reporting of violence, i.e. they may not report it if they felt the person who was violent didn't mean it, or it was a result of them having a difficult day, or they were a vulnerable person.

Action research and fourth-generation evaluation

You may remember that earlier we discussed constructivism and the view that research can be treated as an active learning process in which knowledge is accommodated and reframed continually by ourselves and others. Constructivism has been used to inform action research and fourth-generation evaluation methods. Figure 3.7 shows graphically the cyclical process that is involved in action research in which the research is carried out, action is implemented and there might be further pieces of research and further actions as a consequence.

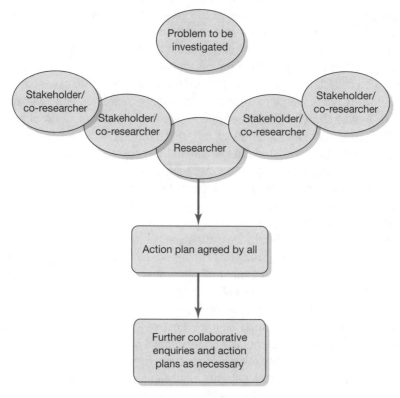

Figure 3.7 An action research method.

Action research is a process whereby researchers seek to research a problem by being involved in a collaborative process with a number of other 'interested parties'. These interested parties, usually called stakeholders, are representative of agencies or organisations who are interested in the 'problem' being researched. Therefore, if an organisation (a hospital) was interested in researching a problem in a patient group (i.e. providing support for people who had cancer), they might, rather than research it themselves, hold meetings with some of these stakeholders (e.g. academics who have studied cancer care, representatives from patients and relatives who are affected by cancer, health professionals who provide cancer care) to organise and develop the research, so that it meets the needs of everyone who has a stake in the outcome of the research. The point is that for these different stakeholders, knowledge of an area will be improved if it is not just based on the knowledge and experience of a few expert researchers, but on the knowledge and experience of a number of co-researchers who will have different knowledge and experience of the problem to be investigated. This also means that there is more ownership among the stakeholders (and, by definition, co-researchers) when the research is completed and actions are recommended as a result.

One specific example of action research has been put forward by Guba and Lincoln (2001) who suggest a certain framework for a certain type of action-based research, called fourth-generation evaluation. Fourth-generation evaluation emphasises that research needs to be participatory and collaborative and we will use a summary (now called constructivist evaluation) put forward by Guba and Lincoln (2001) to illustrate what this type of research method looks like. A constructivist evaluation would suggest that the researcher considers the following:

- The possible number of stakeholders, and to invite as many as possible to take part in the research process.
- What information can be gained from the stakeholders about the current perception of the problem to be researched and the research process they think should be undertaken.
- A research design which incorporates all these different perceptions.
- To facilitate agreement from the group of stakeholders about what research design(s) should be used.
- The development of agreement from the group of stakeholders about what phenomena should be explored.
- Where there is no agreement, to recognise competing aspects of the research and incorporate the consideration of this within the study.
- Ensure that stakeholders are fully aware of issues and where they are not aware of an issue, perhaps because they are not experts in the area, the researcher will help develop that awareness through training.
- Establish a suitable forum for discussion between the different stakeholders that will enable people to share information and concerns about the research.
- Provide written information that communicates the general agreement among stakeholders and highlights the solutions to any issues that have been raised.

- Where unresolved issues remain, the researcher is to look at these and see how they can inform further work.

The main thing to remember about action research and fourth-generation evaluation is that they emphasise collaboration between a number of stakeholders, there is ownership of changes that are implemented, and there is more chance of sustainable change through having such collaborations.

An example of the way action research is used in nursing research was recently carried out by Dineke Vallenga and colleagues (Vallenga, Grypdonck, Tan, Lendemeijer and Boon, 2008). In this study the researchers were interested in improving some of the decisions made by carers of people with epilepsy and a learning disability in terms of the risk posed to them. The challenge for carers of residents in this particular long-stay unit centred on the perception that caregivers often had to find a balance between risk-taking and protection, as both can have a negative effect on quality of life for patients. Vallenga and colleagues identified the various stakeholders – the clients, their representatives and caregivers – that are involved in this decision-making process. By investigating the problem together, the co-researchers managed to reach an agreement about risks and obtained a commitment to risk management between all involved. This agreement was used to adjust caregiving to more fully meet clients' needs and capacities.

Self-assessment exercise

Which research methodologies and methods could be used to look at the following?

A research unit is undertaking a study to describe life on acute psychiatric wards from the point of view of patients. It aims to bring a new perspective to our understanding of the current state of acute wards. The underlying premise is that solutions to current problems must be informed by a good understanding of what actually happens on the wards and what it feels like to be a patient there (Quirk and Lelliott, 2002).

Summary

In this chapter, we have introduced you to some of the important considerations when deciding which qualitative methodology to base your nursing research on. We have shown you the nuances of doing research through the approaches of phenomenology, symbolic interactionism and grounded theory, to name but a few. There is also a wide array of tools that are available to you when doing qualitative research, and we have shown you some of the common methods that exist, which include one-to-one interviews, participant observation, focus groups, ethnography and action research. In the following chapter, we are going to get you into doing research by covering how to develop research ideas and how to start to find out the state of play in the literature through effective and efficient searches of electronic databases and other bibliographic resources.

Chapter 4

Reading the literature and generating research ideas

KEY THEMES

Literature review • Search strategies • Keywords • Library databases • Internet searches • Brainstorming

LEARNING OUTCOMES

By the end of the chapter you will be able to:

● Develop a strategy for searching the literature

● Distinguish between the different approaches that are needed when searching Internet and electronic library databases

● Make effective use of keywords and search terms, like Medical Subject Headings (MeSH)

● Read abstracts efficiently and effectively to decide whether it is worth looking at a resource in more depth

● Pull together the literature to generate research ideas through brainstorming.

Introduction

IMAGINE THAT . . .

You are a student nurse who is on a placement in general practice and you are con-
tributing to the work of the district nursing team that is based in the general practice
surgery. You have found, when going out on the visits to patients' homes, that many
of the patients are older people who seem to have varying levels of quality of life. You
are concerned that some of the older patients appear isolated and lonely and are
sometimes restricted by their physical health problems too. You mention your concerns to your mentor and your mentor identifies an article (Coubrough, 2008) about
the government asking people to take part in a debate on the future of the care and
support system in the United Kingdom for older people with a view to helping older
people stay active, retain their dignity and respect and have a good quality of life (if
you want to read the article it is at: **http://www.nursingtimes.net/whats-new-in-nursing/
minister-calls-for-londons-views-on-care-for-older-people/1744134.article**). This gets
you thinking about the older people that you have encountered on the visits and how
district nurses might be able to enhance these patients' quality of life. It may be that
you can find research into this area that can help you to improve district nurses' current practices and make the situation of these older patients a lot more manageable
for them.

This is one example of how evidence-based practice works and how you can inform
your practice by looking to see what information is out there in the research literature. This chapter is going to pick up on this theme and show you ways of collecting
information that can inform your practice. Formally, this is known as a literature
search.

In this chapter, we will be returning to this example of looking for research into the
quality of life among older people in community settings.

4.1 Starting out

OK, so you've read the article by Coubrough (2008). Where to go next? You've realised you know nothing about these areas. You are sitting down next to a computer,
so perhaps start there. You fire up the computer and type **www.Google.co.uk** into the
address section of the Internet web browser to use Google as your starting point.
Then, when in this search engine, you type 'What information is out there on older
people and their quality of life in community settings' and you then select 'Google
Search', you will get the following screen as in Figure 4.1 (though note if you actually
did this now you wouldn't get a screen like this).

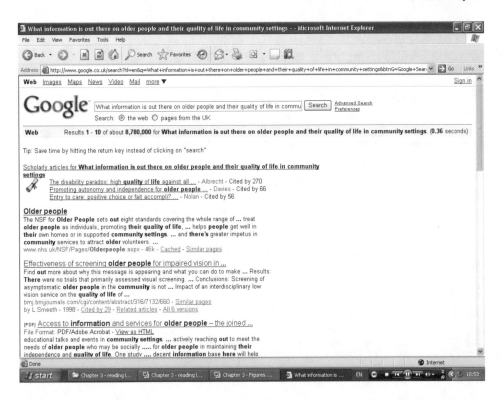

Figure 4.1 Output from a search on Google for 'What information is out there on older people and their quality of life in community settings'.

Excellent. 1 out of 10 of 8,780,000 results were found for your query. That's quite a lot! OK, you could click on the first few links and some of them look promising, such as a webpage on the National Service Framework for Older People that the Department of Health has developed. However, maybe it might be better to see what scholarly articles have been written in the area of quality of life among older people. You could click on the link that says 'Scholarly articles for what information is out there on older people and their quality of life in community settings'. This brings up a search engine known as Google Scholar, which sources more academic publications. Let's look at some of the first few resources that can be found by using Google Scholar (See Figure 4.2).

The first article on the list is entitled, 'The disability paradox: high quality of life against all odds', there is a list of the authors (Albrecht and Devlieger), it was published in *Social Science and Medicine* in 1999. There is also a brief excerpt from the article; this doesn't look like it's the abstract/summary but it gives a quick insight into what's being discussed (i.e. coping with disabilities and still having a decent quality of life). It has been cited in 265 other resources and you could click on the 'cited by 265' link to see who has referred to the article in their own work. By clicking on the title of

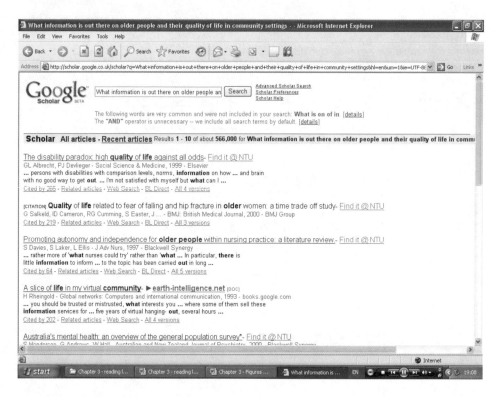

Figure 4.2 A typical screen dump from Google Scholar with a search of *'What information is out there on older people and their quality of life in community settings'.*

the article, this will often take you to the full article (see Figure 4.3a). There is also another article that looks potentially useful for the purposes of examining quality of life among older people in community settings. It is by Davies *et al.* (1997), was published in the *Journal of Advanced Nursing* (see Figure 4.3b), and is a review of the literature. This looks potentially more useful to meeting your aims of exploring quality of life among older patients than the first journal article. There is also another article (Parker *et al.*, 1998) that came up as one of the first few resources listed with Google Scholar and this deals with looking at the health status for older people using a tool called the SF-36, which assesses quality of life (see Figure 4.3c). Overall you are making progress in finding some answers to your questions about the quality of life among older patients in the community, but there is no one article with the initial search that seems to stand out as being the major resource to use.

Overall, we know there is information out there by using Google Scholar but this is only the tip of the iceberg as there was still only another 566,000 articles to go . . . Even if you just click the next few pages, this might all seem a little overwhelming. How do you know what information to gather, what is useful to you? To be honest your head is spinning a little and you're wondering whether this is a good idea? Don't panic, don't give up. What you need is a Search Strategy.

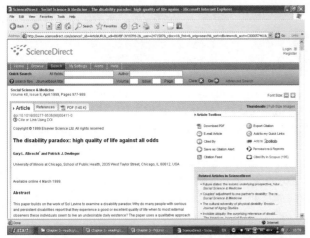

(a)

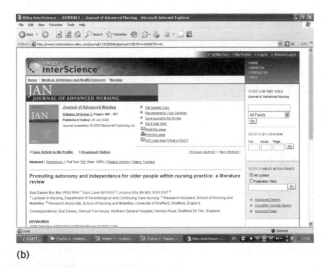

(b)

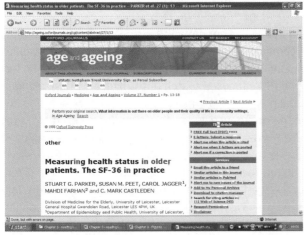

(c)

Figure 4.3 Some of the first few links from Google Scholar on *'What information is out there on older people and their quality of life in community settings'*.

4.2 Search strategy

A search strategy is quite simply a way of you defining your research to make sure you can quickly and efficiently condense a huge amount of information into a manageable quantity for your purposes. It's not only in the scenario above you might be asked to search the literature. You might be responding to a question that has been set as an essay or exam question. You might have been asked to do some extra reading, or prepare yourself for a discussion in a seminar or presentation. In all these activities you will be searching the literature in some way.

Defining your topic: more is definitely not better

It will save you a huge amount of time if you actually give yourself a general definition of what you are looking for. The results may not point you in exactly the right direction straight away, but they will give you confidence in rejecting some (in fact most) of the information you will come across. This is one of the key things you can do in a literature search: rather than collect information upon information until you end up with hundreds of pages of information that are unmanageable, concentrate on a key area that you have defined, if nothing else but to keep your sanity. For example, there is little point in identifying 50 research resources when you've been asked to do a 10-minute presentation in class. There is no way you are going to get all that information into 10 minutes.

Outline what you already know about the topic. If it's very little, or nothing at all, then you might try to be a little more general in your search strategy so you can get to grips with the key ideas. If you know something about the topic then you may already have a good idea of what you are looking for. If you are an expert, then you perhaps need to find some key sources that support your current thinking.

In terms of our current search for older people, up to now we've been a little wild with our search strategy, typing in the equivalent of 'tell us everything you know about older people and quality of life in community settings'. This is probably because it would be fair to say that we are starting out, and really are non-specialists in the area. So let us instead define our topic by using more focused search terms by typing in synonyms for community settings like 'general practice' or 'primary care' or 'patient homes' to include patients who are treated in the community. When searching for things to do with older people, we might need to use words that are used in everyday language and perhaps in research, but some of these terms are not necessarily advisable to use in everyday clinical practice (e.g. talking about 'the elderly' when the acceptable term is 'older people'); however terms like 'elderly', 'geriatrics' and 'gerontology' are very useful for finding highly relevant resources. As we have found from our original search of Google Scholar, one of the resources that popped up had identified 'health status' as being similar to quality of life so perhaps this term might also be used when you do your search, along with other related phrases like 'life satisfaction'. You can begin to see how readily we can develop a list of words that might help us get a clearer idea of the state of the literature into the quality of life among older people in the community. We can do this through using keywords and subject headings.

Keywords and Medical Subject Headings (MeSH)

Keywords are absolutely crucial to your research strategy. They are really useful in honing down your searches. When Google was used to do an initial search, it will have zeroed in on certain phrases and disregarded others that were much too common to help with your search. The terms that Google will have focused on will be the following underlined phrases:

What information is out there on older people and their quality of life in community settings?

Google will select certain key words ('information', 'out', 'older people', 'quality', 'life', 'community settings') and will disregard other terms that are often used as conjunctions to join up with other words (e.g. 'what', 'is', 'there', 'on', 'the', 'and', 'their', 'of', 'in'). In a certain way this is what you must do – identify the keywords in your search. We would argue that the keywords important to our search are:

older people

community settings

quality of life

Therefore we must start making these words important when putting in search terms into any search engine in the future, and worry less about the other terms, because essentially search engines like Google reject them. Another thing to note is that Google doesn't really recognise 'quality of life' as one word. It saw it as quality and life, and though it identified links to quality of life, we might do better in future to put the phrase in speechmarks, "quality of life", because this will only identify sources with this phrase. So we've now developed our keywords, but you might also want to see whether there are other terms that a database uses to categorise things. In the field of nursing, there is a common set of headings, known as MeSH, which stands for Medical Subject Headings. We will have a quick look at what you could do with MeSH by drawing on a search of PubMed, the free online version of MedLine. PubMed is hosted by the National Library of Medicine and the National Institutes of Health for the United States of America. It is similar to search engines like Google Scholar. However, PubMed also has the additional features of specialising in the health field and being able to set limits to your searches, such as only looking for resources published over the most recent decade, for instance, or exploring resources to do with health care for a specific age group. MeSH is also another way of limiting your searches. In Figure 4.4 you can see the main screen that is used in PubMed to find out more on what MeSH is all about. There are some tutorials to help you search using MeSH terms and how to combine these terms to make for a more sophisticated scouring of the literature.

Entering the weblink **http://www.ncbi.nlm.nih.gov/sites/entrez?db=mesh** into your Internet browser takes you to the webpage illustrated in Figure 4.4. We can then find

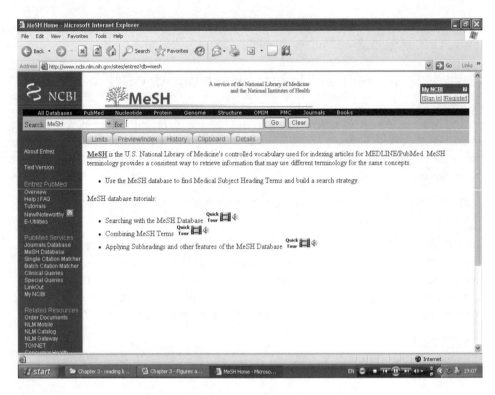

Figure 4.4 How to find the Medical Subject Headings (MeSH) in PubMed.

out what alternative terms might exist in this veritable feast of subject headings known as MeSH! For the purposes of our literature search, we have typed in the term quality of life in the blank space to the right of 'Search MeSH for' that is shown in Figure 4.4. We obtained the following list (Figure 4.5) of search terms that are encompassed within quality of life and there is a definition of what quality of life entails.

It is clear that we could get some potentially helpful results if we entered in 'life qualities' or 'life quality'. There are other terms as well, such as 'Life Style' and 'Sickness Impact Profile'. If you click on the links for each of these alternative terms, you can get more information on each of them. It seems, however, as if 'quality of life', 'life qualities' or 'life quality' might be the terms that could be the most fruitful as other terms don't seem to capture the essence of what we would like to uncover. It's also a good idea to note that some other synonymous phrases, borrowed from psychology in this instance, might be useful, for example using a term like 'life satisfaction'. How about the MeSH for older adults? Could this throw up some interesting alternative terms? From following the same process of typing 'older adults' into the space to the right of 'Search MeSH for', we found the following (see Figure 4.6a, b). Please note that this information on the MeSH for older adults filled up more than one page so the two images show what it would look like as you scroll down the page. Again, there seems to be a definition of older adults, and yet it isn't! When typing in 'older adults', we got a definition for 'frail elderly' and alternative terms such as

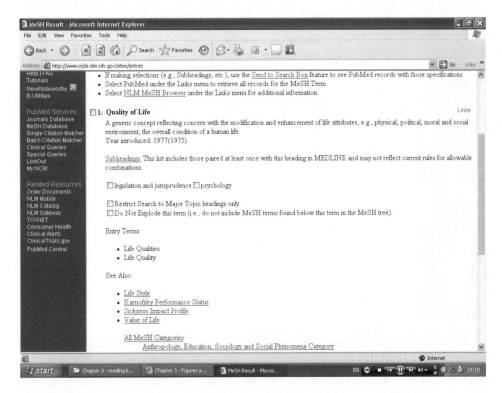

Figure 4.5 Medical Subject Headings (MeSH) related to searches on quality of life.

'Elderly, Frail' and 'Frail Elders'; it would seem as if there is a special interest in medical circles concerning the health needs of older people who seem to have multiple health problems – surely nurses will be more enlightened than this and be looking for older adults who don't just have all these many health problems. What about the healthier older adults too? It would seem that there are also other search terms that might be more relevant and have fewer assumptions about the frailty (or otherwise) of the older adults. Have a look at the link for 'Health Services for the Aged' – this might be a better route. An interesting insight into the search terms using MeSH is what had been used previously; from 1991 onwards, PubMed and MedLine had used MeSH with the term 'frail elderly' whereas before that time other phrases had been used, such as 'Aged' (for 13 years) or 'Aged, 80 or over' (for only 3 years). As we can see, the phrases that are used to explore the medical databases seem to have altered over time and with changing interests in specific age groups or health needs.

In Figure 4.7a, b, we have attempted to take our journeying into the world of MeSH one step further to find out more about combining searches with MeSH terms related to older people and quality of life with a specific focus on the home. To do this, we typed in home care to find out what terms are used in the MeSH thesaurus. As you can see in Figures 4.7a and b, it looks like 'Home Care Services' and 'Home Nursing' show the most promise, which are numbered 1 and 9 respectively on the list of terms most closely allied to the concept of home care.

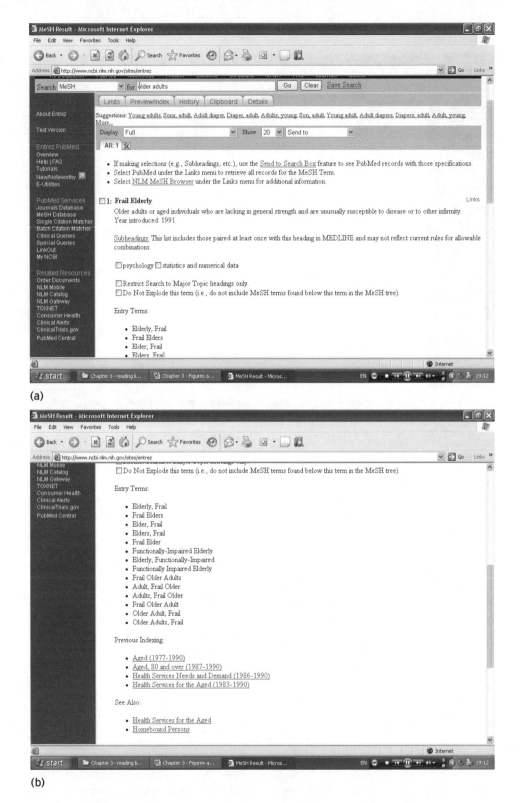

(a)

(b)

Figure 4.6 Medical Subject Headings (MeSH) when searching on older adults.

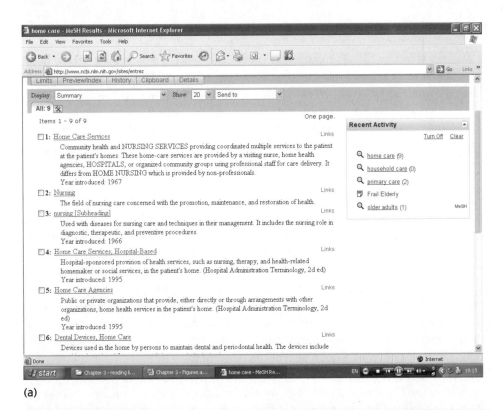

(a)

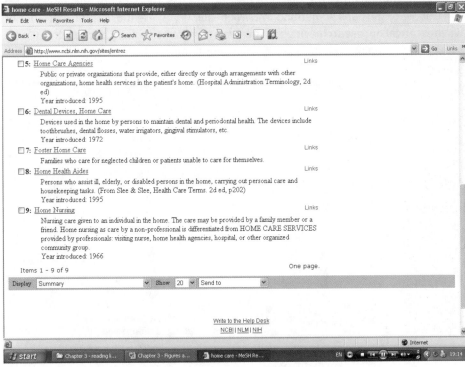

(b)

Figure 4.7 Medical Subject Headings (MeSH) when searching on home care.

Another thing to bear in mind when conducting searches on the electronic databases is that some terms might be commonly used in the United States, such as 'Home Nursing', whereas other allied terms are more commonplace to the United Kingdom, like 'primary care nursing' or 'district nursing'. As a result, do be prepared to deploy a range of terms to explore the literature and allow for different types of jargon being used, depending on the health care system to which the research is referring.

What to search

OK, there are a number of sources out there that can give us information, including Google, Wikipedia, or electronic databases such as MedLine or PubMed, CINAHL (which stands for Cumulative Index to Nursing and Allied Health Literature) and the many books or journals within your institution's library. This is a lot. All of these areas can give you information, but the key is to know how best they can be used and when they should be used. Therefore we're going to outline in this chapter how you could carry out a literature search using a number of sources to get the best information without spending endless hours searching the database and at the end you can be confident you've covered a good deal of the relevant literature.

Figure 4.8 represents our first time-saving idea – giving you a breakdown of how you should see these resources. What we would suggest is that if you are looking for general understanding of a topic, or a part of an area, then a good place to start is with Google or perhaps something like Wikipedia. If you are looking for more definitive theoretical or research evidence then you need to be looking at academic library resources, be it online (via databases) or in your library.

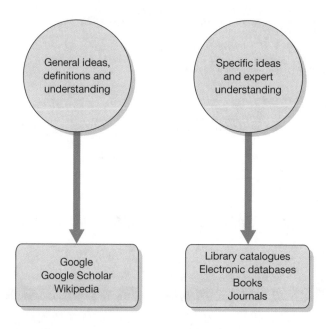

Figure 4.8 Contexts for searching Internet and library databases.

It is important to understand that using Google or Wikipedia as the main source for all your literature is a very bad idea. It's not so much that they can't give you interesting information, and save some time, but it might give you too much information that is unmanageable or leads you to lose focus; it might not also give you the best-quality information as these resources are sometimes not subjected to the same kind of scrutiny by peer reviewers as, say, in an academic journal. We would suggest using these sources to only get background information before moving on to the more specific sources to get an expert understanding of a topic.

Wikipedia

Wikipedia is basically is a free online encyclopaedia. It can be quite useful for getting general information about topics and give us clues about the major areas to consider. Some academics use Wikipedia, some do not. Most of all you should *never* use it as a source of information in an academic piece of work, but rather as a background source. Like a newspaper reporter writing a ground-breaking story, you always treat Wikipedia as your background source. You never cite it in your final work, but it may help you come a long way in developing your story and point you in the right direction.

How could we use Wikipedia with our current search? Well, we know about older people and the home setting, but we are less certain what people actually mean by quality of life. If we search for this in Wikipedia we get a Quality of life page, some of which is presented in Figure 4.9.

Now this is a good example of a typical Wikipedia page. It's very general and has a lot of information. There are no citations to academic authors on the page. It is also a

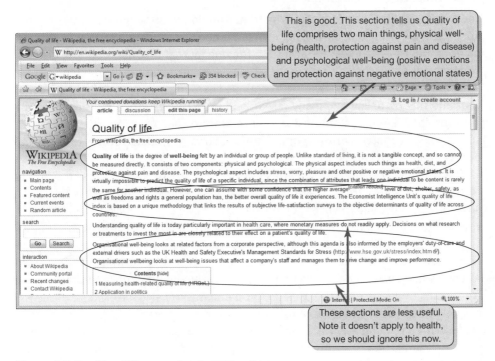

Figure 4.9 Quality of life according to Wikipedia.

summary of everything you need to know and touches on many areas, e.g. measurement, politics. However, what it does is give us some crucial information about quality of life, but it also gives us some irrelevant information. What we need to do now is have some confidence, see what information is useful to us and take away only that.

Look at Figure 4.9 in a bit more depth. The first paragraph provides some definition of quality of life and there is some useful information. Here we now know that quality of life is basically defined as having two components – health and psychology. So as we progress with the topic, we need to be able to see whether any of this can be applied to the situation of older people living in their homes. All the other information is irrelevant to us, it looks at quality of life from an economic and organisational perspective. Although sometimes older people might experience economic hardship, these aspects are not directly relevant to our main concern and so can thus be ignored for our purposes. It is tempting to think 'oh this might be useful' or 'I've found this, I've done the extra work, my goodness I'm going to use it'. Ignore it; it doesn't fit our search strategy which is older people, and their quality of life in the home. What we do know from this page is that essentially when we're talking about older peoples' quality of life at home we're talking about their health and their psychological well-being. However, using Google, or similar Internet databases, can leave us with a wealth of information that we are unable to manage, and Wikipedia gives us some insight, but nothing big on quality of life in terms of older people. We need to turn to where the real expertise exists, which is in the electronic subject databases.

Electronic subject databases

Today there is little need for students to go running into the library searching the library catalogue for that elusive book. In times gone by, students would wrestle each other in a 16-round contest for access to the one journal that has all of the articles. The time has gone when dishonourable students would move a useful textbook to another part of the library for their own continued use. These days you can find most of your information online and many research journal articles are also available online via your library. You can do most of your literature searching from the comfort of your own home (particularly if your institution allows you outside access to its facility by way of an Athens account).

There are many electronic databases like MEDLINE (there is a free version available on the web called PubMed, CINAHL and ASSIA, among others). Your course tutors will have introduced you to the ones you need to use. However, one main library database your institution might have access to is Web of Knowledge (WoK). The ISI Web of Knowledge Service for UK Education provides you with a single route to all journal subscriptions that your institution possesses. It allows you access to abstracts for many resources and links to journal content, if your institution subscribes to that journal. We're going to illustrate the use of electronic databases by using the example of accessing WoK; through this route, we can show you the major strategies to use when searching an electronic database. We're not going to show you how to log on to WoK, as each institution will have different methods for this. Instead, what we are concerned with here is the way you use a library database to effectively search the literature.

Searching a library database: an example using Web of Knowledge

Searching a library database can be a lot of fun. You get to explore a whole world of literature. However, to get the best out of it you need to be adaptable and think about things. What you enter into the database in terms of keywords, search terms, really determines the quality of what comes out. The quality of what you get out of the search is dependent on the amount of work and thought you put into the search. It is not just a matter of typing some things out into the search box and getting some re-sults, reading through and leaving things as they are. You have to be inventive, and think about what you are typing in. Most of all you need to think about your search terms, your keywords, and be adaptable, continually think 'do I need to broaden out these terms?' or 'do I need to be specific?'. In the next four sections, we're going to show you five ways of breaking down your search via:

- Title versus topic
- Looking for general resources
- Looking for recent resources
- Looking for highly cited resources
- Stop, consolidate, review and STOP!

THINGS TO CONSIDER

Other resources for your literature search

There are other resources to find out more about what research has been done apart from journal articles, but do remember that reports of many of the top-quality research studies will have gone through a peer-review process and will be published in journals that have used this process. However, research is published via books, conference papers, dissertations, government publications, NHS/Department of Health publications, indexes/abstracts printed. It may be tempting to go for the other sources first. For example, if you found a book/report in the area, that would be an excellent find, so do check places like the book catalogue in your library, or book pub-lishers, particularly large booksellers, on the Internet to see if there is anything out there.

However, try not to spend too much time on this, usually if there is a definitive re-port or book it will be relatively easy to find. Other sources, such as conference papers and poster presentations or dissertations and theses, are less useful in the first in-stance as getting hold of the full conference paper or thesis may be very hard to do. Overall, with these types of resources you might often be left with just the abstract/summary of the study unless you're able to track down the authors and re-quest a copy of the paper presentation or you're able to get a digital copy of some-one's Masters or Ph.D. thesis.

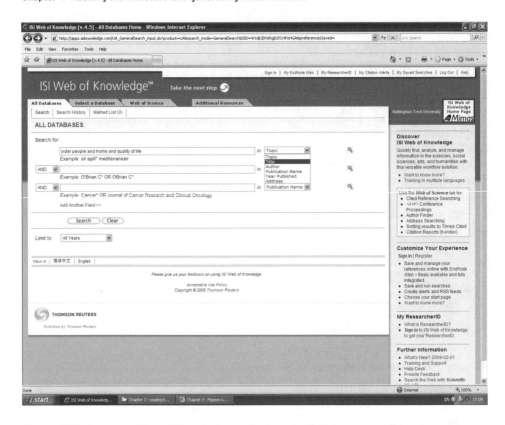

Figure 4.10 Searching Web of Knowledge by topic and title.

Title versus Topic

The first thing we want to point out is that what literature you might get from a library database can be very much different depending on whether you search databases via 'topic' or 'title'. The 'Title' search looks at Title information only, and the 'Topic' option searches the Title, Abstract and Author Keywords. Take a look at Figure 4.10.

The first thing you will note here is that we've put in the following search terms 'older people', 'home' and 'quality of life' with 'AND' in between them. This is telling the library database that we want only those articles that have older people AND home AND 'quality of life' in them. We've run that search term for Title and Topic, and in Table 4.1 you'll find the list of the first eight resources that came out of the database. Resources come out of the database as most recent first.

The main thing that should leap out at you is the two search strategies provide very different findings. In fact, there is no overlap between the two lists, which is surprising as we used exactly the same search terms but just alternated searching in the 'Title' or 'Topic' part of all of the references stored by Web of Knowledge. We have highlighted in bold some of the resources that might be of interest for the purposes of the literature review into quality of life among older people in community settings (i.e. item 1 in the topic list and item 4 in the title list) and we can see from both lists

Table 4.1 Different findings on 'older people and home and quality of life' depending on search by topic or title

When done by topic (609 references found)	When done by title (8 references found)
1. Impact of health education on health-related quality of life among elderly persons: results from a community-based intervention study in rural Bangladesh	1. Seniors at Risk: The Association between the Six-Month Use of Publicly Funded Home Support Services and Quality of Life and Use of Health Services for Older People
2. Protecting Personhood and Achieving Quality of Life for Older Adults With Dementia in the US Health Care System	2. Health-related quality of life and depression among older people in Yerevan, Armenia: a comparative survey of retirement home and household residents aged 65 years old and over
3. Making Meaningful Connections A Profile of Social Isolation and Health Among Older Adults in Small Town and Small City, British Columbia	3. Quality of life and symptoms among older people living at home
4. Developing community in care homes through a relationship-centred approach	4. PEARLS home based treatment significantly improves depression, dysthymia, and health related quality of life in older people.
5. The impact of social support and sense of coherence on health-related quality of life among nursing home residents- A questionnaire survey in Bergen, Norway	5. Quality of life among older people in Sweden receiving help from informal and/or formal helpers at home or in special accommodation
6. Rehabilitation for older people in long-term care	6. Predictors of quality of life in older people living at home and in institutions
7. Growing old in a new estate: establishing new social networks in retirement	7. Health-related quality of life and health preference as predictors of mortality among older people at veteran home
8. Case management by nurses in primary care: analysis of 73 'success stories'	8. Functional and quality of life outcomes in elderly patients following discharge from hospital

that both these options in the library database provided us with potentially interesting resources. It is intriguing to note that some of these studies have compared the quality of life among older people in residential or nursing homes versus those still living in their own homes (see items 3 and 8 in the Search 'By Topic' list and items 2, 3, 5, 6 and 8 in the title list). It is also noteworthy that there are as many as 609 resources that crop up when we do the search 'By Topic' and only 8 resources are found when doing the search 'By Title'. Therefore, the lesson to learn from this is that you must use different ways within the menus for the electronic databases to do a systematic and comprehensive search of the material. Depending on what database you are using, the search terms you use and the areas within the reference citation that you are searching (i.e. title vs. topic), you may come up with very different kinds of information. It is all too often that we have found students will come to us with the age-old complaint 'I've searched everywhere for literature and can't find anything!' However, as you can see from this example, you can very quickly identify a range of interesting and potentially handy resources by being flexible in the strategies you utilise when searching the literature.

THINGS TO CONSIDER

Using abstracts/summaries

In any database, most resources listed (unless they are cited conference papers) will have an abstract. An abstract is an overview of the resource and lists the main points and findings from the resource. Therefore when you find a resource that you think might be of interest, click on the title and it will take you to a full reference for the resource, including the abstract. This way you can find out more about the research before you read it. For example, using our lists from Table 4.1 let's look at two of the following resources that we thought might be of interest; 'Case management by nurses in primary care: analysis of 73 "success stories"' and 'Functional and quality of life outcomes in elderly patients following discharge from hospital'.

Case management by nurses in primary care: analysis of 73 'success stories'

Author(s): Elwyn, Glyn; Williams, Meryl; Roberts, Catherine; Newcombe, Robert G; Vincent, Judith

Source: Qual Prim Care **Volume:** 16 **Issue:** 2 **Pages:** 75-82 **Published:** 2008

Abstract: BACKGROUND: There is interest as to whether case management reduces unplanned patient admission to hospital. However, very little is known about how the intervention is delivered and what the most salient outcome measures are. DESIGN: Qualitative study embedded in a wider evaluation. SETTING: Primary health care. METHOD: Analysis of case manager case reports in a service innovation evaluation study. RESULTS: Case management provides home-based care to frail elderly patients using a process of assessment and medication review. This often leads to new diagnoses, to the co-ordination of further care and the tailoring of services to suit the needs of individuals. The benefits reported are complex and relate to improving a patient's quality of life more than the prevention or otherwise of admission to hospital. The type of attention provided by these roles seems to be absent from current NHS arrangements. The role enables time to be spent assessing the individual needs of patients who live at the margins of independent living. CONCLUSION: The case managers describe having the time and the skills to assess a mix of clinical and social problems, and then accessing the correct networks to help elderly people with multiple illnesses navigate a complex system of providers. More weight should be given to the ability of this intervention to result in improved quality of life for patients, and to the investigation of costs and benefits.

Functional and quality of life outcomes in elderly patients following discharge from hospital

Author(s): McEvoy S, Blake C

Source: EUROPEAN JOURNAL OF PUBLIC HEALTH **Volume:** 15 **Page:** 140
Supplement: Suppl. 1 **Published:** NOV 2005

Times Cited: 0 **References:** 0

Document Type: Meeting Abstract

◀

We can see the first resource seems interesting by examining the clinical and social problems experienced by older people, whereas the second resource is just an abstract from a meeting; it is a very short note and gives away little information as to what is covered. Unless you are looking for an exhaustive list, it might be best to exclude this second resource from the list.

Looking for general resources and reviews

Another way of breaking down your literature review is to look for major resources in the area. 'Review', 'meta-analysis' and 'meta-synthesis' are all terms used in research that describe resources combining the results from several studies to provide an overall review. Meta-analyses and meta-syntheses have specific ideas attached to them that are used in research, the details of which we're not going to get into, but nonetheless the point is that these types of resources provide us with potential overviews of an area. To see whether meta-analyses have been done in the area of quality of life among older people in the community, we could enter this term, 'meta-analysis' as part of the search (see Figure 4.11). The list of seven resources below outlines what we obtained with our original search terms, along with the addition of 'AND meta-analysis' to these terms.

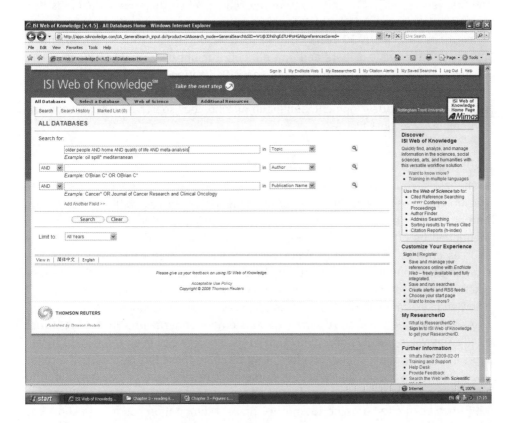

Figure 4.11 Finding meta-analysis-type resources on older people, the home and quality of life.

- Locomotor disability: meaning, causes and effects of interventions
- Physical activity programmes for persons with dementia
- ACNP white paper: update on use of antipsychotic drugs in elderly persons with dementia
- Meta-analysis: protein and energy supplementation in older people
- Occupational therapy for community-dwelling elderly people: a systematic review
- Predictors of efficacy in depression prevention programmes – meta-analysis
- Institutional versus at-home long-term care for functionally dependent older people.

Again, we've shown in bold the resources that look interesting from just reading the title, although a read of the abstract/summary might help. These approaches have thrown up a number of useful resources for examining the quality of life of older people in their homes.

Looking at recent resources

From our examples above we have highlighted six resources (five resources from the title and topic search and one from a meta-analytic search), and these were only from the first few resources to emerge from the search, when there were hundreds that could possibly be extracted. Databases cover many years. Web of Knowledge, for example, goes back nearly 30 years – that's a lot of resources! So you can see how much information there is out there and how difficult it might be to handle. One excellent strategy is to limit your search to recent years. By limiting your searches to the most recent five years could help you concentrate your attention on the most recent research and theory development, and aid in making your search as cutting edge and contemporary as possible.

Looking at frequently cited resources

In the last section, we told you about limiting your search to previous years, but a question remains – are you missing out on influential resources? Well, you can always find out which resources are the most influential by exploring how often they are mentioned by other researchers. However, there is a way of finding influential resources on Web of Knowledge quickly and efficiently. With each entry there is a citation count and this tells you quickly how influential the resource is. For example when we did a search for 'older people, home and quality of life' via topic in Web of Knowledge we came across the following five resources (see Figure 4.12).

As you can see for each resource, there is a note underneath, which says 'Times cited'. This value denotes how many times this resource has been referred to by authors in another publication. Therefore, if we compare these five resources, the reference 'Ongoing work of older adults at home after hospitalization' has been cited 10 times, the next reference has been cited 43 times, whereas one reference (Farquhar, 1995) has been cited a grand total of 119 times! High citation counts can show you that this resource might be worth investigating, particularly if the title fits your key

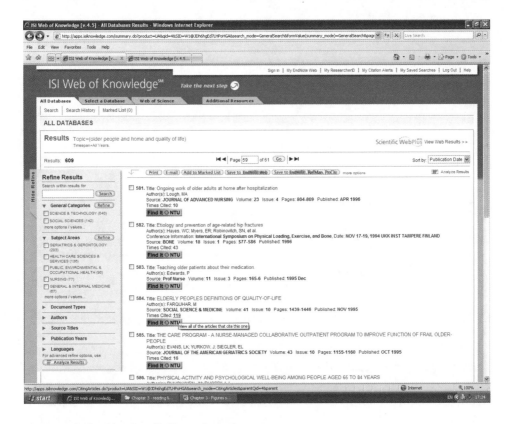

Figure 4.12 Looking for citations of papers.

searching requirements. The Farquhar (1995) reference does look particularly promising, as the title seems to suggest that the article is dealing with what older people
understand as being a good quality of life. We then place our mouse pointer over the
'Times cited' part of the reference and this takes us to the screen that you can see in
Figure 4.13. Although high citation counts are no guarantee of the overall validity and
reliability of the resource itself, it is an indicator that other researchers think the resource is worth mentioning. Therefore it's certainly worth following up resources that
are highly cited.

Also you can further help your literature search by clicking on the number of times
cited as this will list all the resources referring to this work (see Figure 4.13). Do bear
in mind that number of citations for each resource you find might be skewed a little
by how new the resource is; if a resource is relatively old (e.g. published 10 years ago),
it might be referred to by many more authors than if the reference was only two or
three years old. Another thing to be cautious about is whether the resource has
mainly been cited by the authors themselves in other work (known as self-citation).
This is something to be wary about as you should mainly be researching whether people other than the authors themselves see the work as invaluable. By clicking on each
of the resources that have cited the one that you're interested in, you should be better equipped to discover whether there are many self-citations. Overall, citation

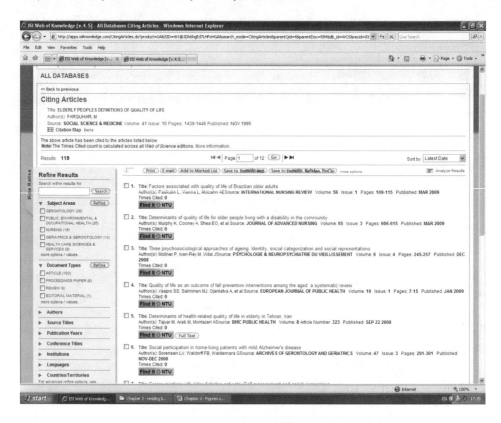

Figure 4.13 Finding out who has done the citing (an example of Farquhar, 1995).

counts is a fantastic tool, because it provides you with some additional resources that have followed up on this work and some may be relevant to you.

There is one thing to note here. So far we've emphasised looking at the most recent resources around and to some extent looking for comprehensive resources. However, the citation count provides you with another way of doing a literature research. Imagine that you have a resource or a key theory that you want to follow up. Using the 'Times cited' part of Web of Knowledge you can see what other work has been done in the area by looking at all the resources that cite that original resource. The list provided by 'Times cited' will reference all the research work that has cited that article and therefore you can very quickly obtain a large overview of the literature in that area. This feature is something that is now becoming increasingly common in many electronic databases (e.g. Google Scholar) so make sure you check to see whether it is included in the database you're currently using.

Stop, consolidate, review and STOP!

Even with this cursory review we've generated 9 resources (7 from topic/title, 1 from using meta-analysis as a search term, and 1 from looking for highly cited resources). As you can see we've already got a substantial number of resources, with relatively little work. We also know, from using our criteria, we've got very recent resources, we've got some general review resources and we've got resources that are highly cited. This mixture of literature would provide a firm basis for any review. So the next skill is about knowing when to stop.

You could endlessly look for resources, but at this stage, perhaps when your number of resources has got into double figures (i.e. around 10), this would be the time to start reading. Clearly, this won't be a complete literature review but reading these first few resources will give you a good idea of whether you are on the right lines or not. If you're on the right lines, great! If you're not, then you might need to think about broadening out or narrowing your search terms. Check your search words against a thesaurus, like MeSH, to see if there are other keywords you could use. For example:

● You might broaden out the term 'older people' to include 'older persons', 'elders', 'elderly', 'old age,' or 'retirement'.
● You might change the term from 'home' to 'community'.

Most importantly, be sensible in your searching. It is most likely that your early experiences of literature searching will have entailed a large-scale collection of any possible resource relevant to the topic area; by contrast, being sensible would mean not doing an exhaustive review but rather a selective overview of the recent, relevant literature. Hopefully all the strategies discussed above will help you achieve this - just remember it is important to know when to stop searching and actually get on with reading the resources and writing about them.

THINGS TO CONSIDER

Know your journals!

The advent of the ISI Web of Knowledge Service for UK Education is useful for many clinicians because there are links between each citation and the resources available in your institution's library. However, you may not have ready access to Web of Knowledge and the resources available via this route. If this is so, it might be a good idea before starting your library search to get a list of journals held in your library or available as an electronic journal. It will also be crucial to find out which important journals are the best in the nursing field that you can access via this route; you will then know which journals you can access and which ones are highly esteemed by those in the field. This might shape what articles you select in your search.

If you know there is a book or article you need but your library doesn't have it, your library will usually have an inter-library loans system that will get you any article/book after you complete a request form and submit it to your institution's library. After a short time, the article/book will arrive at your library. In some cases, articles can be emailed to you via secure electronic delivery. You may need to find out from your library how many inter-library loans you are entitled to and whether you have to pay for this service.

Effective and efficient reading

OK, so you have your 10 articles to start with. This is a lot of reading, and there may now be the tendency to panic. However, you don't have to read all these articles from beginning to end. In research you need to gain information very quickly about that article, then if you think it is one of the most useful you might return to it later for full consideration when you have read others. Below we have outlined a ten-point plan to approach each resource to read.

Point 1: read for a purpose

Remember why you are reading the article. You will have set aims, be it to answer a question, or to find out about an area. Therefore as you have a number of articles to read, only worry about information that informs the areas you are interested in. Remind yourself of this before reading. For example, using our search above, we would only be interested in information from a resource that informs our understanding and knowledge of older people's quality of life in the home.

Point 2: overview – read the abstract first

For many research articles the main findings and conclusions of the resource are presented in the abstract, so always read that. What do the authors say they found and what were their main conclusions?

Point 3: record the full reference

Record the full reference and where you found it. Nothing is more annoying that forgetting where something is, particularly when it is crucial to your literature review. This is also important so you can reference your ideas properly in any write-up of the literature review you do. It is a well-known fact that in many plagiarism cases, students are reprimanded because they have failed to record where they got their ideas from properly. Making these notes early and clearly will not only improve the academic quality of your work, but also stop you making mistakes and errors.

Point 4: why has the research been done?

Often in research there is a problem that has been looked at. Often in nursing this will be for two reasons. The first reason will be to solve a problem. For example, this might be to report on the usefulness of a drug, or to solve an issue in nursing. Therefore the research is designed to address or inform us about how to 'solve' this problem, whether to solve it directly or to add to the debate. The second reason might be to test some sort of theoretical proposition. For example, a nurse researcher could be evaluating if a certain approach in nursing is successful, such as applying person-centred approaches and person-centred planning in learning disability care. The problem or approach being researched will always be stated clearly in the introduction of the resource.

Point 5: what is the central research question?

At the end of the introduction will be a main statement about the aims of the research. This is also sometimes called the **hypothesis**. Record this information so you can focus on central ideas being tested in the research information. Also, this statement might be accompanied by a rationale for the research. This is also useful to make notes on because it tells you about the authors' thinking and what assumptions they are making when carrying out the research.

Point 6: what methodology and methods were used?

It is important to record what type of methodology and methods were used. Much of this information should be in the 'methods' section. There is no need to write out everything from the methods section, but make a quick note of the type of study. What methods were used (e.g. questionnaires, conversation analysis, interview, participant observation)? It might also be useful to record whether the work was largely quantitative or qualitative in nature. If it's not clear, have a quick look at the results/findings section; if this section is full of statistics, it is probably a quantitative study, whereas if it's full of quotes from interviews or everyday interactions between nurses and patients, then it's likely to be a qualitative study. If it has both, then it's probably a mixed methods study.

Point 7: what are the main findings?

Usually full details of the findings are listed in the results section, but there is no need to repeat it all. In the first (few) section(s) are a summary of the main findings. Therefore it is useful to make a note of the main findings using these, as they are obviously the findings the author(s) found most important for meeting the research aims/questions of the study.

Point 8: what is the main contribution(s) of the research?

After the reporting of the main findings, the authors will try to establish the importance of the findings. That is, what is the reader expected to take away from reading the resource as being the key implications of the study for theory or health care practice? The author(s) may suggest that the work has solved the problem, or supported or refuted the idea being tested. They will also identify how the finding fits in with the current literature or practice. Therefore a quick summary of the main contributions will be useful to note. If you've read a resource and you're still not sure, then look at the abstract or the final paragraph of the discussion, this is sometimes the point at which the authors will emphasise the main contribution of the research.

Point 9: what recommendations/directions are made for the future of this research? Have the author(s) pointed to any weaknesses in the study?

In the discussion, the authors will try to make recommendations for future research, to guide the research onwards. So what recommendations do the authors make and what future directions do the authors identify? Also, did the author identify any problems with the research or shortcomings? What weaknesses did they identify and do they suggest how the research might have been improved?

Point 10: your own reflections

What did you think of the resource? More importantly what ideas did you come up with while reading the resource? How did this resource compare with other resources in the area? Did you think of a research idea, or a better research project while reading the resource? Or did you think of a way that the research might be improved?

Finally, we think it a good idea if you rate the resource in terms of your aims, i.e. give it a mark out of 10 in terms of how well the resource would help you with your literature review; with '1' being 'not much help' and '10' being 'a great help'. Now this might seem strange, but after having read through 30 articles and having a limited number of words to write your literature review, it will give you a brief, at-a-glance template for condensing and understanding the most important research around in the area. With limited time and space to write your literature review, this template can give you the best way of choosing which references make the most difference in helping you to develop a viable research question. You can then look at your rating system and choose the best resources that fit in with your work.

EXERCISE 4.1

Unearthing the key points from a paper

Read the following research paper by using our '10-point plan' form on p. 95 and fill in the sections. Also time yourself – you might be surprised as to how quickly you can collate information from the paper using this technique.

Case study 1 Falls among older people

Ward, F., Williams, G.A., Maltby, J. and Day, L. (2008) Assessment of nutritional problems and risk of falling in hospital-based older person care: Brief research report. *Optimal Nursing Research*, *25 (3)*, 25-29.

Abstract:
Falls among older people are problematic in the hospital environment and a cause for concern among administrators, patients, relatives and health professionals alike. In the current study, the views of 31 nurses on falls' risk assessment were obtained from a randomly selected sample of 50 nursing staff working in three Care of the Older Person wards. We focused on nurses' consideration of poor nutrition among patients as being a major factor for making falls more likely and hypothesised that there would be a relationship between the type of ward that a nurse was based on and acknowledging nutritional problems as being implicated with falls. No significant link was found between ward type and nurses looking at nutrition. We outline the implications for staff training with needing to ensure that more nurses see nutrition as a falls' risk factor. It is also recommended that this education does not need to be targeted to those working in only one type of Care of the Older Person ward.

Introduction:
Falls among older people contribute greatly to mortality and morbidity throughout this country and the government (Department of Health and Health Care, 2003) has been

implementing action plans to target this growing problem. The Dietetic Society (2007) has claimed that one of the major risk factors for falls among older people is that many of them are undernourished, thus leading to dizziness when older people are mobilising. In the hospital environment, there should be less chance of older patients not having sufficient nourishment, as there should be more control over what food is administered to them. However, there is evidence that the older patient has problems with diet and feeling hungry due to polypharmacy (i.e. needing to take a cocktail of prescribed drugs throughout the day) (Jefferies and Dealer, 2006). In the current study, we were aiming to see whether nurses involved with care of the older patient were taking poor diet/malnourishment into account when considering a patient's risk of falling. This study focused on the reported falls' risk assessment practices of a sample of registered general nurses working at three Care of the Older Person wards in a community hospital based in a city within the New Pleasant state. We also sought to explore whether there was a relationship between the type of ward that the nurses worked on and the reported assessment practices. It was hypothesised that there would be a link between ward and assessment of diet when examining risk of falling. This hypothesis was grounded in observations by the research team that one of the wards (Spondlebury) appeared to have patients with higher dependencies than in the other two wards, which dealt mainly with rehabilitation, and that staff would thus have less time to consider nutrition as an issue.

Method:

Participants – A random sample of 50 nurses was approached out of the population of 75 full time and part time nurses employed by the hospital. Agency nursing staff were not approached, as the permanent staff would govern all induction and training in patient assessment and we viewed them as being vital to driving the methods and ethos of patient assessment. Out of the nurses that we sampled, 33 replied to the invitation letter with a completed questionnaire (66% response rate), although only 31 of the forms were useable with complete data.

Materials – We used the Stanislav Falls Assessment Procedures Index (Stanislav, 2005). This comprised a 35-item form that requires respondents to identify the factors they consider when assessing an older person's risk of falling. This questionnaire has been mainly validated with hospital-based older person care (Stanislav and Spector, 2004) and has been found to have subscales tapping into three main concepts – physical health, psychological well being and the mobilisation process. These three subscales have internal consistencies of 0.89, 0.65 and 0.85 respectively.

Analysis – As we were primarily interested in the relationship between type of Care of the Older Person ward and nurses' reported assessment of nutritional problems when examining patient risk of falling, we conducted a chi-squared analysis on these two variables.

Procedure – Posters advertising the study were placed on staff notice boards near the three wards and the agreement of the staff unions and the hospital management was obtained before commencing the study. Local Research Ethical Committee approval was also granted in November 2005. The research team sent the questionnaire to the sample of nurses via the internal post during the week commencing 12 December 2005. The forms had a self-addressed, stamped envelope for participants to send their completed returns to the team by a two-week deadline.

Results:

Table 1 outlines the distribution of nurses who said that they either did or did not consider nutritional problems among their patients when assessing risk of falling on the wards. It is noteworthy that only 16 out of the 31 (51.6%) nurse respondents reported looking out for nutritional problems when assessing falls' risk.

Table 1 Nutritional problems as a risk factor for falls among older patients

'Which ward do you work in?'	'Consideration of nutrition problems?'	
	No	Yes
Spondlebury	5	6
Wickham	7	7
Hesham	3	3

A chi-squared analysis showed that there was no significant relationship between the type of ward that the nurses worked on and their focus on nutritional problems among patients when conducting falls' risk assessment, $X^2(2) = 0.059$, $p > 0.05$.

Discussion:

It can be seen from the results that only half of the nurses who responded to our survey of falls' risk assessment practices said that they considered nutritional problems among their patients. This trend is in line with prior research (e.g. William and Hill, 2003) showing that nutrition is a neglected part of inpatient care for the older person and that nutritional well being tends to be left to the dietician to monitor (Tidy and Meal, 2000). Unexpectedly, there was no link between type of ward and evaluation of nutritional problems as a risk factor, thus indicating that nursing practice seems fairly consistent within a community hospital setting. There are some potential limitations that need to be considered. Although our sample of 31 respondents was a sizeable percentage of the population of nursing staff within the three wards, it needs to be recognised that there may have been fewer senior nurses obtained with random sampling as they constitute a relatively small percentage of the total number of nurses employed in the study sites. Given that it is likely the senior nurses would be more involved with patient assessment (and falls' risk assessment) than junior nurses, this could explain why only half of our sample had considered nutrition as a factor. Further research could aim at replicating the administration of our questionnaire to staff at other similar wards, but through the use of a stratified sampling method. Nevertheless, the current trends seem to suggest the need for nursing practice to routinely incorporate the nutritional status of an older patient and for nurses to be educated to the impact that poor nutrition among older patients can have on making the patient disorientated and weak when mobilising. As we did not find a link between type of Care of the Older Person ward and reported assessment practices, we would recommend that this education should cover the training of all grades of nursing and in all types of wards.

10-point research paper summary sheet

1. Purpose: why you are reading the article?

2. Overview/abstract: main points of the paper

3. The full reference.

4. Why has the research been done?

5. What is the central research question?

6. What methodology and methods were used?

7. What are the main findings?

8. What is the main contribution(s) of the research?

9. What recommendations/directions are made for the future of this research? Have the author(s) pointed to any weaknesses in the study?

10. Your own reflections:

How long did you take to read the article? _____ minutes

How long did you take to write your summary of the article? _____ minutes

How useful is the paper for your literature review? _____ /10

4.3 Generating research ideas

There comes a time in all research projects when you will need to come up with your own research ideas. Unfortunately, ideas for nursing research are sometimes difficult to generate as you might think that other people have done all of the relevant research and that it's tough to come up with anything new. There are a couple of ways you can generate research ideas and this is through brainstorming ideas. We're going to show you two ways of brainstorming – on your own and with others.

Brainstorming research ideas on your own

Brainstorming is a technique for generating new ideas and in essence it is a matter of you writing down as many ideas as possible. The technique is particularly useful when you are out of ideas or you want a new way of looking at things; i.e. thinking up new research ideas. Most usefully you can effectively use the information you got from your 10-point literature review above.

To brainstorm on your own, get a few pieces of blank paper, a pen and start to jot down as many ideas as possible to the following questions;

1. From your literature review, what areas have been investigated and what areas have not been investigated. You might find point 9, what recommendations/directions are made for the future of this research?, would inform your brainstorming here.

2. What general explanations are provided or concentrated on in this literature? Are there any ideas here that interest you, or should form the basis of any consideration in this area?

3. Are there any variables or aspects of the research literature that have not been looked at together before?

4. How have other research projects defined and measured key concepts in the study? Could these concepts be looked at in a different way?

What you should now have is a list of brainstormed ideas about how to move the work forward. Now take all your ideas and list them. These are your possible ideas for research.

Brainstorming research ideas in a group

Another way to brainstorm is with other people. This might be a tutor at work, some classmates or fellow nurses and other health professionals, managers and service users. Brainstorming in a group will potentially increase the richness of research ideas. It may concentrate the research around the literature and may draw on problems/issues encountered in nursing or clinical practice.

When working in a group you ask the same sort of questions as above. You may have to introduce them to the topics, and to get a brainstorming group working well you might need to do the following things.

1. Define what you want to come out of the session and establish what needs to be talked about and what doesn't need to be talked about.

2. Appoint someone to write down ideas, preferably on a flip-chart so that everyone is reminded about what ideas have been developed so far.

3. Suggest that the session is non-critical. That is, you are not there as a group to evaluate ideas, but to generate as many ideas as possible in an enthusiastic manner.

4. Try to keep all the participants in the group focused on the issues.

5. Try to have fun, allow them to come up with silly ideas as that will clear their heads, and allow them to move on to other ideas.

6. Try to ensure that no one aspect is considered for too long. If this occurs people may shift the debate away from your objectives and into a particular topic.

7. Try to ensure that everyone gets the chance to contribute. If you are having problems in giving everyone an opportunity to generate ideas, try to shift from one group member to the next and get them to shout out any concepts that come to mind. The more you emphasise in the brainstorming process that ideas won't be edited until as many ideas have been 'splurged' onto the flip-chart paper as can be managed.

At the end of this session you also need to make a list of possible research projects and there is no reason why you can't get the group to provide some opinion on what research projects would be the best ones to do.

Your final ideas

After your brainstorming sessions you might have at least a couple of research ideas, and some opinion of which one you could do (if not one that you would like to do). It is definitely worth noting down at this stage some of your thinking about coming to that decision, particularly if it is led by some of the ideas in the literature. Often in any academic resource there is some rationale to the study, and therefore making some notes now will be useful in any write-up you do.

With that done, you need to finally make a statement about the aims of the research. This needs to be a clear and simple statement. Sometimes this is done in the form of a statement, and a lot of research. Whatever the statement, it is worth making it clear to yourself at this stage of the research process what exactly it is you want to look at in your research study. It is worth making clear to yourself what you want look at because it will help you develop your reading into a good study, help you make decisions about what methods to use, and most of all keep you focused throughout your research.

Self-assessment exercise

Let us bring these ideas together by you doing something on your own. Think about your current practice, and think about something you want to know more about from the research literature. Write this topic in the box below.

Now give yourself 20 minutes on the Internet. Use 5 minutes to find out what you can from Google, Google Scholar and Wikipedia about your topic, and 15 minutes to find out what you can from the electronic databases in your library about your topic. Now write down the main things you found out about your topic from these difference sources.

How do you think you did? We think you probably found out a number of things about your topic, and more things than you expected to. It is just a matter of dedicating some time to the literature search.

Summary

In this chapter, we have introduced you to methods of finding out more about the literature before conducting your nursing research. We have shown you how to develop a search strategy and the different methods that can be used to delve into Internet and electronic library databases such as PubMed and Web of Knowledge. You should also be more aware of the types of search terms that you can use to explore these databases, especially with a list of words that the databases use to do the searches (e.g. MeSH). You should also be more confident in being able to generate research questions having done this literature search and engaging in brainstorming activities either by yourself or with others. In the following chapter, we will take you through some of the processes you need to undertake to set up your own nursing research study.

Chapter 5

Setting up your study: Methods in data collection

KEY THEMES

Data collection methods • Questionnaires • Interviews • Question types •
Bias • Error • Sampling • Ethics

LEARNING OUTCOMES

By the end of this chapter you will be able to:

- Identify many of the key considerations when planning a research study,
  including being aware of issues relating to bias, error, sampling and
  research ethics

- Know when to use questionnaires, one-to-one and focus group interviews, or
  clinical/health assessment tools and how to plan appropriately when using
  these data collection methods

- Distinguish between various kinds of questions that can be posed in a
  questionnaire or interview, such as closed and open questions, and you will be
  able to identify the advantages and disadvantages of using these questions

- Distinguish between different types of interview schedules (i.e. sets of
  questions to be asked) and know the difference between unstructured, semi-
  structured and structured interview schedules

- Appraise and critique data collection methods used by others.

Introduction

In the previous chapter, we looked at developing effective research questions through searching the literature and using methods such as brainstorming, to generate ideas. In this chapter, we are going to take one further step by matching research questions with an appropriate research method.

IMAGINE THAT . . .
You are that student nurse from the last chapter who was interested in the quality of life among older patients cared for in the community; you have generated research ideas and questions as a result of your literature searching and you have typed up a summary of what you found and the areas still to be researched and you have put this in your professional portfolio. Your personal tutor has seen this entry in your portfolio and has told you that you've made some good progress in identifying interesting research but these ideas are not going to solve any problems unless they're translated into action. Your personal tutor mentions to you that you have a research proposal to do for one of your modules and you could put some of the literature review in the proposal but you still need to identify how you're going to follow up on some of the research questions you've developed. 'Where next?', we hear you cry! The next step is deciding on an appropriate method to use to address your research questions and to collect data, if your research proposal is seen as acceptable.

In this chapter we're going to look at some of the most commonly used methods in nursing research. We're going to describe these methods in detail so you could set up a good study using any one of them. We are then going to introduce you to some important considerations you need to make before starting any research, which involves the ethical treatment of participants and sampling. Being familiar with a range of methods and data collection will also help you in appraising and reading research in order to develop your evidence-based practice.

5.1 Choice of method

In setting up a study one of the first things you need to do is select the method you are going to use. Figure 5.1 shows how the different methods described in this chapter are related to quantitative and qualitative studies. This diagram is used to simplify the ideas in your mind.

There might be a number of reasons for doing the study that will inform your choice of method. You might have very strong indication of what sort of study you need to run. For example, if you're studying the effects of a new drug then you will need to adopt an experimental approach because you need to run clinical trials. It might be that your research supervisor or colleagues have suggested that they need a survey to be carried out. However, it may be that you are designing and carrying out

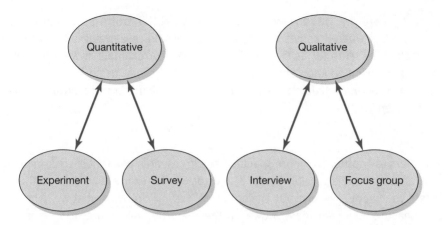

Figure 5.1 Different types of research methods used in nursing research.

the study by yourself as part of a dissertation. Hopefully this diagram should help you weigh up what research method to use when doing your research. For example, you might be interested in taking a quantitative approach to a topic because you want to be looking at adopting a traditional scientific method in which you can compare patient groups or relationships between variables such as a patient's depressive symptoms and suicidal intentions. Therefore you know that the methods open to you are experiments or surveys. Or you might know that you want an in-depth examination of patients' experiences and therefore a qualitative approach might be more appropriate.

The importance of guarding against bias and error

However, before we move on, we need to introduce you to two concepts that drive much of the good practice we describe in this chapter when doing quantitative research. The quantitative researcher's enemy, so to speak, is bias and error.

Bias

Bias is a major concern for nurse researchers doing quantitative studies. Bias exists in our everyday life, sometimes it happens naturally, sometimes it happens deliberately. Certain newspapers have a bias toward certain political thought. Some we might consider more closely aligned to right-wing thought, and some more closely aligned to left-wing thought. You are biased in terms of what type of clothes you wear, whether you would prefer to take a friend or a stranger out for dinner, unless of course that stranger was Brad Pitt or Angelina Jolie. Therefore, we have certain biases towards certain strangers. We show bias in our choice of TV programmes we watch. We would like to watch a programme that interests us rather than bores us. Bias in life is an exciting part of our life. It helps us understand about ourselves (shopping or the library?). However, when it comes to establishing the truth, bias can sometimes distort that. Take for example our politicians. All politicians claim to act in our best interests, but we know that sometimes politicians are biased and may try to spin the 'facts'. Therefore, we can never be certain of what the 'truth' of the matter is. This is also an issue when it comes to research methods. In research it is important that we establish the truth (or as close to it as we can). For example, if we are trialling a new drug, we want to know that if people get better when using the drug, it is the drug that is actually helping people. Therefore, researchers are always guarding against potential bias.

Error

Error refers to another and more specific issue in research and that is error in measuring: an area where it is possible to make an error. Say for example we ask you the question 'are you happy?' we give you the option of 'Yes' or 'No'. Now what we're hoping to do is measure your happiness. However, there are possible sources of error in this measurement. For example, you may say 'Yes', therefore you are happy, but you may not be totally happy, you may just be happier than you are unhappy, but our measure just determines that you are happy. Therefore there is possible error in our measurement because we've not assessed the correct level of happiness exactly, so our assessment of your happiness is not wrong (you've said you're happy) but has a degree of error to it. There are many sources of potential error. Perhaps if we asked you two questions; are you happy in 'work' and 'life in general' to determine your happiness. If you answered yes to both then you are happy, but it is perfectly possible that you are not happy in specific areas of your life, such as a relationship. Again, there is potential for error here because our measure of happiness, when measuring happiness, might be open to possible error because it misses out a question on relationships.

There are many sources of possible error and bias in research. It is important to note that these are often not measurable on their own and are often unknown quantities. For example it is impossible to know what real happiness is, therefore asking people are they happy and determining on that whether they are happy or not has a huge possible amount of error, because the extent and depth of happiness is probably unknown and would make your head hurt just thinking about how to measure it. However, rather than simply giving up, researchers persevere. As a researcher it is almost impossible to eradicate all possible sources of error from research, but researchers try to guard against possible biases and error so they can establish confidence in their work. For example, when you write an essay there is the risk of bias and error. You may read only a certain section of the literature and give one side of an argument (i.e. a bias) or you may not account or document a particular idea properly (i.e. an error). If you hand in this work with many biases and errors you may not expect to get a good mark. However, if you wanted a good mark, which represents confidence in your work, you would try to read all sides of the literature (by doing a comprehensive literature search) and try to make sure you understood and relayed concepts properly (by checking with your lecturer or colleagues that you properly understood it). You can't remove all possible biases or errors from your work – you haven't got infinite time to read the literature, or space in your essay to put all your ideas down. Nor may you exactly understand every concept, but by reading and checking your work you are trying to reduce the possible biases and errors you make.

It is the same for quantitative researchers. They try to guard against possible bias and error to produce confidence in the results. They do this by trying to 'control' the research, and often, particularly in experimental research, these controls are needed to eliminate alternative explanations of research findings. In each of the methods described we will see how researchers try to guard against bias or error. This might be with the quantitative experimental researcher who tries to ensure that they don't influence results by putting only healthy people into one trial group and unwell people into another trial group so a drug doesn't seem to have a positive effect on health when in fact it is due to one of the groups being in greater health. Each researcher is trying to guard against bias and error in their research to boost confidence in their results. Therefore in each description of each method, the good practice we describe will help you as a researcher produce confidence in any findings you get from your research.

THINGS TO CONSIDER

Systematic and random bias and error

We've tried to keep the explanation of bias and error above simple, but it's worth noting some formal terms about error, just so that when you come across it in the literature it doesn't confuse you. Bias and error are considerations to make regarding the accuracy of the research. Both these concepts are regularly split into two ideas, random bias/error and systematic bias/error.

Random bias or error are the result of unpredictable factors affecting the research. For example a random error might be that you are carrying out your research among clinical out patients suffering from seasonal affective disorder during January and on one day of your research the sun may be out, so everyone you see on this day is in a particularly good mood, when normally everybody has complained about the weather. This might affect the answers they give. This is an unpredictable factor and you may not realise, or even be able to assess its effects.

Systematic bias or error results from factors which consistently affect the research. For example it may be that your research has been carried out among another sample of outpatients while noisy building work has been going on in the hospital. Regardless of *when* the study was being conducted, people's answers may have been affected by the noise. For example, all your participants may have given you short and concise answers to interview questions so they could get away from the noise and go back home.

5.2 Experimental methods

In Chapters 2 and 3 we covered a number of experimental designs: experimental, quasi-experimental, clinical trials, randomised controlled trials, case-control design and cohort studies. We are not going to describe all these research designs again, but you should consult the descriptions of them when thinking of an experiment so you can explore possible different ways of running an experiment. In this section we are going to describe some of the common steps that need to be taken or considered when running an experiment. Overall we are going to describe what aspects should be 'controlled' for in any experiment by using the 'gold standard' of randomised controlled designs. This is because randomised controlled designs are designed to control as many variables as possible in the research design. Randomised controlled trials (RCTs) are the most commonly used in nursing and medicine across all types of clinical trials described above.

The main aspect of RCTs is the idea of controlling against potential bias and error so as to establish greater confidence in the result and present the strongest consideration of a study, treatment or intervention. Though there are many developed aspects of RCTs we are going to introduce you to three concepts that are common features of these trials that control against bias. Here, we are going to introduce you to the following issues of: (1) the placebo effect, (2) randomisation of participants and (3) 'blind' administrations.

The placebo effect

One phenomenon that occurs in research is the placebo effect. The placebo effect is an effect felt by an individual of improvement in health that the individual feels is the result of an intervention (i.e. medication), but the improvement in health is not due to the intervention.

An early example of the placebo effect came from the French pharmacist Émile Coué, who lived between 1857 and 1926. Coué worked as a pharmacist in Nancy and was horrified when he discovered that he had dispensed the wrong prescription to one of his customers. He was then surprised to find that the patient recovered. Coué then found that he could show an improvement in the efficacy of a medicine among patients simply by praising its effectiveness to the patient. This later led to Coué devising the phrase 'Tous les jours à tous points de vue je vais de mieux en mieux', which you may better recognise as 'every day, in every way, I'm getting better and better'. Coué used this method in psychotherapy and was able to show that this positive thinking led to better health and recovery from illness.

A well-documented example is the reports of Dr Nelda Wray (professor in the Department of Medicine, Baylor University) and Dr Bruce Moseley, team physician of the Houston Rockets (a US basketball team) and a member of the Association of Professional Teams. These researchers became suspicious of the effectiveness of arthroscopic surgery ('keyhole' surgery of joints which involves some cutting and manipulation) for arthritis of the knee. In this surgery the surgeon rinses out the joint with fluid, shaving any rough cartilage and other torn fragments, getting rid of the cartilage, crystals and cells that cause inflammation thus reducing mechanical stress. Bruce Moseley and colleagues (1996) started out treating ten former military male patients suffering from arthritis. Two of the men underwent the arthroscopic surgery, three just the rinsing alone and five had no recognised surgical procedure - instead

Moseley stabbed their knee three times with a scalpel. Six months later all 10 patients still didn't know whether they had undergone surgery or not, but all reported less pain. Furthermore, none of the patients reported being unhappy with the outcome of the operation. This led to a larger and more detailed study among 180 patients (Moseley *et al.*, 2002) in which a number of different variations of the surgery were tried. The researchers concluded that there were no differences in patient satisfaction or clinical outcome between any of the patient groups, with all three groups showing improvement, though in the long term conditions returned to preoperative levels. Moseley and colleagues concluded that the observed improvement was due to the placebo effect.

There is some debate about how powerful and permanent placebos are. Hrobjartsson and Gotzsche (2001) looked at 114 clinical trials and found little evidence that placebos had powerful clinical effects. However, the introduction of a placebo control can provide an effective insight into what a treatment or intervention can accomplish. With randomised controlled trials, a researcher could try to compare the effectiveness of a medical treatment against a placebo to control for possible effects and to make the experience for the participants as close to the experience of the person undertaking the intervention or treatment. In clinical research, a placebo effect occurs when an intervention has no medically known effects but beneficial effects might still have arisen due to the person taking the placebo believing that the intervention is meant to have positive effects. To use an example of testing a new drug, administration of the new drug to one group will need to be accompanied by the giving of a placebo intervention to another group (i.e. the **control group**). Therefore, any beneficial effects of the drug can be compared to the effects of someone taking a placebo.

There is one thing to note about the use of placebos: in some clinical trials the use of the placebo may not be ethical. For example, in testing a new contraceptive pill, it would not be ethical to administer some participants in the clinical trial with an effective pill and others with a sugar pill.

Randomisation of participants

The first aspect is that there is some **randomisation** of patients in clinical trials. Imagine you are testing a new drug and have the intervention group of people who are taking the drug and you have the placebo group of people who are taking a sugar-coated pill.

In all RCTs a central aspect is the random allocation of participants to the different groups. This is the only sure way to control for possible bias. A popular example of a problem of possible bias in participant bias is the problem of participant self-selecting bias. In this example imagine you were running a trial for an antidepressant (A-D 800) and you were recruiting volunteers at a local university by advertising the study around the campus. Say, for example, you allocated the first 20 people to arrive to the placebo group, and the next 20 arrivals for the treatment drug A-D 800. You then carry out the clinical trials and actually find that there is no difference in the level of depression in the groups. Therefore, you would conclude that there was no evidence

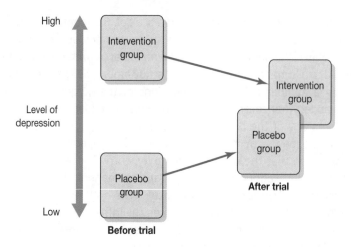

Figure 5.2 The need for random allocation in clinical trials.

for the effectiveness of the drug. However, now imagine that there actually was a problem with your sample selection. The first 20 people who came along were perhaps more eager and active than the last 20 people. Certainly, the first 20 people were more likely to be up earlier, they were certainly more enthusiastic about taking part in the study, while the last 20 people may have dragged themselves along to the study. Therefore, the failure to find any difference between the placebo group and the treatment group may not be down to the failure of the drug, but instead to the differences between the samples. For example, depressed people sleep in later and are less enthusiastic and, therefore, the last 20 people may have been more depressed. There may have been a positive outcome for A-D 800 but it is masked because though the drug helped people become less depressed, the treatment group before the trial was more depressed and although the drug lowered individual's depression in this group, it was no different to the placebo group after the trial (see Figure 5.2).

This is a rather simple example. Nonetheless the randomised allocation of people to different subject groups, whether to treatment groups or placebo groups, is a feature of RCTs. For example, Stotts *et al.* (2003) used a randomised clinical trial of nicotine patches for treatment of spit tobacco addiction among adolescents. In this study, they researched three groups and participants were allocated to each group randomly. The control group received some counselling and then a follow-up phone call two weeks later. The two intervention groups received a six-week behavioural intervention; one of the intervention groups received active nicotine patches while the other intervention group received placebo patches. The authors found that behavioural intervention proved successful but the nicotine patch offered no improvement to the rate that the adolescents cut down (or eliminated) spit tobacco use. What is important here is that because you know people were allocated to each group randomly, you have increased confidence in their findings. There is one thing to note about randomisation: it does not guarantee fairness or equality in allocation; it just makes it much more likely.

'Blind' administrations

The physician's belief in the treatment and the patient's faith in t
a mutually reinforcing effect; the result is a powerful remedy that is a.
teed to produce an improvement and sometimes a cure.

(Skrabanek and McCormick, 1994, p. ι_

An important aspect of RCTs is that those involved in the trial do not know what treatment individuals are receiving, be it a real treatment or a placebo. First of all it is important that the participants in the trial do not know what treatment they are receiving. If individuals knew they were receiving a treatment drug the researchers would not be able to control for the placebo effect, because those taking the treatment drug may influence the effects of the drug because they believe it will work. Therefore, in RCTs researchers do not reveal to the participants what and which type of treatment they are taking. This is known as a **single-blind** trial, where the researcher knows the details of the trial but the patient does not.

However, many researchers have pointed out that it is important that they, or the person administering the study, also do not know what treatment participants are receiving. This is because the researchers might consciously or unconsciously treat the participants differently when administering the drug. They may, for example, feel guilty for administering a worthless pill to those participants who are only receiving the placebo and be additionally nice to these patients. Equally, they may really want the treatment drug to work, because they are desperate for a cure to be found and so may act differently with those people taking the treatment drug. Regardless, if the researcher knows which drug they are administering then they may influence the results in many different ways. Therefore, RCTs are often **'double-blind'** operations, where the participants and the researchers (particularly those administering the treatment) are unaware which participant is getting the study treatment and which participant is getting the placebo. Usually another researcher, not involved in the administration of the drugs or the day-to-day running of the study, will, through randomisation, allocate who is getting the treatment drug and who is getting the placebo.

In nursing the most common form of experimental design is a clinical trial. These can be prevention trials, screening trials, diagnostic trials, treatment trials and quality of life trials. Each of these has a different function. However, common to all these trials is the use of RCTs in which the possible bias that can occur in any treatment or invention are attempted to be controlled for through randomisation, 'blind' administrations.

5.3 Questionnaires and survey research

Questionnaires and surveys can be used to collect quantitative and qualitative data. However, a lot of questionnaire and survey research will contain measures that use quantitative ways of scoring of questions to assess whatever the person is measuring.

n this section we're going to introduce you to commonly used ways of constructing a questionnaire or survey, including some advice on making up your own questionnaires.

What is a questionnaire or survey?

A questionnaire, also known as a survey, a measure or a scale, usually provides a set of questions from which the person chooses one of many options in answer to a particular question or statement, or asks the respondent to provide some written information about a particular area or a number of different areas. Types of questions and possible responses can vary wildly, but at the heart of most questionnaires and surveys is the need to collect information that can be quantified.

There is no golden rule for when to use a questionnaire, but there are a number of factors about a questionnaire which suggest when it might be useful to use a questionnaire/survey as your research method:

- *When you need a large sample.* Questionnaires are relatively simple to administer and the research does not necessarily need to be supervised, or the researcher present, when the questionnaire is being answered. Therefore you can administer questionnaires to many people at the same time.

- *When time is limited.* Questionnaires tend not to be a time-consuming method of collecting data. Usually questionnaires and surveys are brief, particularly due to the way questions are asked, therefore allowing a lot of information to be collected in a relatively short period of time.

- *When resources are limited.* Questionnaires are not expensive. Though all research can be expensive in terms of preparation, in terms of each person the administration of the questionnaire is relatively inexpensive when compared to an interview. Many questionnaires can be photocopied and sent in a matter of days, while a series of interviews will need to be taped, administered separately and involve people (be it the researcher or the participant) travelling to and from interviews.

- *To protect the privacy of participants.* Questionnaires can be relatively anonymous, particularly if when the questionnaires are returned there is no way of identifying the respondent (i.e. through the mail or a postbox). This can be useful when there are embarrassing questions of a personal nature that the participant might be happier to respond to anonymously rather than face to face.

Designing a questionnaire or survey

There is some general good practice and specific knowledge you need when designing a questionnaire. Consider the following two questionnaires that examine a patient's satisfaction with waiting times following admittance to an A&E unit (Example 5.1, below). The aim of this research for both of these questionnaires is to find out the visitors' experience of the A&E unit and to somehow assess how positive the experience was for them.

Example 5.1 Two questionnaires compared: their items and response formats

Patient Experience Questionnaire 1

1. Gender: Male/Female

2. How did you happen to be in the A&E unit?
_____

3a. Overall, how would you rate your experience in the A&E unit?
_____

3b. If you had to give your experience a rating out of 10, what would it be?

(a) 0 (b) 1 (c) 2 (d) 3 (e) 4 (f) 5 (g) 6 (h) 7 (i) 8 (j) 9 (k) 10

4. Think about the times when you've visited other A&E units as a patient or accompanying someone. Also think about when you've had a similar injury. Also think about a time when you had (or the person had) a similar injury to the one you recently experienced. How would you rate your current visit out of 10?

(a) 0 (b) 1 (c) 2 (d) 3 (e) 4 (f) 5 (g) 6 (h) 7 (i) 8 (j) 9 (k) 10

5. During your visit at the hospital you will have met some of our very helpful staff. Just how helpful were they?

(a) Only sightly helpful (b) Quite helpful (c) helpful (d) Very helpful

6. Overall how would you rate the treatment given to you/patient during your time in the A&E unit?

(a) Extremely poor (b) Very poor (c) Poor (d) Quite poor (e) Slightly poor
(f) Neither poor or good (g) Slightly good (h) Quite good (i) Good (j) Very good
(k) Extremely good

Patient Experience Questionnaire 2

1. Sex? _____

2. How did you happen to be in the A&E unit?

(a) As a patient (b) Helping a patient

3a. Overall, how would you rate your experience in the A&E unit?

(a) Very negative (b) Negative (c) Neither negative nor positive (d) Positive
(e) Very positive

3b. Are there any other comments you would like to make about your overall experience in the A&E unit?
_____

4. How does the current experience compare to your experiences of A&E units in other hospitals?

(a) Much worse (b) Slightly worse (c) Neither worse nor better (d) Slightly better
(e) Much better

5. During your visit to the hospital how well would you rate the helpfulness of our staff?

(a) Very unhelpful (b) Slightly unhelpful (c) Neither unhelpful nor helpful (d) Slightly helpful (e) Very helpful

6. Overall how would you rate the treatment given to you/patient during your time in the A&E unit?

(a) Very poor (b) Poor (c) Neither poor or good (d) Good (e) Very good

Let us consider these two surveys within a number of factors important to questionnaires.

Closed versus open questions

The first thing to consider is that many researchers make the distinction between two different types of questions: open-format or closed-format questions.

Open format are questions that asked for some written detail but have no determined set of responses. Therefore any answer can be given to these questions. These types of questions lead to more qualitative data because the number of possible responses that could be obtained is large. Take, for example, Question 2 in Questionnaire 1 'How did you happen to be in the A&E unit?', which could lead to a large number of different responses. However, this wouldn't lead to getting the rich qualitative data that you might get from an interview, mainly due to there being limited space to write responses in a survey and the pressure to respond relatively quickly.

There are problems with open-format questions in a survey. Given that they produce a large number of possible answers, each potentially different, they may cancel out the advantages of a questionnaire which can be time-consuming for the participant if it takes a long time to fill in. This contrasts to an interview situation where the respondent speaks. Open-ended questions in a survey will make research participation seem like an exam, making the participant bored and perhaps less inclined to spend as much time as they could on the question. Open-format questions are also time-consuming for the researcher, who has to analyse all the different answers.

However, open-format questions can reveal high-quality data, particularly when there is no other way of asking the question. Therefore to be truly useful in a survey the use of open-format questions need careful consideration. It is often suggested that researchers limit or avoid the use of open-format questions in a survey, and if they do use them, they will usually put the question at the end of the survey.

Therefore in surveys you will tend to see a lot of closed-format questions. Closed-format questions are those where there is a short question or statement followed by a number of options. For example Question 3a in Questionnaire 2, 'Overall, how would you rate your experience in the A&E unit?' is followed by a number of options; (a) Very negative (b) Negative (c) Neither negative nor positive (d) Positive (e) Very positive. You can see from this question that the respondent cannot just write their opinion, but is instead asked to indicate their experience in terms of their positive or negative experience.

However, this highlights a potential issue with closed-format questions: they do not look for a wide range of experiences or information, but a specific piece of information. The main aim of closed-format questions is to break down respondents' surveys into data that can be quantified and that supplies the information you want to know (i.e. you can say that so many people choose option a, so many choose option b etc. etc.). However, you also need to be mindful that respondents may have other things to say about their experience. You should ask the question you want simple answers to, but if you feel there is a need to obtain slightly more information, i.e. give you a little more data on why people found the experience positive or negative, or if you want to give people room to express their opinion, you can always ask a supplementary question such as 3b in Questionnaire 2, 'Are there any other comments you would like to make about your overall experience in the A&E unit?'. This allows people to express opinions if they wish, but if they have nothing further to say they don't feel obliged to add to their answer, allowing them to move on to the other questions.

In most surveys, you will tend to see closed-format questions, with either no use of open-format questions, or if they are used they will appear at the end or are supplementary questions.

Clarity of questions

Whether you are asking open- or closed-format questions, you have to ensure that the wording of your questions is clear. Good practice says that questions must be clear, short, and unambiguous. Compare question 4 in both questionnaires. Clearly the author of question 4 is trying to get the respondent to compare their experience with an occasion and injury that was similar, and a recent experience. This is an admirable aim, but the question is so long that it is confusing and leads people to perhaps think of many occasions. Question 4 in the second questionnaire would be a more typical question to ask, it is shorter and the meaning is clear. It may not be as exact, but it is unlikely to cause confusion. That said it's not perfect, some people may have never been in an A&E unit before, and would be unable to answer. This highlights how hard it is to write survey questions.

The main aim of writing a good survey question is to make sure that the question will not mean different things to different respondents. This is very important. If your questions are ambiguous (the meaning can be interpreted differently) then your participants will in fact be answering different questions. This will muddy your results because you will never be sure what interpretation respondents have been answering. For example, the question 'Did you see the patient in a bad mood?' could mean 'Did you see a patient who was in a bad mood?', or 'Did you yourself see a patient whilst you were in a bad mood?'

There is other good practice for writing survey questions. Try to consider language or culture and make sure that all of the questions can be understood by all sorts of people. Remember those who may have a poor reading age and try to make the questions as simple as possible. Some of the questions may seem patronising, but people who have a high reading age will still be able to understand the question. Also try to avoid jargon or technical language, particularly abbreviations. Not everyone knows that A&E means accident and emergency and ENT means ears, nose and throat.

Leading questions

Leading questions are those that try to steer the respondent to a particular answer, or in the direction of a particular answer. Take for example question 5 in both questionnaires 1 and 2 above. Let us first consider question 5 in questionnaire 1. There is no doubt that all hospital staff are helpful at all times, but to a larger extent this example is trying to lead the respondent to (a) assume during their time in hospital the staff were helpful (b) indicate only the degree of the helpfulness. Respondents, in answering this question, are unable to indicate that the staff were unhelpful. Let's take questionnaire 2 which, though rather less upbeat in its questioning, means respondents are able to indicate whether their experience of staff helpfulness was either positive or negative.

However, leading questions can arise inadvertently and can occur due to the phrasing of the question. For example:

A. Do you agree with recent government attempts to oppose increased funding of the NHS?

B. Do you agree with recent government attempts to support decreased funding of the NHS?

There are possible different interpretations or opinions based on the positive and negative use of oppose/support and increased/decreased because essentially they are asking different things, even though you've just swopped the wording around. However, such differences do not become apparent until you actually write the questions out.

Good point

Other types of questions to avoid

There are other types of questions.you should try to avoid or at least be aware of:

- *Embarrassing questions.* Generally, questions dealing with personal matters should be avoided. This is because this may make your respondent feel embarrassed or uncomfortable and doing research that causes this type of feeling in participants is not good practice, indeed it is frowned upon. Equally it is not good for the researcher because it may lead the participant to give incorrect or misleading information, or fail to complete the rest of the questionnaire. That said, research in nursing will sometimes have to ask potentially embarrassing questions, particularly about things such as their health, medical history, their diet and even sometimes their sexual health. This is where survey research can be useful, because it can allow individuals to fill in questionnaires anonymously or at least in privacy and so they may be more likely to reveal this information. Great care should be taken when asking personal or potentially embarrassing questions, and you should spend a lot of time thinking about how to best ask them.

- *Hypothetical questions.* Hypothetical questions are those that place the individual in a situation they may never experience and ask for their opinion on something. So for example, you might ask 'If you were Prime Minister of the country, what would you do about the National Health Service?', or 'If you were a hospital administrator how would you allocate funding to hospital departments?'. These types of questions might produce colourful answers, but are considered bad research practice because answers will be in response to a situation the person may never have considered rather than their real view or feelings about something.

- *Questions that involve the participant's social desirability.* Within research there is a term called social desirability that suggests that respondents can respond to questions that make them look or sound good. For example, no-one is likely to respond 'No' to the question 'Do you give regularly to charity?' even if they don't, unless they have particularly strong views. That is because answering yes makes the person look good and answering no makes them look bad. As a researcher you should try to avoid questions with a potential prestige bias as you may never be sure whether you are getting a true reflection.

Response formats

The final area to consider for good survey design is response formats. All closed-format questions give a series of choices, and there is good practice in terms of response choices to use. The general guideline is to use simple rating scales or lists of choice, and where possible minimise the number of choices. If you look at question 6 for our two questionnaires you will see two sets of responses to the same question 'rate the treatment given to you/patient during your time in the A&E unit'. Which of these two questions would you find easiest to answer? You can see in the first questionnaire there may be quite a lot of possible confusion, and possible redundancy, from the responses for the first questionnaire. If you can, make the set of responses as simple as possible.

You also need to clear about the responses. Look at question 4 of our two questionnaires and the response format. In questionnaire 1 the answer has 11 choices, while questionnaire 2 has 5 choices. Out of these two questions which would you find easier to answer? Look at the questionnaire 1 version again. Do you actually know what 'out of 10' means? Would all respondents know that 10 meant a better experience on this occasion?

There are a lot of things to think about when writing surveys!

Health and clinical assessment instruments

In the last section we discussed how you might create a survey. However, what you will find in nursing research is it is very unusual that you will have to create a whole survey. This is because people will have had to ask questions in your area of research interest before, so it is always a good idea to get copies of surveys that other people have done before you start out on your own - existing surveys might already be suitable for your needs. In this section we're going to highlight some surveys that are already use in health and clinical assessment. This is so you can see how health and clinical aspects are sometimes surveyed and assessed in nursing. These types of assessment are surveys that have been developed over time and have been found to very useful, reliable and valid and are therefore commonly used in practice.

One example of a clinical assessment instrument is the Edinburgh Postnatal Depression Scale (EPDS). The scale was developed by Cox, Holden and Sagovsky (1987) as a way of assisting primary care health professionals to detect postnatal (or postpartum) depression, thought to affect at least 10 per cent of women, among mothers who have recently had a baby. Before using the scale, researchers need to be aware of three things:

1. Care should be taken to avoid the possibility of the mother discussing her answers with others.

2. The mother should complete the scale herself, unless she has limited English or has difficulty with reading.

3. The EPDS may be used at 6–8 weeks to screen postnatal women. The child health clinic, postnatal check-up or a home visit may provide suitable opportunities for its completion.

The scale has ten questions, but before reading the questions, any respondent has to adhere to the following procedure.

1. The mother is asked to underline the response which comes closest to how she has been feeling in the previous 7 days.

2. All ten items must be completed.

Respondents then need to respond to the items in the EPDS (see Example 5.2, below).

Example 5.2 The Edinburgh Postnatal Depression Scale

As you have recently had a baby, we would like to know how you are feeling. Please UNDERLINE the answer which comes closest to how you have felt IN THE PAST 7 DAYS, not just how you feel today.

1. I have been able to laugh and see the funny side of things.
   As much as I always could
   Not quite so much now
   Definitely not so much now
   Not at all

2. I have looked forward with enjoyment to things.
   As much as I ever did
   Rather less than I used to
   Definitely less than I used to
   Hardly at all

3. *I have blamed myself unnecessarily when things went wrong.
   Yes, most of the time
   Yes, some of the time
   Not very often
   No, never

4. I have been anxious or worried for no good reason.
   No, not at all
   Hardly ever
   Yes, sometimes
   Yes, very often

5. *I have felt scared or panicky for no very good reason.
   Yes, quite a lot
   Yes, sometimes
   No, not much
   No, not at all

Example 5.2 **continued**

6. *Things have been getting on top of me.
   Yes, most of the time I haven't been able to cope at all
   Yes, sometimes I haven't been coping as well as usual
   No, most of the time I have coped quite well
   No, I have been coping as well as ever

7. *I have been so unhappy that I have had difficulty sleeping.
   Yes, most of the time
   Yes, sometimes
   Not very often
   No, not at all

8. *I have felt sad or miserable.
   Yes, most of the time
   Yes, quite often
   Not very often
   No, not at all

9. *I have been so unhappy that I have been crying.
   Yes, most of the time
   Yes, quite often
   Only occasionally
   No, never

10. *The thought of harming myself has occurred to me.
    Yes, quite often
    Sometimes
    Hardly ever
    Never

(EPDS; Cox *et al.*, 1987)

Translations of the scale, and guidance as to its use, may be found in Cox, J.L. and Holden, J. (2003) *Perinatal Mental Health: A Guide to the Edinburgh Postnatal Depression Scale.* London: Gaskell.

Answers are scored 0, 1, 2, and 3 according to increased severity of the symptoms. For question one 'I have been able to laugh and see the funny side of things', the response 'As much as I always could' would be scored 0 and 'Not at all' would be scored with a 3, meaning that a higher score of '3' would mean the respondent had not been able to laugh and see the funny side of things at all, indicating that they had a symptom of depression. Items marked with an asterisk are reverse scored (i.e. 3, 2, 1, and 0), although these wouldn't be marked on the scale, and a total score for the scale is then computed by adding together the scores.

In terms of scoring, possible scores then range from a minimum of 0 (not depressed at all) to 30 (very depressed). It is unlikely that many people will score 30 on the scale. Indeed Cox et al. (1987) suggest that anyone scoring above 12 or 13 and higher (practice varies with this cut-off point) may be suffering from possible postpartum depression. They also suggest that any assessment should look at item 10 closely for any possible suicidal thoughts.

The main thing about these sorts of questionnaires is that they are a tool to make an initial assessment. Cox et al. (1987) emphasise that the scale should not be used in preference to using clinical judgement and it is a tool to facilitate discussion between the health professional and the mother; where mothers score above 12/13, a more rigorous clinical assessment should be performed to explore whether postpartum depression can be diagnosed.

There are many types of these sorts of tests available – in fact there are hundreds. Other examples include the SF-36 and the GPAQ. The SF-36 (Ware et al., 1993) is a health survey used in nursing to measure health status. It has a number of scales within the survey. One scale refers to the person's physical functioning (e.g. being able to climb stairs) and another to the amount of pain people are feeling. Other scales ask about peoples' energy levels, or how their health is affecting their ability to perform everyday tasks or relationships with other people. Another scale is the General Practice Assessment Questionnaire (GPAQ) (National Primary Care Research and Development Centre University of Manchester, 2007). GPAQ is a patient questionnaire for use by a number of different health professionals and there is also a version of the GPAQ designed to survey patients who have been treated by nurses in primary care. The main purpose of the GPAQ is to help health practices find out what their patients think about the care they receive and questions focus on access (how do you rate the hours that your practice is open for appointments?), interpersonal aspects of care (how do you rate the way you are treated by receptionists at your practice?) and quality of care (how well has the doctor explained your problems or any treatment that you need?). You can follow the links in the References section to find out more about these tests.

5.4 Interviews

With any interview, the researcher is searching to understand the meanings, experiences and themes that occur for each participant for the topic being explored. Interviews are very useful when the researcher is looking to gain in-depth information from respondents. In this section we are going to outline (1) the types of interviews that can be performed and (2) good practice in interviews to ensure they go well.

Structured, unstructured and semi-structured interviews

Structured interviews are designed to ensure that the interviewer covers the same general areas with each interviewee. Structured interviews will generally comprise a list of specific questions: the interviewer has to ask all questions and would not normally be allowed to ask additional questions. This is done to ensure that the interviewer didn't influence the information given by the interviewee in any way. The interviewer might ask the interviewee to elaborate on something they have said, or clarify what they have said, but the interviewer would not ask a supplementary question. Certainly the interviewer would not give their own opinions on things.

In nursing practice you tend to come across structured interviews in the assessment of patients or service users. A structured interview schedule would be something like the SESCAM (Side Effects Scale/Checklist for Anti-psychotic Medication) (Bennett *et al.*, 1995), which was developed by Bennett and colleagues to check for side effects among patients who were taking antipsychotic drugs. Typical items in the SESCAM can be found in Table 5.1.

The structured interview is designed primarily to gather factual information, give information to patients/service users or to motivate the patient to do something.

Table 5.1 Items from a structured interview schedule (the SESCAM)

Do you have any of the following:	Yes	No	If yes, specify problem
(a) Dizziness			
(b) Drowsiness			
(c) Sexual problems (ejaculatory erectile, libido)			
(d) Constipation			
(e) Urinary problems			
(f) Skin problems (rashes, photosensitivity)			
(g) Excessive weight gain			
(h) Blurred vision			
(i) Feeling restless			
(j) Lack of get up and go			
(k) Other			

Assessment interviews are often given in mental health situations to assess the severity of mental health patients. For example, a psychiatric nursing interview would be used to gain information on a patient. Here, a psychiatric nurse would use a structured interview schedule to assess the patient's mental heath, understand how they are currently dealing with their mental problems and gain information on their current sources of support. Throughout this interview, though it might be difficult, the nurse will try to obtain information so they can best treat the patient, therefore they won't try to discuss issues, but will ask questions to get the patient to discuss things more openly.

Formally, within structured interviews there is a further distinction. There are standardised open interviews, where the same open-ended questions are asked and respondents answer questions freely. However, some interviews are closed fixed response interviews where interviewees are asked the same question but only choose an answer from among the same set of alternatives.

Unstructured interviews are much more informal and are conversational in nature. There may or may not be predetermined questions, but if there are questions their order and presentation would not be as rigid as a structured interview. For example, the researcher may follow up questions with new questions if they feel they are discussing something of interest. On occasion the interviewer might even give their own opinion, or a contrary opinion, so that they can explore the interviewee's view of something or to stimulate their thought in the area. When used in nursing, the unstructured interview might be used to produce a shared understanding of the patient's health. That is, the assessment interview which is used to diagnose a patient is one in which the nurse or practitioner will tell the patient about their health issue. An unstructured interview might be used to allow the patient to realise their health concerns and get them to act on them.

Formally, within unstructured interviews there is a further distinction. There are informal conversational interviews, where no predetermined questions are asked by the interviewer; rather the question asked is decided by the interviewer as the interview progresses. There are also interviews that have a general interview guide approach in which the interviewer devises a guide to ensure that the same areas are visited for discussion during the interview, but by using a guide rather than set questions it allows for a certain amount of freedom for the interviewer.

Finally, the researcher is able to mix up these different types of interview techniques, and have parts that are structured and parts that are unstructured – this is often referred to as a semi-structured interview (see below for an example) and is a more flexible way of approaching the interaction between interviewer and interviewee. The interviewer has a schedule of topics that needs to be covered and there is generally no major set order but rather responsiveness to what the interviewee is saying. For instance, in the sample semi-structured interview schedule in Example 5.3, below, the interviewee might say how they are affected psychologically by neurofibromatosis (NF) and then go on to say how they have attempted to cope with NF (question 9). The interviewer would not be worried that the questions are not following the order that is listed in the interview schedule but would instead be focused on making the interaction as much like a natural conversation as possible. In this specific example, the interviewer would only be aiming to revisit question 9 in the interview if they thought that all of the areas of interest had not been covered when the interviewee had started to talk about coping after being asked about the effects of NF.

Example 5.3 A semi-structured interview schedule

Main questions are numbered, with potential prompts/guidance notes listed underneath in bold. Initial exploratory questions are intended to get more information to contextualize the participants' life histories and to start to link this to the syndrome of Neurofibromatosis.

After the initial questions (up to, and including, question 3), the interviewer will attempt to ask questions in turn although flexibility with this ordering is encouraged so as to be responsive to interviewee responses.

1. Please tell me a little about yourself.

Age, marital status, profession, ethnic origin, home-town, whether the participant has children

2. When were you diagnosed with Neurofibromatosis (NF)?

3. Do you have a family history of NF?

Who is affected? Briefly, how are they affected?

4. Describe how NF affects you physically

5. How does it affect you psychologically?

6. How are your relationships affected by NF?

Family/friends/sexual

7. How do you feel about having NF?

8. Do you feel as though you face obstacles due to NF?

Anything on: Pain/suffering; People's reactions; Uncertainty; Having children; Relationships; Missing out on things; Lack of confidence; Perceptions of self as a 'sufferer'

9. How do you cope with NF?

Optimism (defence/functional); Realism; Social support; Culture; Inspiration; Challenges set by NF

10. Tell me about your goals and ambitions in life

Hopes and fears regarding the future; Compare the life you have with the life you imagine if you didn't have NF – what would be worse? What would be better? Opinions on quality of life

11. What do you enjoy about life?

What gets you through the bad times? What occupies your time?

12. Has having NF changed your outlook on life for the better?

Example 5.3 continued

13. Tell me about the good that might have come out of having NF

Meaning-making; Spirituality Community of those with NF (social support); personal strengths; things to be grateful for; Milestones; Making friends through NF; appreciating 'smaller things'.

14. Do you feel well-informed and supported regarding your NF?

Knowledge of doctor, information available, sources of support. Differences in cases where there's no family history and cases where there is family history.

15. In your opinion, is there enough awareness around NF?

Thank interviewee for taking part and debrief so that interviewee knows what to do regarding any queries/concerns/further information requested about the study and its findings.

(Used for a study by Dheensa and Williams, 2009)

Good practice in interviews

Of course, despite writing different questions, the whole process of the interview needs to go well. After all you need your interviewee to talk, and if they don't feel comfortable or confident they are unlikely to do so. There are a number of things you can do before and during the interview to ensure that it progresses in the best way possible that orientate around the questions to be asked, the setting, things to done before the interview and things you can do during the interview.

Choosing and devising your questions.

When coming up with your questions for an interview you need to plan them very carefully. The first thing you need to plan is what you want to find out, therefore you need to write down a list of things you are hoping to find out. While doing this you also need to think about other related areas that might inform what you want to know. When you have finished that list you need to write a list of questions that will allow you to get the information you are looking for. Again, like survey questions, keep them as simple as possible. When doing this you would do well to check the questions carefully, perhaps getting one or two people to look at them to see if they think they are appropriate or whether they could be worded more carefully.

Choosing your setting and equipment.

When setting up your interview, make sure you choose a private area that should have no distractions. For example, try to position the interview where there is very little noise and where people are unlikely to be seen (i.e. through a window). Most certainly the room should be private and people shouldn't access the room during the interview. To this end, it is advisable that you put a note on the door stating that an interview is underway and you should not be disturbed. Also work out how you are going to record the interview. In almost all cases you will need to record the conversation, so make sure you have a good recorder that can record *clearly* two people talking in the room. You might want to have a go with a friend before setting up your interview to test it out.

Starting the interview.
When starting the interview first of all you need to explain what the purpose of the interview is and how long it is likely to take. This is also a good opportunity to ask the interviewee if they have any questions because it allows you to reassure them and make them feel comfortable. Also explain the general format of the interview and you might mention the areas that are going to be explored.

During the interview.
During the interview it is not just a matter of asking questions, you have to manage the interview. Ask one question at a time and encourage a full response. Yes or no answers are not usually good answers for a qualitative researcher as they provide little data to work with. Researchers need to encourage much longer responses or ask people to elaborate on points. One way to do this is to be careful about your body language when the person is talking. Look as if you are listening (i.e. lean forward) and nod as if to say I understand what you are saying, tell me more. Don't be too eager to move on to the next question. One useful technique in any interpersonal situation to get the other person to talk is not to feel uncomfortable with a silence. People are uncomfortable in silences, so when the person has finished talking or you have just asked a question, always give it 5 to 10 seconds before speaking again. The other person might feel uncomfortable in the silence and talk some more or start talking. Try also to keep the person on track. It is easy for interviewees to move the interview on to another topic therefore bring them back (after they've finished talking) to the main point. Also provide transition statements between topics ('Now we've talked about X . . . . I would like to move onto Y'). This will also keep the interview focused.

Focus group interviews

A **focus group** interview is a method by which a number of individuals share their thoughts, feelings and experiences around a certain topic. In many ways it is an extension of the interview but differs because the method is thought to encourage a free-flowing discussion around the area being studied. Focus groups are a particularly good way of getting a rich vein of qualitative data because people in focus groups are not only talking about their own views and experiences, as in a one-to-one interview, but also on their responses to others' own views and experiences.

As with an interview there are a number of things the researcher can do before and during the interview to ensure that the focus group session proceeds in the best way possible, by thinking about and preparing the questions and the session and doing particular things during the interview.

Choosing and devising your questions.
Like the interview, questions for a focus group need to be planned very carefully. The first thing to consider is what you want to find out, and you need to write down a list.

When you have finished that list you need to write questions that will allow you to get the information you are looking for. When writing these *all the questions you ask should be open and neutral to encourage discussion*. Also ensure that the phrases you use are likely to be terms that people are familiar with. Again get someone to check the questions carefully, perhaps getting one or two people to look at them to see if they think they are appropriate or whether they could be worded more carefully. Then set your questions out like an agenda for a meeting. You may want to *start on an issue people have strong feelings about* to facilitate discussion.

Choosing your setting and equipment and setting up your study.

When setting up your focus group interview, make sure you choose a private area with no distractions. People should be arranged in a circle so that they are talking to one another and each participant can see each person. Again record the session, but you might place a couple of recorders around the room just in case the main recorder doesn't pick up what someone says, hopefully one of the other recorders will have done. You might also want to get another researcher to record the session and make observations to ensure you don't miss anything. However, you must also record all responses on a visual board (i.e. white board/flip-chart). This provides a good record for you and keeps the session focused on key points or allows you to return to points or navigate around points. You then should invite around 6–8 people to take part in your focus group.

Running the session.

In a focus group the researcher is known as a moderator. Focus groups require a *skilled and experienced moderator* if they are to run well. This is not simply a matter of asking the questions. When introducing the session prepare an introduction explaining the purpose of the session, how the session will run and some of the topics that will be explored. You may want the participants to introduce themselves. However, there are a number of things you need to do during the session apart from enabling participants to answer questions. The following guiding principles could help you:

- *Encourage discussion.* There are a number of things you can do to encourage discussion. You can ask everyone to make a response to a question, and keep going round until everyone has spoken two or three times. It is important that people feel they have been able to express everything they want to express. It is sometimes a good idea to get participants to think about issues for a few minutes (perhaps noting down their ideas) and then get them to speak. If people give a short answer, ask them to elaborate on what they are saying.

- *Give positive feedback.* Let participants know that their contributions to the session are valuable. You can do this through your body language, as well as what you say.

- *Dealing with difficult situations.* You have to remember that you will no doubt be asking people about things they care and/or have opinions about. Disagreement and debate within the focus group is excellent as they will provide you with a rich source of data. However, this may also mean that things will get heated or produce new discussion. Or one person may feel particularly passionate or knowledgeable about a topic and may dominate a session. Therefore it is up to the researcher to keep the session on track. If you feel that things are getting out of hand, take a five-minute break and restart the session on another question.

- *Be aware of concentration levels.* Discussions can be exhausting, particularly when they are about emotional issues, and the researcher should look to provide short breaks if necessary.

5.5 Final important considerations in your study

There are two more important things that underpin any research you do: ethics and sampling. In the next section we will outline some of the major considerations when designing a study.

Ethics (from Maltby, Day and Macaskill, 2010)

Research participants have moral and legal rights and it is important that as nursing researchers we do not violate these rights. Individual researchers may not always share common moral values, and this can result in very different judgements being made about what are acceptable and unacceptable ways to treat research partici- pants. Sometimes enthusiasm for the research topic can lead researchers to pay less attention to the experience of the research participant because they are so focused on answering their research question. A code of research ethics is required to ensure that there are agreed standards of acceptable behaviour for researchers which pro- tect participants. In this section we are going to outline the basic principles for ethi- cal research and we will revisit this in Chapter 13 in terms of the current ethical considerations and processes for nurses.

Research participants

The welfare of all participants must be a prime concern of researchers and all re- search should undergo ethical scrutiny. Research with individuals who are termed 'vulnerable' participants needs very careful consideration. Vulnerable participants can be defined as:

- Infants and children under the age of 18 or 16 if they are employed
- People with learning or communication difficulties
- Patients in hospital or under the care of social services
- People with mental illness
- Individuals with an addiction to drugs and alcohol.

If you wish to recruit vulnerable participants as defined above then you need to con- sider where you will be interacting with them. If you wish to undertake research with vulnerable populations that require you to be on your own with the individual in a pri- vate interview room or the like then you will need to undergo Criminal Records

Bureau Screening (your university will be able to provide you with information about this). This will take some time so you need to plan for it if it is necessary for your research. You may also be required to pay for this screening. It may be that you can arrange supervised access to your research participants. For example, you may interact with children in a public place such as the corner of a doctor's surgery in the presence of another practitioner or some other public venue within the institution where you are not alone with the participant for significant amounts of time. These are issues you will have to discuss when arranging access to your research participants.

Obtaining consent

Where possible, participants should be informed about the nature of the study. All of the aspects of the research that are likely to affect their willingness to become participants should be disclosed. This might include the time it is likely to take, particularly if you require significant amounts of their time. You are seeking to get informed consent from your participants so they need to be adequately briefed. For research involving vulnerable participants getting informed consent may involve briefing parents, teachers or carers about the study.

For some standard questionnaire studies, for example where the topic of the research is not a particularly sensitive issue, it may be sufficient to include a description of your study at the start of your questionnaire and completion of the questionnaire is generally accepted to imply consent. Your university will have rules on this and you must comply with them.

Confidentiality

Here you must conform to data protection legislation, which means that information obtained from a research participant is confidential unless you have agreed in advance that this is not to be the case. This means that you must take care to anonymise data that you obtain from participants in, for example, interview studies. To do this you must change names and any details that might make the person easily identifiable. This should be done at the transcription stage when interviews are recorded. You are required to assure your participants that this will occur. If you cannot successfully anonymise data, for example if you were interviewing doctors and there are only six in your area, you have to make it clear to your participants that they may be identifiable. For example, in a qualitative study their quotes may be recognisable and here you need to come to an arrangement with the individual. They may not mind being recognised but they may wish to see the quotes you intend to use before you make your study publicly available to your university or to the public in print.

Deception

In many clinical studies, deception should not be necessary. Sometimes however participants may modify their behaviour if they know what the researcher is looking for, so that by giving the full explanation to participants you cannot collect reliable data. Deception should only be used when no other method can be found for collecting reliable data and when the seriousness of the question justifies it. A distinction is made between deliberately deceiving participants and withholding some information.

Deliberate deception is rarely justifiable. Rather than being deceptive, some researchers might be a little less forthcoming in what they are expecting participants to say or in not revealing their hypotheses. This might mean for example giving your questionnaire a general title such as *An exploration of patient experiences in the care of the older person unit* rather than saying which specific experiences you are expecting to find. The guiding principle should be the likely and possible reactions of participants if the full picture of the research is revealed. If participants are likely to be angry or upset in some way, then deception should not occur. If deception is involved then you need to seek ethical approval for your study.

Debriefing

When deception has occurred debriefing is especially emphasised, but it should be a part of all research to monitor the experience of the participants for any unanticipated negative effects. This may involve providing participants with written information describing the study and/or the contact details of helplines or counselling services or health care agencies that participants can contact if they want to discuss the issues further. Participants should also know how to contact you after the study, even if it is via a tutor.

Withdrawal from the research

Sometimes individuals may get distressed during an interview, and you must make it clear that they can withdraw from the study at any time without giving any reason. It may be that a participant decides after an interview that they have said things they now regret. Participants should be able to withdraw their interview data in cases such as this. If you are interviewing on sensitive issues, it is good practice to give a cut-off date in the participant information sheet up to which participant data can be withdrawn. This will normally be up to the time when you intend to start your data analysis. Remember your participant information sheet and consent form comprise a contract between you, the research and your participants so you must not make claims in it that you cannot deliver. A common instance of this is where consent forms unconditionally state that participants can withdraw their data. Once your data is analysed withdrawal becomes more difficult, hence it is a good idea to give a cut-off point for withdrawal.

You need to be aware that NHS or social services research, or social care that involves social services, is required by law to go through separate ethical approval and related processes. As mentioned earlier, these procedures were developed to prevent some ethical issues or difficulties arising that might bring adverse publicity to the NHS and to ensure that the research carried out conforms to sound ethical principles. The procedures are complex and time-consuming but full details are available at **http://www.nres.npsa.nhs.uk/**. However, we extend our consideration of ethical considerations in Chapter 13, particularly:

● The four major ethical principles to gauge the acceptability of a proposed nursing research project.

● Understanding some of the processes required to make an application to a local Research Ethics Committee.

Sampling

Whenever you conduct or read about a research study there will be a **sample**. A sample will usually comprise the research participants used in the study, they are so called because they are sampled from the population. All research will use samples. It is important to remember that a population is just a way of describing a group of people. For example, it doesn't just to refer to everyone in a country, rather all the nurses in the UK are a population (the nurse population of the UK), all the patients in a hospital can be a population (the patient population of a hospital), even patients staying in a particular inpatient ward can be a population (the ward's population). In research it is very rare that people can use the whole population for a research study. To get the whole population to take part in a study is time-consuming and expensive and almost impossible because sometimes people don't want to participate in the research, as is their ethical right. Therefore all research studies tend to sample the population for research and try to get a sample that is representative of the population. For example, if the NHS wanted to survey all the nurses about work conditions in the UK, they might use 10 nurses in each hospital in the country so they got a good idea of the picture in each hospital.

Sampling error and its impact on clinical care

However, sampling is not perfect. Let us assume you had limited money and could study only 2 patients out of the population of 30. What effect will the small sample size have on being able to get a representative group? It is likely that there will be a higher risk of *sampling error* being present. Sampling error is an inevitable part of nursing research where we cannot study the target population as a whole.

The following exercise should illustrate the issues of sampling error more clearly. Let us use the example of looking at 30 patients who are thought to have dementia and who visited at a memory clinic (see Figure 5.3), but let us assume you had limited money and could only study 2 patients out of the population of 30.

The number above each person's head is the score they achieved on a memory test; low scores indicate poor memory performance and high scores represent excellent memory. You need to choose just two patients for your sample, so close your eyes and point your finger at two people in Figure 5.3, add up their memory scores and divide the total by 2. What effect will getting only a sample size of 2 patients out of 30 have on being able to get a representative group? It is likely that you will be at higher risk of sampling error being present. If, for example, you chose two patients in the exercise with memory scores of higher than 50 and the population mean for mild dementia was actually 25, you would be overestimating what people with mild dementia could do on a memory test. This is a considerable problem, because if other clinicians wanted to look at the severity of dementia with the same memory test, they may end up seeing people with mild dementia as having worse memory abilities than they really possess. What if you had taken a sample of two people with dementia and found that they had scores of 10 or lower? In this way, you would be underestimating the population mean. This poses another problem, as your memory test would not be

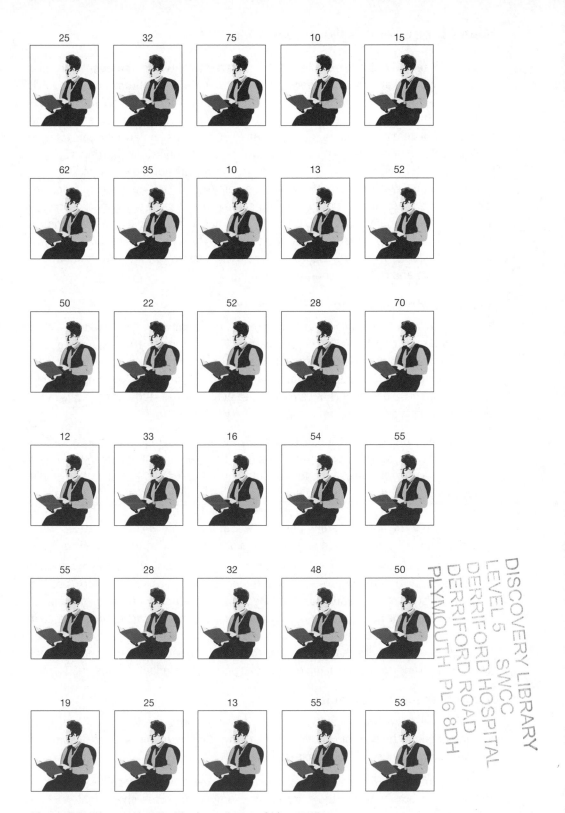

Figure 5.3 'Size matters!' – The importance of big samples.

sufficiently sensitive to be able to tell the difference between someone with mild dementia and someone with moderate levels of dementia symptoms. How about if you were to close your eyes again and point down at 10 different people in Figure 5.3 and add up their scores and divide the total by 10, would that be very different to the population mean (i.e. adding up the scores of all 30 patients and dividing this total by 30)? Overall, we hope this exercise has shown you the complexity of getting a sample large enough for you to know it's likely to be representative of the wider population.

Ideas around bias and error can also be relevant to getting your sample. Researchers therefore always try to obtain a sample that best represents the population. There are many different ways to sample research participants from a population, and we are now going to outline the main types of samples and terms you are likely to come across in research. These are broken down into two main areas, representative and non-representative sampling.

Representative sampling

Representative sampling (also known as probability sampling) is designed in such a way as to be representative of the population. This is done to try to guard against sampling error or bias. As a consequence researchers will try to randomly select participants for the study. Through random samples all the members of the population being studied have an equal chance of being selected for the study. There are a number of different types of random sample:

- A **random sample** would mean that everyone in the sample has had an equal chance of being selected from the population. For example, if the researcher wants to get a sample of nurses among a population of nurses in a hospital, they would get a list of all the nurses in the hospital and then select the sample from that list randomly. That might be done by generating random numbers and choosing the sample from the corresponding position, e.g. a name comes in alphabetical order, or putting the names of all the people into a box and drawing them out at random.

- **Stratified sampling** involves selecting a number of samples from a number of sub-populations within the population. Here the population is assessed in terms of the characteristics of the population and selection is based on that. So for example if 60 per cent of the nurse population is female and 40 per cent is male, and 70 per cent of the nurse population is under 35 years and 30 per cent is over 35 years then the researcher would ensure that the sample contained 60 per cent female participants and that 70 per cent of the sample contained participants under the age of 35 years.

Non-representative samples

However, it is not always easy to sample randomly, therefore it is important that researchers note the type of sampling used. Below are several more types of samples that are commonly used in nursing research.

- **Quota sampling.** With a quota sample the researcher deliberately sets a proportion of different groups within the sample. For example, the researcher might want to get 10 nurses (the sample) from each hospital (subpopulation) in the UK (population) so they can get a wide sample range across all nurses in the country, representing each hospital. Therefore the researcher would randomly select nurses from each hospital, and once they had selected 10 nurses they would move on to creating the next sample.

- **Availability/convenience sampling.** With availability/convenience sampling the researcher chooses participants that are easiest to obtain. Therefore a researcher might just sample the first 50 people they come across, or who volunteer to do the study.

- **Snowball sampling.** In a snowball sample, the researcher will ask each participant to suggest someone else who might be available to do the study. Snowball samples are useful when certain people are hard to contact, for example a person trying to contact drug users might use a snowball sample.

Because these samples are non-representative and are likely to include bias, it is important that you report your sampling technique so you are able to acknowledge possible biases within your research.

5.6 Piloting your study

Before starting your study, it is always worth piloting the methods that you're using. This means trying out the ways in which you collect the data before you actually do the proper study. If you're running a questionnaire study then try out the question- naire with some people beforehand. However, it might also be a good idea to pilot some aspects of the questionnaire before then, when writing the questions. Talking to colleagues and finding out the best way of wording questions or ensuring they are suitable may save you a lot of work in the long run. Also, if you have devised a set of interview questions then it is good practice to run a pilot interview with someone. However, again, before running a whole interview with someone it would be good practice to talk about possible questions and wording of the questions with someone, so you can concentrate on evaluating how the whole of the interview goes, rather than busily rewriting questions. Equally, if you are running an experiment then get some people to carry out the experiment beforehand so you can pick up on any potential difficulties.

This piloting is always done best with colleagues or fellow students and is impor- tant because it will help you identify any problems with the questionnaire/interview/ experiment before you do the 'real thing'. If problems are encountered, do make sure you reflect on why they might have happened and try to adapt your method of data collection accordingly. Don't treat the pilot as a hurdle to be jumped over – use it as a trial run to get some practice in the processes of running the study. Good pilots make for even better larger-scale studies.

Self-assessment exercise

Below are a number of topics with headlines and a short extract from a news article that have been published in *Nursing Times*. Now it's time to use your imagination. Imagine you had to run a research project looking into *one* of these areas. It might be to research something about the topic or to evaluate the issue outlined in the article. Using any of the methods outlined above, design a research project of your choosing. In the box after the articles, describe the main components and procedures of this research project and provide some examples of some of the materials/questions that you might use.

Article 1

> **Summer heatwave health warning**
>
> The Met Office has warned of a heatwave across the Midlands and Southern England early next week. The Department of Health and the Met Office have triggered a heatwave plan warning that daytime temperatures in London could reach 32 degrees Celsius in the daytime falling to only 20 degrees Celsius at night. A Department of Health spokesperson said that this was 'an an important stage for social and healthcare services' who would be working to ensure readiness to reduce harm from a potential heatwave.

(Helen Mooney; *Nursing Times*, 27 June, 2009; http://www.nursingtimes.net/whats-new-in-nursing/specialists/older-people/summer-heatwave-health-warning/5003316.article)

Article 2

> **Yoga and Wii Fit helps Yorkshire step up obesity fight**
>
> More than 150 people took part in an event in Yorkshire last week to help step up the fight against obesity. Change4Life LIVE – held at Doncaster Racecourse – included interactive demonstrations, such as yoga, dancing and a Wii Fit challenge which saw attendees competing against each other.

(*Nursing Times*, 27 June, 2009; http://www.nursingtimes.net/whats-new-in-nursing/acute-care/yoga-and-wii-fit-helps-yorkshire-step-up-obesity-fight/5003328.article)

Article 3

> **Good communication helps to build a therapeutic relationship**
>
> Building relationships is central to nursing work and communication skills can be improved by avoiding jargon and ensuring patients are not labelled. The importance of communication in health care hit the headlines recently at the British Medical Association's annual consultants' conference earlier this month. Jargon, said the doctors, could harm patients' care.

(*Nursing Times*, 19 June, 2009; http://www.nursingtimes.net/nursing-practice-clinical-research/acute-care/good-communication-helps-to-build-a-therapeutic-relationship/5003004.article)

Article 4

> **Midwife helps run breastfeeding course**
>
> A midwife is helping to run a course for new mums that both promotes breastfeeding, and encourages women into higher education.
>
> The 'Breast buddies' course, run by the University of Greenwich's School of Health and Social Care as part of the Sure Start scheme, promotes the benefits of breastfeeding to new mothers in Gravesend, Kent.

(Graham Clews; *Nursing Times*, 27 June, 2009; http://www.nursingtimes.net/nursing-practice-clinical-research/clinical-subjects/midwifery/midwife-helps-run-breastfeeding-course/5003326.article)

Now describe your project in the space below:

Summary

In this chapter, we have covered the essentials when it comes to matching the appropriate methods to use in deciding on your data collection methods to address the research questions and ideas developed out of the previous chapter. We have looked at fundamental issues of whether to use survey or interview methods and we have also focused on the nuances of questionnaire and interview schedule design. We have equipped you with the basic skills for developing tools to collect your nursing research data. In the following few chapters, we will give you pointers on how to analyse the data once you have collected it using these tools.

Chapter 6

Qualitative analysis:
A step-by-step guide

KEY THEMES

Qualitative analysis • Thematic analysis • Qualitative data management •
Qualitative data coding • Interpretation of qualitative data

LEARNING OUTCOMES

By the end of this chapter you will be able to:

- Understand the aims of doing a qualitative analysis

- Be more aware of the different types of qualitative data that could be
  analysed

- Understand the key principles of qualitative analysis, along with the
  processes of conducting such analyses with Ritchie and Lewis' (2003)
  analytic hierarchy of data management, descriptive accounts and explanatory
  accounts

- Understand the issues concerning whether to do a qualitative analysis by
  hand or with a computer

- Understand how different types of qualitative analyses can be done with
  actual datasets by using content analysis, thematic analysis and
  interpretative phenomenological analysis (IPA).

Introduction

IMAGINE THAT . . .

You are a nurse who has met a patient with a rare, chronic health condition known as neurofibromatosis type 1 (NF1). You know very little about what it is like to have this disease and some of the issues that this patient might encounter on a daily basis. A potentially fruitful way of understanding this patient's experiences could be to try to look at the world through their eyes using the phenomenological approach that we introduced you to in Chapter 3. Imagine also that you are now part of a research team that is conducting a project into exploring the experiences of people with NF1. You have carried out semi-structured, in-depth interviews with seven participants and you have the content of the interviews transcribed. You have a complete record of what was said, who said it, who responded to which questions, etc., etc. . . You have the transcripts and you have heard about an analysis technique known as interpretative phenomenological analysis – perhaps this is appropriate for using on your interview data. However, everything all seems a bit vague and muddled – there's so much information to analyse! Where do you start?

Perhaps you thought that doing qualitative nursing research will not be as difficult as dealing with quantitative studies. After all, qualitative studies don't have all of those statistics to get worried about! However, doing high-quality qualitative analyses is not without its challenges. You might read a journal article that reports on a qualitative study that has been conducted and wonder how the authors came to their conclusions in relation to the data they reported on; there may not seem much of a clear connection between the findings and the conclusions. Qualitative analysis is often shrouded in mystique; it is something that just happens and some of the researchers who use qualitative approaches make the analysis seem vague and bombard the reader with plenty of jargon.

In this chapter we aim to demystify the process of conducting qualitative data analysis and will provide you with a step-by-step approach to make it clearer to you and those who read about your analyses. We will give you a taster of the kinds of qualitative analyses that can be done using health care-related qualitative information and show you three levels of analysing qualitative data at various stages so that you can distinguish between surface-level analyses and much deeper ways of examining the data.

To make qualitative data analysis more vivid for you so that you can see the relevance of these kinds of studies for your nursing practice, we have compiled a few real-life examples. To focus on doing content analysis, we will look at stress and coping among 191 health professionals working in community settings (Laungani and Williams, 1997). Through these participants' responses, the researchers were able to find out how stress showed itself in a range of ways including physical symptoms, problems in thinking and problem-solving, emotional problems and behavioural difficulties in coping. A second example from real-life research is McGarry and Thom's (2004) exploration of getting users and carers to help educate nursing students; this example will show you the processes involved in doing a thematic analysis and also in looking for similarities and differences across three different participant groups. To look at the phenomenological approach, specifically using interpretative phenomenological analysis (IPA), we will cover the example of people's experiences of coping with neurofibromatosis type 1 (NF1) that we covered at the start of this chapter. Drawing on real-life data (Dheensa and Williams, 2009) that have been analysed using IPA, we will show you the techniques that will give you a deeper understanding of this methodology. More about the data from these studies to come later . . .

6.1 Aims of qualitative analysis

Overall, the principal purpose of qualitative analysis is to explore information on a deep level. It is possible for qualitative data to be examined superficially, but this method of treating the data will not likely lead to substantial benefits in understanding a patient's experience, why health care professionals act in a certain way when trying to build up a rapport with patients, etc. Superficial analyses do not require as much expertise or time but it may be that the research needs to be done with a minimum of resources and is constrained by limits on when the research should be completed. However, for competent, deeper analyses it is not an easy process to undertake. Good, proficient qualitative researchers need to move through varying levels of depth in their analyses. This is essential before they can obtain meaningful and clinically useful findings, make transparent and justifiable interpretations and draw insightful conclusions from their analyses.

Transparency in qualitative analysis

For a qualitative analysis to step beyond the realm of being just competent, it needs to show evidence that the research was needed and that the researchers were not merely forcing their expectations of the subject area to come to the fore. The process of analysing qualitative data should be clear to readers and it may help to provide an example of how the findings were obtained. It will help to ensure the analyses are verifiable; for example, is it clear how the researchers have arrived at developing a theme of 'positive coping' from the patient interview transcripts? Could the theme be called something else instead? Do the researchers point to some of the raw data (e.g. an interview quote, an excerpt from minutes of a meeting, examples of a patient's expressions of their feelings through art) to illustrate the theme/category that is said to have emerged from the data? To show that the data analysis is rigorous, it is also important for the researcher to demonstrate that different interpretations of the data have been considered too. What helps in raising the possibility of multiple interpretations of data is having more than one person look at it and see if they can come up with similar or contrasting perspectives. If the co-analyst arrives at a different view of the data, it is important to show how these differences are reconciled. All too often, articles that report on a jointly authored qualitative study state that consensus was arrived at through discussions between the researchers, and this may be due to restricted space being available in a journal. However, good practice would be to regularly consider how you report your findings if an agreement is not reached; this will make for an interesting portrayal of the complexity of analysing qualitative data and demonstrate that the subject matter is not black and white.

The methodological basis for qualitative analysis

A final requirement for good qualitative analysis is for there to be a coherent research question, or set of questions, that the data set is meant to answer. Although we could look at an interview transcript and see the extent to which an interviewee is answering each interview question, it is also especially important to consider whether each answer is helping to answer the questions that the entire study is concerned with (i.e. the 'bigger picture'). This is often tied up with method of analysis and methodology (i.e. underlying philosophical approaches to studying a particular topic). For example, a nurse researcher may look at interview data obtained from adults who have started to experience epileptic fits from adulthood where the researcher is examining how people try to cope with these fits. The analyses that follow could adopt IPA to understand what it feels like to have symptoms that precede the epileptic fits and how the person tries to cope with them. IPA could also explore how that person feels the epilepsy affects their identity and their sense of incorporating or rejecting epilepsy into their sense of self.

With the same data set from these interviews of people who are having epileptic fits, qualitative researchers could adopt a different strategy of looking at the language that is used by the interviewees and how this discourse allows the interviewee to take a physical position with their language about themselves and their situation. A qualitative researcher using discourse analysis might look at how the person with epilepsy could imprison or empower themselves with the language that is used.

Another approach with the same data might entail taking a narrative analysis and using the data display method (see Miles and Huberman, 1994) to show the sequence of events and decisions made by the person with epilepsy when in different situations. As we can see, it is possible to look at the same data set in various ways and possibly see different things that arise from it. It might depend on how these interpretations are filtered by the assumptions that are made by operating within a methodological framework and this could also affect the types of questions that are asked before doing the analysis. The main thing to bear in mind when deciding how to analyse qualitative data is that it might be possible to only use one or two analysis methods as the way in which the data will have been collected or arranged could restrict the types of analyses that can be used with the data. For instance, it may be virtually impossible to do discourse analysis on a series of one- or two-word responses to open-ended questions, whereas content analysis (i.e. mainly counting the number of times that a certain concept or topic is mentioned) may be the main option available for this type of data.

6.2 The value of a competent qualitative analysis

Qualitative analysis can offer insights into what things cause people to think, feel and do certain things. It can also help us to understand why patients might not access health care services and why they don't take their medication or check their health on a regular basis (e.g. diabetic patients checking blood glucose levels). This method of analysis can help us to find out more of the perceptions and the meanings that are attached to using certain words in the health care environment (e.g. Becker's 1993 exploration of what medical professionals meant when they called a patient 'a crock' and how this influenced the professionals' perceptions of these patients). Qualitative analysis also gives opportunities to listen to the narratives that patients, service users and carers offer when asked about a range of things from their experiences of having a specific disease to their passage through the health care system and sometimes feeling like they are being passed 'from pillar to post'.

6.3 Qualitative analysis of uniqueness versus commonalities

Qualitative analysis is also used to search for the uniqueness of a participant's experiences as well as the commonalities that might exist between one participant's viewpoint and another's. These commonalities are what researchers are looking for when they are searching for shared themes or categories (see Things to consider) during the analysis of research participants' narrative accounts or interviewees' responses.

THINGS TO CONSIDER

Do we call them 'themes' or 'categories'?

The term 'theme' is often used when researchers are using IPA, whereas researchers who are applying a grounded theory analysis sometimes call it 'category'. Essentially, they are very similar in focus and mainly just represent the idea that there are common areas of experience or perceptions that have arisen from analysing the participants' data.

Qualitative analysis is also used to understand the power dynamics that are portrayed through language. If you are interested in knowing how the language people use gives away clues about the differences in power between health professional and service user you might want to use something known as 'Foucauldian* discourse

---

*This approach to qualitative research comes from the French philosopher Michel Foucault (2003), who was interested in power dynamics in a range of settings in society, including health care and in prisons.

sis'; this approach would focus on how patients might adopt a 'sick role' and be-
passive recipients of health care, but it could also reveal the opposite in terms
how patients assert some of their own influence over how they are cared for by
establishing territory/personal space through the words that they use. Overall, qualitative analysis in nursing research has a series of strengths including helping to
build theory to understand the dynamics of health care, promotion of healthier living, why people don't comply with health advice and so on. It can also be used to test
theory; although one type of grounded theory, advocated by Barney Glaser (1978),
has highlighted the importance of going into qualitative research with no prior expectations or hypotheses, Strauss on the other hand (e.g. Strauss and Corbin, 1998)
has allowed qualitative researchers to test out their expectations and ideas with
their research participants. As you can see, there appears to be confusion among researchers as to what is the best way to analyse qualitative data. However, when we
look at the different types of qualitative data that are available and can be analysed,
it is not surprising . . . In the next section, we will give you an overview of the kinds of
data that are amenable to this approach – contrary to popular expectation, this isn't
just interview data!

6.4 Different types of raw data in qualitative studies

Although the common assumption about qualitative research in nursing is that the
main type of data will be taken from an interview (Silverman, 2007), there are many
other kinds of qualitative data sources. Qualitative data analyses could be applied to
the following types of data (see Table 6.1), which we have split up into three main
kinds – text-based, pictorial/audiovisual and observational. It is important to remember when handling these kinds of data that the rights of the research participants
should be respected at all times. Some of the data to be analysed could be in the public domain (e.g. minutes from meetings held by a primary care trust might be displayed on the Internet). However, other forms of data will often be collected after
participants have consented to take part provided that the researchers have given re-
assurances about data security (e.g. storing the data in a password-protected computer file) and that the data will be used in a responsible manner (e.g. not using a
person's real name when quoting from them and not making the person identifiable
to others when giving background information about that person).

6.5 Qualitative data handling decisions

Right! Now, you've collected the data and you need to decide what to do with it to
store it appropriately and to make it manageable for the process of coding it into
something more coherent. What do you use to help – a computer or plenty of paper?

Table 6.1 Examples of raw data that can be analysed with qualitative methods

Textual materials (coded as text only or by using the Jefferson system*)	Pictorial or audiovisual format	Observational
Naturally occurring dialogue – this could between health care professional and service user (e.g. Bysouth, 2007; Silverman, 1987). It could be a tape-recording of a meeting between health professionals, a service user and a carer in a case conference.	**Poster content** – these could be posters in hospitals, GP surgeries or clinics by: promoting uptake of a service; or checking one's health; or taking up specific behaviours; or avoiding less healthy behaviour. Examples could include anti-smoking posters, promoting breastfeeding among new mothers, getting checked for hepatitis C, etc.	**Participant observation** of dialogue and practices witnessed in the clinical setting and also where health professionals carry out some of their work (e.g. watching what nurses do in their offices or during team meetings). Typical of this approach is ethnographic study of district nurses' practices and interactions with patients in their homes and in other work settings (McGarry, 2007a).
Scripted dialogue or dialogue with a formal agenda such as that between health care providers and the service user's non-scripted responses (e.g. NHS Direct telephone conversations that need to stick to a protocol of questioning depending on the caller's set of symptoms). Alternatively, dialogue that emerges from a set agenda (interviewer with interviewee)	**Visual products** of persons engaged in artistic activities that are being used as therapy (e.g. for people with mental health problems). This could also include a commentary on the process of taking part in a type of art therapy through keeping a video diary (e.g. the kind of things that you might see on YouTube)	**Behavioural observation** such as using a behavioural checklist for observations of inpatients' symptom expressions within a mental health unit, for example.
Formally prepared textual material (e.g. weekly typed minutes from a meeting between members of a district nursing team)	**Audiovisual messages** such as television advertisements (e.g. TV adverts on keeping more active to combat childhood obesity; the Green Cross Code on crossing the road safely; anti drink-driving campaigns; promotion of a smoking cessation helpline)	

*The Jefferson system is one that clearly indicates who is speaking, whether there are pauses before utterances, people are talking at the same time, or there is overlap between one person finishing their speech and another person starting to talk. This system also helps identify whether certain words are being emphasised more strongly than others; it also shows if the pitch of the voice goes up or down at the end of utterances.

The decisions on whether to use a computer to help code the data or rather use paper and pens are something that you will need to consider. When using a computer package like NUD*IST or NVivo, there is the convenience of being able to use quotes more than once to represent different themes. There is certainly more versatility with ruter than using paper and needing to make multiple copies of certain quotes ə applicable to various themes. You can also re-label themes on the com- .reas after several cycles of coding and recoding your data on paper, things ,uuk quite messy and potentially unmanageable as themes are given different labels from those they had originally and various code numbers are scratched out and re-allocated. By contrast, using the coding method on paper is more portable and is often easier to visualise; you can spread out the quotes on the floor to see how the themes are emerging and get a sense of how some of these themes might interrelate with each other. You can also physically arrange the themes to create hierarchies in which some themes are more dominant than others and start to subsume some of the more minor sub-themes. Granted, you can still create hierarchies of data in quali-tative analysis computer programs, but some qualitative analysis purists might still prefer being able to visualise the bigger picture rather than be confined to what can only be seen on the computer screen.

6.6 The three stages of qualitative data analysis

Analysis of qualitative data is not to do with sticking to a set formula of blindly follow-ing distinct stages. Instead, it is an interactive, ongoing process of shifting in and out of different phases of data collection and analysis (Davies, 1999).

In practice, this involves identifying emerging themes and concepts, often whilst collecting the data or being knee-deep in reading and re-reading transcripts or ob-servational diary entries. Identification of gaps in the data and areas for further ex-ploration and clarification are then highlighted and pursued in subsequent observations and interviews. An iterative (i.e. cyclical) approach involves constantly moving between data collection and analysis, with each stage informing the other. This is imperative, as Hammersley and Atkinson (1995) highlight, in order for the re-search to become increasingly focused rather than remaining at a broad and ill-defined level.

Although carrying out data collection and analysis at similar times throughout the research would appear to be very demanding and time-consuming, this process is es-sential to ensure that the theory and practical insights being developed are justifiable to others. As Hammersley and Atkinson (1995) point out:

Some reflection on the data collection process and what it is achieving is essential if the research is not to drift along the line of least resistance and to face an analyt-ical impasse in its final stages.

(Hammersley and Atkinson, 1995; p. 206)

There are a number of conceptual frameworks that can guide the process of qualita-tive analysis (Miles and Huberman, 1994). By 'conceptual frameworks', we mean that you would be using a systematic method of thinking and questioning about the data that have been collected. In this chapter, we are using the analytic hierarchy model (Ritchie and Lewis, 2003), which essentially has three stages: (1) data management (i.e. filing and sorting your data), (2) descriptive accounts (i.e. coding your data and looking for patterns) and (3) developing explanatory accounts (i.e. interpretation of patterns and how they might be organised) (see Table 6.2). Each phase is dependent on the other being executed to a competent level before moving on to the next phase. The ultimate goal of flitting between all three stages is to get to a state of deep interpretation. Your interpretations of how the qualitative data are structured would need to be verifiable; to do this, readers of your analyses should be able to see illustrations of the interpretations that you've made when you have used a selected quote or other piece of evidence (e.g. an excerpt from the minutes of a meeting, a section identified from health promotion materials, etc.) as examples.

Table 6.2 The analytic hierarchy in qualitative analysis

		Iterative process throughout analysis
Seeking applications to wider theory/policy strategies		
Developing explanations (answering how and why questions)	EXPLANATORY ACCOUNTS	Assigning data to refined concepts to portray meaning
Detecting patterns (associate analysis and identification of clustering)		Refining and distilling more abstract concepts
Establishing typologies		
Identifying elements and dimensions, refining categories, classifying data	DESCRIPTIVE ACCOUNTS	Assigning data to themes/concepts to portray meaning
Summarising or synthesising data		
Sorting data by theme or concept (in cross-sectional analysis)		Assigning meaning
Labelling or tagging data by concept or theme	DATA MANAGEMENT	
Identifying initial themes or concepts		Generating themes and concepts
RAW DATA		

Source: Ritchie and Lewis, 2003

Although the framework is described as a hierarchy there is also explicit recognition of the iterative nature of the analysis:

> The analytic process, however, is not linear, and for this reason the analytic hierarchy is shown with ladders linking the platforms, enabling movement both up and down the structure. As categories are refined, dimensions clarified, and explanations are developed there is a constant need to revisit the original or synthesised data to search for new clues, to check assumptions or to identify underlying factors. In this respect, the platforms not only provide building blocks, enabling the researcher to move ahead to the next stage of analysis, they also make it possible to look 'down' on what is emerging, and to reflect on how much sense this is making in terms of representing the original material.
>
> (Ritchie and Lewis, 2003; p. 212)

While this model has been developed by Ritchie and Lewis (2003) it has also been recognised by some as having similar properties to Carney's (1990) ladder of analytical abstraction (Miles and Huberman, 1994) so you can see that qualitative researchers use similar methods to get a deeper and more comprehensive understanding of their data.

In order to capture the social worlds of study participants adequately, analysis of qualitative data might often mean the nurse researcher needing to organise many forms of data (e.g. themes, sub-themes, an overall theoretical model being developed), whilst still being very familiar with the raw data and revisiting it to check for alternative interpretations. In addition, although there are a number of ways in which data analysis can be carried out, generally all methods of qualitative analysis tend to include most of the following activities: (1) data management, (2) indexing or coding and the recognition of patterns or themes and (3) the development of explanations and insights provided by the data collected. Each stage of the analysis is described in detail in the following sections.

Data management

In keeping with the analytic hierarchy framework, the first step in the analysis process involves revisiting and familiarisation with the data, examining the underpinning assumptions surrounding the rationale for undertaking the research and the salient literature. The next step is the process of coding or indexing the data. This involves creating an indexing system (conceptual framework) by grouping the main themes recurring within the data and associated sub-themes. Each of the sub-themes is then assigned a code number. Data are then indexed using the predefined numerical codes, thus linking themes and concepts with the data. A thematic chart (Ritchie and Lewis, 2003) for each main theme is developed in order to consolidate the data as a whole under the themes identified. In this way it is possible to consider the similarities and opposing views within the data as a whole, while also providing a clear outline of the process through which the analysis has progressed. However, it is also recognised that these initial themes are not set concepts and as the study progresses these need to be continually revisited and refined as appropriate. At this stage of analysis the themes are directly evolved from the data, for example, brief quotes or descriptive statements, rather than at the level of interpretation.

Descriptive accounts

During the next stage of the analysis, the process of moving from description to interpretation of the data begins to take place. The key dimensions of this stage of the analysis have been described by Ritchie and Lewis (2003) as detection, categorisation and classification. In practice, utilising the thematic charts it is possible to move from the original text to interpret the data in a more conceptual way, described by Ritchie and Lewis (2003) as 'unpacking' the data. In practice this may involve constructing a series of charts with three columns. The first column (column A) containing the original statement or quote from the data, the second column (column B) containing the first stage of abstraction but where description remains close to the original data, and finally the third column (column C) where the data begin to be interpreted in a more conceptual way. As such, in the final column, labels which move beyond the original data can be assigned. Grouping and summarising segments of data which although described by participants in different ways have a similar or related meaning is also untaken at this point. Table 6.3 shows an example from real-life data (McGarry, 2007a) on how the three columns are used.

This study by McGarry (2007a) involved analysis of district nurses' negotiations of psychological and physical boundaries within patients' homes. In the final column of Table 6.3, labels that moved beyond the original data were assigned. Grouping and summarising segments of data which, although described by participants in different ways, had a similar or related meaning was also carried out. Once all of the data had been charted and investigated thoroughly, cross-referencing with other category charts was undertaken which enabled McGarry (2007a) to identify similar concepts that could be developed under a broader classification (e.g. the theme 'place of care'). This again

Table 6.3 Using the three columns to 'unpack' the data

Column A	Column B	Column C
Data charted in column 7.2	Elements and dimensions identified	Categories
RN12: Interview 1 . . . seeing people as they really are in own home . . . (p3) (7.2)	Holistic care - seeing the 'whole person' - hospital care only part of the 'jigsaw'	Place of care - central to defining the individual as a person - hospital 'fragmentation' Caring ideology
RN13: Interview 1 . . . they exist in their homes (p1) (7.2)	Hospital as 'alien' environment - people 'live' in their homes - links to own values	Individuality - defined through artefacts/history of home Professional belonging Place of care central to professional identity and caring values

was undertaken using sheets of A3 paper where all the elements identified through-out the data were listed in 'blocks' of a similar nature. Finally, the 'blocks' or sets were individually 're-sorted' into subcategories under each main theme (Ritchie and Lewis, 2003) for example, within the theme 'the place of care' RN13 (the pseudonym for one of the district nurses) described older people as 'they exist in their homes', and this has been developed and placed in the subcategory 'coming home: the place of care'. Another nurse, RN12, spoke of seeing 'people as they really are in their own home' and while described differently, exhibited the same features in that the place of care is perceived by nurses as being central in defining the older patient as an individual and recognising this when delivering care to them. As you can see, McGarry (2007a) used the coding of these columns as a way to get closer to developing explanatory accounts of the data, which is the next phase.

Explanatory accounts

As highlighted by Ritchie and Lewis (2003), the final stage of analysis, though pivotal, is not easily described and involves a number of different processes:

> The search for explanations is a hard one to describe because it involves a mixture of reading through synthesised data, following leads as they are discovered, study-ing patterns, sometimes re-reading full transcripts, and generally thinking around the data. It involves going backwards and forwards between the data and emergent explanations until pieces of the puzzle clearly fit. It also involves searching for and trying out rival explanations to establish the closeness of fit. (p. 252)

During this stage of analysis there are a number of ways of developing explanations, distinguishing between explanations developed through explicit responses given by participants, for example, through interview or questioning, and those developed im-plicitly through interpretation of the data. As highlighted by Ritchie and Lewis (2003), throughout the study the development of explanatory accounts will need to be in-formed by the salient literature and existing **empirical** studies. Throughout the analysis it is also vital to be aware of the original research question, how the data are answering the research questions and the implications of the findings (e.g. applying the findings to the delivery of health care or enhancing a patient's experience of health and illness).

6.7 Qualitative data analyses in action

In this section, we will demonstrate what goes on when conducting qualitative analy-sis of data relevant to nurses and other health professionals. We will introduce you to different methods of analysis, some of which might only look at the surface of the data whereas others might require deeper insights and interpretations. We will touch on the following in turn: content analysis, thematic analysis and interpretative phe-nomenological analysis (IPA) using data that were part of published studies.

Content analysis

This method of analysis entails looking for patterns in the data but this often involves mainly looking on the 'surface' of the data. For instance, a study of 191 health care professionals by Laungani and Williams (1997) involved analysing interview data obtained from semi-structured interview questions. These health professionals were asked about an organisational change that had recently been introduced to their workplace, which was called patient-focused care. Participants were asked to tell the interviewer about their perceptions of patient-focused care, their overall feelings whilst at work, their relationship with patients and relations with management and other factors such as what mainly motivated them when they were at work. The sample of health professionals were also asked about their levels of stress, whether the stress levels had altered significantly since the organisational change, whether they had experienced any effects from the stress incurred by the change and the main strategies that they used to combat their stress. Unlike with a structured questionnaire or interview, these health professionals were not given any set categories to use when responding. Their responses were analysed using content analysis, which mainly involved looking for patterns to their answers and then grouping them accordingly. The following has been adapted from Laungani and Williams' (1997) study (see Table 6.4) and it shows how the responses to a question were classified according to how often certain phrases were uttered by participants.

One thing to note in Table 6.4 is that the percentages won't necessarily total 100 per cent as multiple symptoms might have been mentioned by participants during the interviews, rather than just one symptom being reported by each participant. As you can see from Table 6.4, the process of content analysis might primarily be one of counting frequencies which might mean converting qualitative data into a more quantitative form to enable the readers to see the major trends at a glance. This is one reason why there is some debate as to whether content analysis is truly a qualitative method of analysis. Another way in which content analysis might be a little more quantitative, rather than qualitative, is that some researchers who use content analysis might already have predefined criteria of phrases or ideas that they're

Table 6.4 Physical effects of stress among community health professionals

Symptom	% of sample
Feeling tired ('I'm tired', 'I'm weary', 'exhaustion', 'exhausted', 'knackered')	42
Headaches ('my head often is fit to burst', 'many migraines', 'splitting headache')	12
Hypervigilance ('can't sleep for worry', 'always alert', 'restless')	8
General sickness ('my body can't cope', 'I come down with all sorts of bugs')	7
Tenseness ('my neck's muscles are taut', 'stiff back')	7
Lethargy ('just can't be bothered', 'my body and mind are just not motivated', 'lethargic all over')	4
Other physical symptoms (e.g. 'irregular periods', 'I lose my appetite')	4

expecting to find; as a result, they will mainly count how often these criteria have been met within the content of the spoken data and the analysis is mainly confined to how far the data meet with the researchers' expectations. Overall, content analysis might seem to some a more superficial mode of qualitative analysis, so let us move on to other examples of qualitative analyses. With the next method, thematic analysis, we will now be able to focus less on how often something is said by putting the researchers' prior assumptions to one side and letting the data 'do the talking'.

Thematic analysis

Content analysis might seem a little superficial but it does provide opportunities to extract patterns quickly in qualitative data. This analysis tool might be something that you need to use, as a busy nurse researcher, when contending with the demands of getting in-depth qualitative data from patients or service users and being driven to get answers from all of your data as soon as possible. However, there are other methods, like thematic analysis, that offer an added dimension to your qualitative data analysis. We will use, as a case study, McGarry and Thom's (2004) focus group research with three different groups of people who are affected by users/carers being involved in educating nurses – users and carers, nursing students and the staff who teach the nursing students. In Table 6.5, you can see the themes that emerged from the data analysis, with a representative quote used to illustrate each theme.

You should be able to see that some themes were common to more than one focus group whereas other themes were unique to just one focus group. Both students and service users saw the experience as positive and both groups saw it as beneficial for the users or carers. Students saw it as an opportunity for users/carers to express their thoughts and feelings and the users/carers saw it as a chance to let the student nurses know about things that would make life easier and more pleasant. By contrast, the teaching staff seemed to have different perspectives compared to the students and users/carers, with teachers focusing more on the logistics of organising these taught sessions led by users or carers. However, it's possible to see from the fifth theme for users or carers in Table 6.5 that the organisation of the sessions was also of concern to them, particularly in making sure the taught sessions had a structure to them; in a way, it would seem as if the teachers and the users/carers have a shared agenda, particularly with the arrangement of the actual taught activity itself.

As you can see, the thematic analysis is a more in-depth method of understanding and representing qualitative data than content analysis sometimes is. Let us now look at another in-depth qualitative analysis method – **interpretative phenomenological analysis (IPA)**, which attempts to look at people's experiences through their eyes and is aimed at interpreting the psychology of their experiences.

Interpretative phenomenological analysis

The following account has been drawn from telephone interview transcript data collected for a study by Dheensa and Williams (2009) of six adults who have neurofibromatosis type 1 – a chronic, genetic disorder that includes symptoms like curvature of

Table 6.5 Themes of perceptions of users/carers being involved in nurse education

Teaching staff	Nursing students	Users/carers
Users'/carers' experience as a resource ('It's about putting people in a different role, the user is the helped person. In the classroom the role is changed, you can learn from them rather than the other way around. It is a reversal of power'.)	Opportunity for the user/carer to give his/her perspective ('I think it changes your perception, it's valuable, it's positive in the sense that they [the user/carer] get a chance to say what they think.')	Things to be gained from teaching student nurses ('I think the thing I enjoy is you can actually tell them the little things that would make your life easier.')
Careful planning of sessions ('I think the main points are preparation for all. Tighten up the feedback, tell people clearly what you want of them. Treat people fairly and enter into a contract with them but equally the individual needs to know what is expected of them'.)	Positive experience ('. . . you get this different perspective of what it's like for them [user/carer] to come and talk to the student nurses about how it feels to be in that situation.').	Positive experience ('There are people a lot worse than myself obviously, but it gives me confidence to stand up in front of trainee nurses . . . it's a learning stage for me going into the school.')
Support for users/carers and their well-being before, during and after, the session ('We [lecturers] are often not very well prepared for this [user/carer sessions] and there are concerns about doing damage and I think you have to have a realistic view of what you can achieve.')		Reasons for involvement ('I got involved because X [a charitable organisation] asked me because what I've got is a rarity so they're [student nurses] not likely to have come across it . . .')
		Contributing to knowledge ('It's the practice that is needed, not the theory. I mean the doctors have got the theory but they haven't got the practice . . . Now if you get someone like us who can come to the fore and speak out, it's very credible.')
		Structuring of sessions ('It's about being standardised in terms of when you actually go and speak to nurses and I think there needs to be guidelines, like confidentiality . . . I think sometimes you're not quite sure when you go to talk what we're supposed to be doing.')

Source: Adapted from McGarry and Thom, 2004

the spine, musculoskeletal difficulties and disfiguring tumours over the body. In this excerpt, we will attempt to make sense of the narrative from one of these participants by using IPA (Smith, 1996), which is aimed at gaining an understanding of a person's subjective viewpoint and their ability to make sense of their world. The key task for the researcher using this technique is to interpret and contextualise that person's views from a psychological perspective (Larkin *et al.*, 2006). There are four key stages to doing this (Willig, 2001): (1) the researcher's initial reactions to the text, (2) identifying themes, (3) clustering themes, (4) summarising the themes and interpreting them. We will do each of these in turn when approaching the task of analysing the text of this interview transcript.

Narrative from 'Grace':

1 I don't want my NF to stop me from doing things.

2 I don't use it as a crutch, or as something 'well I got this, it means I have to

3 be on disability, and I shouldn't work' and I don't take advantage of it.

4 I like going to work, I've worked for twenty-five years . . . there hasn't really

5 been a time where I wasn't working! I don't work a lame job, you know.

6 I work a pretty good job . . . I mean, I know that people think I can't do things,

7 or by looking at me [they form] an opinion, but I do what I can do to prove

8 them wrong if I can.

Initial reactions

Upon initial reading of this excerpt, we have noticed the way 'Grace' uses medical metaphorical imagery when talking about how she perceives her experiences of NF (e.g. 'crutch' symbolism in line 2). She contrasts this use of a crutch with a dialogue she might be having with someone if she had decided to accept the assumption that having a disease like NF is equated with low capability to do things and mainly be worthy of claiming support from the state (lines 2-3). Grace talks about being 'on disability'. (Is this an American term? We are aware that Grace is American from the background information collected on her, so this brings to mind questions as to whether there might be differences between the USA and UK in how people with chronic health conditions are treated by the benefit and health care systems. Perhaps it's similar. Either way, it might affect her perceptions of how she thinks others see her.) Grace also talks about not taking advantage of the label of having NF (line 3); this seems to suggest that such a label can be used to get others to do things for her and that potentially it could be misused but she is adamantly against doing this. Being in employment seems to be very important to Grace as she refers to her length of time in work ('twenty-five years', line 4) and also the type of job that she currently does ('pretty good job', line 6). She also contrasts being in a 'pretty good job' with what she thinks people might expect of her, given her condition of having NF (a 'lame job', line 5). Grace seems attuned to how others might see her ('people think I can't do things', line 6); she talks about people forming opinions about her from looking at her (line 7) although she doesn't say whether these opinions are favourable or not. From the look of the preceding text, it seems likely that these opinions are not good, but we can't take this for granted. Perhaps

Grace is mainly commenting on people judging her worth and her abilities and that often these assessments are not true to how she sees herself. In lines 7-8, it seems as if Grace is up for a challenge as she appears to be going through a process of estimating how others see her (from their initial reactions to her) and then deciding on what activities she could do to disprove their perceptions.

Identification of themes

After outlining this initial reaction to the text, we can then progress to approaching the text again in a more systematic way. The main thing that we want to achieve in this stage is to identify whether any of the elements in the text that we've identified so far can be given thematic labels. Through line-by-line analysis, we were able to pinpoint the following themes:

1. Feelings of ownership and uniqueness ('my NF').
2. Perceptions of being impeded or dependent ('crutch', 'stop me', 'shouldn't work', '. . . I wasn't working', 'I can't do things').
3. Other people's perceptions of herself (lines 6-8).
4. Perceptions of self tied into working (contrasting 'pretty good job' and 'lame job' as if good jobs and lame jobs are tied to one's very identity as being a worthy and capable person, 'I like going to work').
5. Rejection of passivity (actively works against following a script of 'well I got this, it means I have to be on disability, and I shouldn't work').
6. Disproving other people's perceptions of herself (refusing to use the label of being disabled and to do what Grace sees as taking advantage of the label in lines 2-3; also the quote 'I do what I can do to prove them wrong if I can').

Clustering of themes

The next step is to cluster the themes that appear to share similar features based on their content in which they might point to common psychological experiences, states or perceptions. By using the six themes identified earlier, we began grouping the themes together to try to see whether essentially they shared similar properties in the assumptions and perceptions that the themes conveyed. The following clusters were created as a result:

- Cluster 1: Self and identity (themes 1, 3 and 4)
- Cluster 2: Dependence and passivity (themes 2 and 5)
- Cluster 3: Empowerment (theme 6 and possibly themes 1 and 4).

As you can see by the way in which the clusters have been arranged, it's possible to acknowledge that labelling some of the clusters might not fit neatly into very separate entities; there might be slight overlap with how the themes and clusters are organised and this recognises that people's perspectives are rarely black and white, with many shades of grey when analysing the nuances of what a person is thinking, feeling and saying.

Table 6.6 A summary table of clusters, themes, quotations and locations of quotes

Cluster and theme	Quote	Source
Cluster 1: **Self and identity**		
• Ownership and uniqueness	'my NF'	Line 1
• Other people's perceptions of oneself	'I know that people think I can't do things, or by looking at me [they form] an opinion'	Lines 6-7
• Perceptions of self tied into working	'I work a pretty good job'	Line 6
Cluster 2: **Dependence and passivity**		
• Being impeded or dependent	'I can't do things'	Line 6
• Rejection of passivity	'I don't use it as a crutch, or as something "well I got this, it means I have to be on disability, and I shouldn't work" and I don't take advantage of it'	Lines 2-3
Cluster 3: **Empowerment**		
• Disproving other people's perceptions of oneself	'I do what I can do to prove them wrong if I can'	Lines 7-8
• Ownership and uniqueness	'my NF'	Line 1
• Perceptions of self tied into working	'I like going to work, I've worked for twenty-five years . . . there hasn't really been a time where I wasn't working!'	Lines 4-5

Summarising the themes and interpreting

We now move on to the final stage of summarising the key themes and clusters by producing a summary table and then interpreting what this is telling us about Grace's perspectives on living with NF. With this summary table (see Table 6.6), what we're aiming to do is make the process and outcome of the analyses as transparent and justifiable as possible. This is why we need to clearly and systematically identify each cluster and constituent theme, along with where to find relevant keywords or quotes to verify the researchers' interpretations of the data.

When writing up the findings, it is useful to acknowledge some of the clusters and themes when interpreting and explaining what is going on with Grace's perceptions. The interpreting part is very important because, without it, your analyses would mainly be to do with analysing people's phenomenological experiences but there would be little beyond mere description. When you interpret the themes that have arisen, you are starting to take on a deeper appreciation of what the person is saying, thinking and feeling. The following is an example of what we could have written about the themes that emerged from the analysis:

Grace's use of the crutch metaphor implied that she does not rely on NF1 to excuse her from usual duties, such as employment, which is something she enjoys. Her hesitance

to let NF prevent her from being 'normal' appears consistent
Nevertheless, she understood that chronic pain does not fit
cept of normality, leading to her thoughts that others are for
based on her perceived inability to 'do things'. Resiliently, sh
perceptions where possible. It would appear to be quite piv
people who have NF (like Grace) might perceive themselve
see them. It would appear that Grace's identity was more ne
worker rather than having her identity subsumed as being an 'NF su
unable to do things for herself. Granted, Grace acknowledged that she had NF and e.
she called it 'my NF' but she seemed to be making active efforts to go against what
she thought people might assume her to be able to do when comparing herself with
someone who also has the same medical condition. Grace saw it as 'her NF' and that
wasn't the only part of being who she was. Instead, she saw that she could hold multi-
ple identities such as someone who was able to hold a 'pretty good job', despite her
thinking that others might see her 'disabled'. She saw that she had a choice with her
reactions to knowing that she had NF and how to cope with societal expectations to
this part of her identity. She saw it as her role to confound these expectations and
appeared to see her reactions as empowering.

Overall, we have shown you a strategy for using IPA when analysing textual data and have given you some tips on how to approach this task in a systematic way by using a four-step approach. We are now going to give you seven more tips on general good practice when doing qualitative analysis.

6.8 Seven steps to a successful qualitative analysis

To recap some of the key pointers for doing qualitative analysis well, we have compiled a list of seven steps for success in this activity. The following practices are ones that we have found useful over the years (and some of them we wish we'd done more often!):

1. Make the process of data collection, data analysis and your interpretations as transparent as possible. Give complete information on what you have done. Don't just state when writing up your study that saturation was reached when analysing the data. Explain how you knew that no further themes could be obtained from the data analysis.

2. Revisit the data on many occasions. You might find that the themes that you have extracted seem to make sense on the face of it but your interpretations might not stand up to scrutiny if you haven't shown that you have accounted for different interpretations of the data. Could the themes be called something else?

3. Tie your analysis to your methodology. Make sure that you have an appropriate way of 'packaging' the raw data so that you're not spending excessive time on tracking information that you're not going to analyse in the long run. For example, it would make sense to use the Jefferson system of transcribing interview data and

ing the pauses and the shifts in conversation between speakers if you're
ng discourse analysis but it would not be as useful for doing IPA. This is because
PA would mainly rely on *what* research participants are saying, rather than *how*
they are saying it.

4. Be clear about what stage/phase of the analysis you are on. Are you at the data management or the description or the explanation stage?

5. Decide on what method you are going to use to handle the data once you have got it transcribed. Are you going to use a computer or do the data handling by hand? Do you need to get further expertise to do computer-based qualitative analysis? Do you have sufficient space in a room to spread out plenty of pieces of paper with various bits and pieces scribbled on them, code numbers, different sections of the text cut out and identified with highlighter pen?

6. Get someone else to look at the data and go through a process of data analysis by using the methodology that you are using. This is restricted by you knowing another person who has a similar level of knowledge on the methodology you're using. If you are studying qualitative analysis on a course, it might be helpful to share your data with other students and get them to code the data 'blind' from your own analysis of the data. It is quite likely that you both might not come up with the same themes as a result of the analysis. This is where the real discussions (and the deeper analysis) begins!

7. Decide on an appropriate time to stop doing the qualitative data analysis. The concept of 'saturation' is a bit vague. It seems to suggest that the researchers have gorged themselves on data and are now feeling too 'full'. You may need to be practical, especially if you are restricted with time and resources to only conduct a certain number of interviews, get them transcribed and go through the transcripts with a fine-toothed comb as well as write up your analyses. Doing this properly might take several months but you need to be up-front with your reasons for stopping any further analyses. Don't say you've reached saturation when you've actually started to run out of time. Instead, only claim that saturation has occurred when you have gone back to the same pieces of data and you can't come up with any other angles on how the data can be understood. If you have been working with a co-researcher and that person can't come up with any further perspectives on the data, then you have truly reached a saturated state!

Self-assessment exercise

Have a look at the following excerpts of data drawn from interviews with two different research participants (Harper, 2006) who were diagnosed with having epilepsy when they were in adulthood. See if you can spot any common themes from the excerpts in terms of what the participants are saying and experiencing.

Excerpt 1

```
 1  Interviewer: OK, tell me something about your epilepsy experience . . .
 2
 3  Participant: I think that stigma is a big problem. Epilepsy is a condition where
 4  there is limited information provided to epileptics, which can cause anxiety,
 5  fear and panic. I think it's important to bond with others about this.
 6
 7  Interviewer: Empathy is beneficial with others in the same position?
 8
 9  Participant: Yes, to know it is normal.
10
11  Interviewer: What other problems do you think you face in your epilepsy
12  experience, or what other concerns do you have?
13
14  Participant: Well there is the concern over taking anti-epileptic drugs for too long.
15  There are long-term worries of osteoporosis.
16
17  Interviewer: what do you mean?
18
19  Participant: Taking anti-epileptic drugs for long periods of time you can develop
20  bone problems. There are two hospitals in my local area and they are both treating
21  epilepsy in various ways, there's no continuity. My epilepsy is medically treated
22  but I don't have anything given to me to help the social side of things.
```

Excerpt 2

```
23  Interviewer: You don't feel affected by any stigma, whether it [seizures from
24  epilepsy] happens or not?
25
26  Participant: No I'm not. That I think is probably because of my age. I do think
27  when you are older you are less affected by what people think. Though I'm sure
28  some people can feel picked on more than other people about their epilepsy. I
29  guess everyone is different and some people need more support than others.
30
31  Interviewer: Yeah, that probably is right. I think that some people seem to adjust
32  and cope to it more naturally than others. So what others say doesn't bother you?
33
34  Participant: I can take jokes about me, and my epilepsy. I can certainly make them
35  too. You have got to laugh about some things. It doesn't get you anywhere being
36  angry.
37
38  Interviewer: You find it easy to take it with a pinch of salt?
39
40  Participant: Well to be honest it isn't really something that I can control or stop so if
    someone wants to criticise me for that well . . . what can I say? That is just pathetic.
```

Summary

In this chapter, we have examined some of the essential issues to consider when conducting analysis of qualitative data. In the following chapter we will be looking at a methodology known as action research, which offers the nurse researcher an opportunity to obtain qualitative and quantitative data, and there is also the chance to bring about substantial changes to the actions that are taken around people's health and health care delivery. This can involve making changes to how health care is organised, the support that health service users (or carers) are given, and can also help in shaping how health-related messages are communicated to the general public. Doing action research is also not without its challenges. We will introduce you to some of the main considerations involved in the next chapter.

Chapter 7

Blending qualitative and quantitative methods: Action research

KEY THEMES

Collaboration • Quantitative data • Qualitative data • Cyclical process • Change

LEARNING OUTCOMES

At the end of this chapter you will be able to:

- Understand that action research is a philosophy and an approach to guide research and development in applied contexts

- Identify the four major stages involved in planning and carrying out action research in nursing

- Evaluate the situations during which the application of action research approaches may be most suitable

- Identify the types of activities that may impede the successful implementation of the findings from action research into more practical situations.

Introduction

Have a look at the following situation, which we will return to at various times throughout this chapter. This imaginary scenario illustrates the sorts of things you might encounter in practice and may be an appropriate starting point for deciding whether or not to use an action research approach in this context.

IMAGINE THAT ...
You are a nurse working on a Care of the Older Person ward in a community hospital. You know that poor nutrition among older people within the hospital setting as a whole has been an issue for a number of years; you also know that a number of policy initiatives have attempted to address this deficit and that it is a continued priority within care delivery (The Healthcare Commission, 2007). However, while the nutritional value of the food that is prepared and served on the ward has improved as a response to national guidelines on patient nutrition, you have also noticed that the supervision of mealtimes and helping patients to eat continues to be devolved to staff with less experience. This seems to signify the continued lack of importance attached to this part of caring for older people. Patients are still not always eating their food and some of them are expressing dissatisfaction with it. Some patients may not be eating their food because their medication regime is upsetting their appetite. As a result, some patients still have poor nutritional health.

> *There are known knowns. These are things we know that we know. There are known unknowns. That is to say, there are things that we know we don't know. But there are also unknown unknowns. There are things we don't know we don't know.*
>
> Donald Rumsfeld

This now legendary quote by the ex-American Defence Secretary Donald Rumsfeld, though open to scrutiny on a number of points from a linguistic perspective (Donald won an award from the British Plain English Campaign for this gem), is an appropriate way to introduce this chapter on action research for two reasons. The first reason is that it highlights the need to *embrace uncertainty* and to acknowledge the 'unknown' and exploratory nature of many types of research, especially action research. Often in the process of doing action research we might end up somewhere different to where we anticipated being. This is not to suggest that action research should lack direction; although we might have a rough idea of the desired outcome of the proposed research, the path of action research is directed by a collaborative approach between researchers and participants and is sometimes open to changes in direction along the way. The second reason the quote is apt is due to the need to be *flexible and open* to input from a variety of perspectives. There should also be openness in our approach to bring about actions as a result of the ideas that we take from the multiple viewpoints ranging from the opinions of staff to those of patients and their relatives. As a result, action research requires a more fluid approach to the research endeavour which may be subject to change over the course of its lifetime; this is very unlike the traditional research method used in some nursing research, particularly with quantitative studies that have a clear hypothesis and highly focused boundaries for the research are already drawn up.

In earlier chapters, we have looked at what theories and pieces of evidence are. There is experiential evidence, such as the types of experiences that you might get on the wards (like in the above scenario) and there is evidence based on quantitative or qualitative research, like the recommendations made nationally on what is acceptable practice. There is also theory in terms of what we would reasonably expect to happen in general cases. In theory, we might expect patients to feel happier when eating healthier food. In theory, they might like more choices, or do they? In theory, we might expect staff to give patient nutrition a similar level of priority as other types of nursing care, but this doesn't look like it's the case. To what extent do all levels of nursing staff see it as part of their role? Overall, it seems there is a gulf between what we might expect in theory and what we're seeing in practice. Perhaps action research is one way to address this gap between theory and practice.

7.1 Identifying the problem: the tensions between theory and practice

If we translate these observations into the context of a potential research question or areas for further exploration we can begin to reinterpret the potential problem in the following ways. First, the current practice that you have observed in this scenario highlights how the accumulation of evidence and the practices that continue to be carried out by nurses could be at odds with each other. Bear in mind that a sizeable percentage of clinical practices might not be evidence-based – one study, for instance, has shown that a worrying percentage of registered nurses had a low to moderate level of knowledge about evidence-based practice (Alspach, 2006). Second, the problem in this scenario seems to centre around the issue of how to change the current routine of mealtimes from one which places the needs of the ward at the centre to one that focuses on the needs of the older patients. This therefore means that a cultural change could be required – the culture of having mealtimes at a certain time, the culture of how meals, and nutrition in general, are perceived by staff and by patients. Cultural change can often be very difficult to bring about and we will cover the relevant things to consider if change is needed to current practices. Thirdly, and finally, in order to bring about change there needs to be some recognition by various parties that the change is needed. The involvement of significant people, like managers, patients, front-line staff and patients' relatives may need to be sought so that change can be implemented more smoothly. Just knowing that change is needed may not be enough to bring about change; instead, there needs to be a way of pulling everyone along with the process of making people aware of the need to change before planning it and bringing it about. Later on in this chapter we will be covering methods of involving all the people who are vital in making changes to practice happen.

7.2 What is action research and what does it involve?

Before deciding whether or not to adopt an action research approach to the problem or issue at hand, it is essential to have a clear understanding of what action research is all about. Very complex definitions could be given on what action research involves. However, rather than trying to compete with Donald Rumsfeld for the Plain English Award, it is best to identify that one of the key elements of action research is that it is an **approach** and a **philosophy** of doing research. In this way, action research could more reliably be described as a research methodology, rather than a research method. To illustrate the major components of action research, Reason and Bradbury (2007) highlight that

> There is no 'short answer' to the question 'What is action research?' . . . It seeks to bring together action and reflection, theory and practice, in participation with others, in the pursuit of practical solutions to issues of pressing concern to people, and more generally the flourishing of individual persons and their communities. (p. 1)

Let us dissect this quote and understand the critical concepts that are covered in it. It is vital to take action, but also to reflect on actions taken and whether these actions are appropriate. There is the recognition that theory and practice are involved but, as we have already noticed, many action researchers would argue that theory itself is not powerful enough to bring about changes in practice and that there is a more complex relationship or interplay between theory and practice (Gustavsen, 2001). In this quote, there is also an emphasis on participation. Participation can be interpreted in a more active form of collaboration. The researcher and the participant both have a major role to play and a more appropriate way of conducting action research would be to see the research participants as collaborators or 'co-explorers' in the research enterprise. Both the researcher and participant are like fellow navigators and are sometimes charting out unfamiliar territory in order to get a shared understanding of the agenda for the study, how to do the research, and what to do with the findings in terms of changes to practice. The metaphor of 'action research as a journey' is very appropriate here.

Another aspect of the above quote is that practical solutions are needed; there is no sense in making recommendations for changing practice if these changes are not going to be workable. Action research as an approach involves looking at how feasible proposed changes are within the culture of a specific organisation. The quote also makes reference to 'pressing concerns'; here there is a recognition of prioritising what is important to be studied with the action research. Not everything can be done, but all people who have an investment in the action research will need to look at what is most important to do. There is also a vital component to the quote that needs addressing when the authors mention 'flourishing'; to flourish is to be reaching higher and higher states of being. In this way, action research should guide the researchers and participants to aim for more improvements in practice and to look at how the status quo can always be improved upon. To do that will often involve many people and this brings us to the final part of the quote that needs discussion, namely the importance of 'individual persons and communities'. The best way to implement changes is through involving individuals and looking at what makes them tick and why they behave in certain ways. It also means seeing how certain groups of people act in a similar way. For instance, it entails asking (in the context of the 'Imagine you are a . . .' scenario) about who are the main people involved in the arranging of mealtimes, getting patients to choose their meals, the delivery of meals, the checking on whether patients eat their meals, etc. There is a lot of emphasis on teamwork when carrying out action research and how the research affects people in practical situations. The famous saying by John Donne, 'No man is an island, entire of itself' is very relevant when doing action research.

If we return to our scenario it can be suggested that action research is well suited to this particular situation, where the purpose of the project is to bring about a change in the ward culture in terms of staff and patient attitudes concerning the importance of mealtimes when gauging how satisfactory patient care is on a Care of the Older Person ward.

What is the overall philosophy of action research?

While the origins of action research have been largely attributed to the work of Kurt Lewin (e.g. Lewin, 1951), who (it is claimed) once said, '*If you want truly to understand something, try to change it.*' The intervening years have witnessed the development of a number of schools of practice, each with differing approaches to the general principles of doing action research. More up-to-date approaches of action research involve valuing the many perspectives that patients, service users, health professionals and service managers may bring to a particular problem in a clinical setting. It is more egalitarian in approach when compared with expert-driven projects that involve a researcher designing a study, collecting and analysing data and making recommendations from the results, often carried out separately from those who have a

THINGS TO CONSIDER

What is postmodernism?

Postmodernism is a complex concept that is hard to define. Essentially, it is a school of thought that arose as a reaction to 'modernism'. Modernism developed during the nineteenth and early twentieth centuries from dissatisfaction in the Western world towards the world view of different kinds of 'authorities'. These authorities could be governments, established scientific and medical opinion, and such like. Although modernists were critical of those who would promote one kind of 'truth', postmodernists went a step further. Postmodernists thought that the modernist approach was still too linear (i.e. step-by-step) to fully understand a rapidly changing, technological world. Instead, the philosophy of postmodernism sees the world as complex and unpredictable; as a result, the postmodernists would argue that conventional boundaries around what constitutes 'real', 'valid' and 'true' knowledge should continually be questioned.

stake in what is done in the research (i.e. the stakeholders). With action research, stakeholders have their views listened to and incorporated into the design and running of an action research project. This kind of egalitarian method entails treating everyone as equals and could be seen as postmodern (see box above) by drawing from a variety of sources of expertise and knowledge and not treating one type of knowledge as more important than another.

Action research is also egalitarian because it can also be seen as 'bottom-up'; this involves people at the sharp end of practice-related situations being actively engaged in the action research so that people who may sometimes be seen as at the bottom (or outside) of an organisational hierarchy get more of a say than they might usually do. Bottom-up approaches are in contrast to 'top-down' methods of researching, in which those at the higher levels within an organisation are tasked with making decisions about how to organise systems of care and changes to these systems might be dictated from centralised bodies like the National Health Service's Department of Health. Other important elements of the philosophy of action research are in being adaptable and open to new avenues of enquiry and also in being facilitated to try out a range of different enquiries before deciding on the direction of the action research, the methods of collecting and analysing the data, and the ways of reporting the results and implementing change.

You may come across a number of action research approaches as you read journals and textbooks in this area. Do not worry about the different labels given to these types of action research. They share some similarities but Table 7.1 shows how they differ to some degree.

Table 7.1 Various types of action research

Type of action research	Main focus
Participatory action research (PAR)	There is a focus on bringing about positive social change. This is done via group work, self-reflection and questioning of practices currently being used. A PAR group may ascertain a common concern through discussion and reflection. A common goal is then negotiated in the PAR group and several cycles of planning, acting and observing and reflecting are undertaken.
Emancipatory research	Focuses on people in disenfranchised or marginalised groups. The research is often aimed at empowering these groups and looking at how to address the social structures that are currently oppressing these communities.
Co-operative inquiry or collaborative inquiry	This involves working with other people who have shared concerns or interests. The group has co-researchers who look at their understanding and experiences of their world, along with attempting to change practices that go on in the world.
Action science	The main aim is to get people in groups to gain confidence and skills in creating an organisation/society to help them to become more effective on an individual and group level. The key principle is exploring whether evidence can be turned into something actionable. Action science often entails looking at information that can't be turned into action to make the distinction between actionable and non-actionable data more apparent.

We have shown you that there are different types of action research but, for the purposes of introducing you to this approach, you will only need to be aware of the main principles to adhere to when using it and the steps that are required when wishing to use this methodology. In the following section, we will look at the steps you can take to get started.

Having decided on an action research approach: what next?

As we mentioned earlier, action research necessitates involving people from the beginning of the project. This will involve listening to many different stakeholders who will have a variety of perspectives to the research problem and using their perspectives to set out a research agenda and to plan a project with the expected outcome of visible change.

The process itself will involve working in a collaborative way to plan and carry out a project that may have a series of different and possibly ongoing phases so that inquiry precedes research, which then precedes action, which then precedes further inquiry, research and future change. This may all sound confusing, however a number of conceptual frameworks have been developed to illustrate the process of action research across a range of disciplines. Figure 7.1 shows how this framework has been adapted and used in the field of education, with David Kolb's (1984) experiential learning theory.

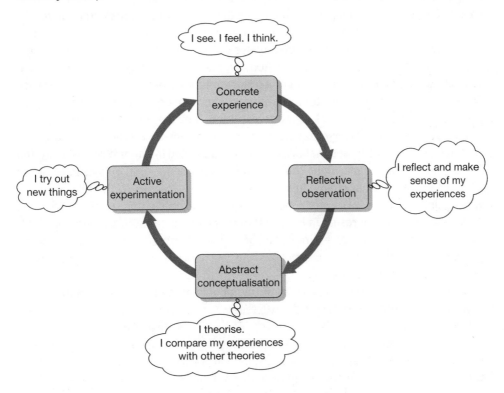

Figure 7.1 Action research frameworks in education (after Kolb, 1984).

With this approach, Kolb has argued that we can learn (and subsequently act) through four main processes of concrete experience, reflective observation, abstract conceptualisation and active experimentation. Let us take you through the four processes in relation to doing action research in nursing. One thing to bear in mind is that the framework is portrayed as a cycle but you are welcome to start at any point, rather than there being just one starting point. For the purposes of this illustration, we will start this example at the process of reflective observation. With **reflective observation**, let us imagine that you are part of a health care team who have found that many of your patients with type II diabetes are not monitoring their blood glucose levels on a regular enough basis and sometimes need to be admitted to hospital with medical complications. As a team, you would reflect on why blood glucose monitoring (BGM) is not being done on a regular enough basis – are the patients finding it difficult to integrate this into a habitual routine? Is it part of the BGM process itself that is uncomfortable or stigmatising? Do the patients get enough support from family and friends? After undergoing that process of reflective observation and gathering evidence on what is happening with your patients, your team can progress to the next stage of **abstract conceptualisation**. In this stage, your team might ask whether there are any studies or theories that could explain lack of compliance in BGM among patients with type II diabetes – what has worked well elsewhere to increase compliance levels? How could you persuade some patients to think of more effective ways to integrate BGM into their lives? Moving on to the next stage of **active experimentation**, your team could get groups of patients and relatives together to find out whether some of the strategies for improving on BGM habits could work well with them. There could be a phase of the patients and relatives trialling a new system of reminders to monitor blood glucose or your team could enable the patients to test out a novel method of doing the monitoring in a discreet way (if privacy was deemed to be an issue by the patients when undergoing BGM). Finally, your team could get to the stage of **concrete experience** by asking the patients and relatives how the new approaches are working and seeing whether there are any teething problems or issues that are not being addressed in integrating BGM into the patient's life. Your team might then go one stage further and collect data about whether the levels of BGM among your patients has increased (**reflective observation** again) and then you're on the next iteration of this cycle, and so on and so on . . . As you can see, action research is something that seems to require a number of different phases and perhaps entire cycles of activity in order to see whether real improvements are being made. Overall, you can make exciting, meaningful changes to practice by using this approach!

While varying slightly in nature, all of the models of action research share a common thread in terms of progression or 'steps' in the process: plan, act, observe and reflect. Indeed you may have noticed the similarities between the stages of action research and some of the reflective cycles that you might use as part of reflections that you undertake regarding your own nursing practice and experiences, such as Gibbs' reflective cycle which we have adapted in Figure 7.2.

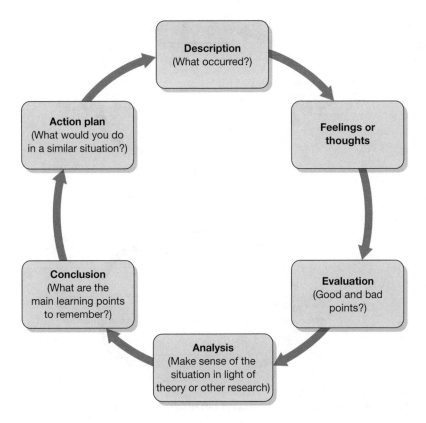

Figure 7.2 A reflective framework (after Gibbs, 1988).

There is also a lot of emphasis in action research on needing to reach higher and higher levels of improvement to practice so there is recognition of a spiral model (Carr and Kemmis, 1986) in setting progressively higher and higher standards of care. Figure 7.3 shows the action research 'cycle' as such a spiral.

What processes (or phases) are involved in action research?

There are several different stages that need to be acknowledged when planning and executing action research. Figure 7.4 shows the main stages (or phases) and also identifies the major questions that you would ask when in each of the stages or phases.

In the earlier stages of the action research, the researcher needs to be receptive and flexible by openly listening to the multiple perspectives and issues that all stakeholders raise. It is really important to get a wide range of viewpoints at this early stage because, without it, you might not be able to anticipate the sorts of things that could get in the way of any changes that need to be implemented later on in the project. The importance of getting a diversity of ideas is epitomised in the old adage of '*A multidisciplinary team without differences is a contradiction in*

163

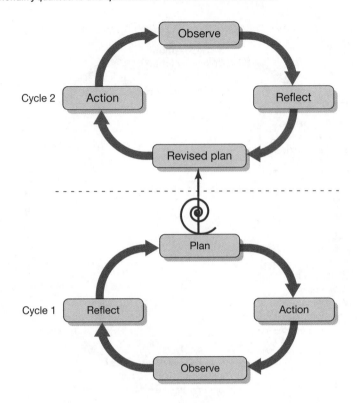

Figure 7.3 A spiral of action research stages (after Carr and Kemmis, 1986).

terms' (Øvretveit, 1995, p. 41). There might be a lot of uncertainty at this stage about whether the project will succeed, whether there are researchable questions to address and whether there is sufficient time to conduct all stages of the action research. At the outset, there might be quite a few things that the action researchers do not know about and the researchers need to be open to, and comfortable with, this possibility. During the early phases of the research, there will be a lot

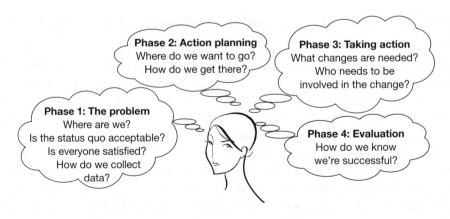

Figure 7.4 A general action research framework with questions to answer.

of 'unknowns' (just like the earlier quote at the beginning of this chapter!) and it will be useful to make these 'known' and recognised by those in the action research group. At the data collection stage, the action research project will be more to do with keeping the data collection on track and keeping to the agreed timetable. The action researchers will need to look at monitoring the progress of the project and ensuring that they will be able to see when the project is achieving specific success milestones.

Once actions have been planned out and changes are due to be implemented, there are a number of considerations that action researchers need to bear in mind. As change is at the heart of action research, action researchers need to weigh up the costs and benefits of changing practice. These costs could be human costs, like any possible inconvenience by getting staff or patients out of their comfort zone, but it might involve costs in terms of financial or time-related issues.

There are other change-related issues that could also be acknowledged during the latter stages of action research. These could include addressing the following questions:

- *Do you want to change people's attitudes and/or their behaviours?* You might have more success in changing attitudes but be less successful in changing people's behaviours. Why might this be so? Could staff or patients be too caught up in habitual ways of acting, despite having a change in their attitudes?

- *What needs changing?* Should there be changes to ways of implementing and documenting care (e.g. person-centred planning, use of clinical protocols) or, rather, changes to the overall ethos of care and how fellow professionals deal with service users or patients (e.g. patient-focused care, essence of care, person-centred approaches)? Do you need to get change in systems of care within a team or throughout an entire organisation? You may need to look at how receptive to change some people are and how you can get their commitment to this change. This may be less of a problem if the key people who will have an influence in the change were treated as stakeholders in the early phases of the project and their views were actively sought out during the entire life cycle of the action research.

- *Who are the 'change masters'?* Change masters (Kanter, 1983) may not always be those who are appointed in a senior/management position. For example, it may be the health care assistants who are the most influential and best able to implement changes at the sharp end of clinical practice. Think about the people needed to lead the change and those required for managing the change; this need not involve the same sorts of people, especially as the leadership of change involves a strategy role, whereas management of change would entail adherence to accepted best practices. In other words, leading is *'doing the right thing'*, whereas managing is more to do with *'doing things right'* (Bennis and Nanus, 1985).

Using the original scenario we have provided an overview of the phases or stages of the action research project. As part of this example we refer to data collection, and this can take several forms, such as through using questionnaires, observations, focus groups and interviews. We will now go through each of the four phases in turn.

Phase 1: identifying the problem

In phase 1 of the project it will be necessary to establish the actual context of the ward routine surrounding mealtimes in terms of current ways in which mealtimes on the ward are organised, who is involved, the context (i.e. the environment), and the stakeholders' perspectives (e.g. staff, patients and carers' views) on mealtimes. Data will be collected and analysed and the data could be quantitative or qualitative in form with the use of surveys, focus groups, or one-to-one interviews, for example. In this phase all participants will be given an opportunity to look critically at practice. There will also be chances for all participants to reach agreement about the need for change and there will be times for stakeholders to clarify any queries or concerns that they might have.

Phase 2: action planning

In phase 2 of the project the data have been analysed and the main trends are reported back to the project team. Based on the findings, an action plan is developed. In the present scenario, it is envisaged that this would entail a change in practices around mealtimes on the ward depending on the issues highlighted in phase 1, for example, environment, comfort and service. However, you will also need to be mindful that there may be a number of different approaches or alternatives to the problem and you will need to be aware of issues such as resources, time available and the learning needs of those involved.

Phase 3: taking action

Phase 3 of the project entails implementing the change. In the present example this may involve for example the general ambience of the dining room, scheduling of medicine delivery times and making mealtimes a 'whole-staff' approach.

Phase 4: evaluation

Phase 4 is the final phase in the first cycle of action research and will form the basis (dependent on findings) of future cycles of work. This can be evaluated in terms of looking at whether significant changes are being made to improve on practices or whether there are issues around the learning needs of staff that need to be involved, among many other possible future interventions with staff or patients.

This example provides one approach to the problem scenario that we presented at the beginning of the chapter. However, this is not the definitive answer and you may have thought of some other components that you would like to add to the project yourself. The following scenario will give you an opportunity to think more deeply about action research and the things to consider before setting out to do it and things to worry about whilst you're doing it. We have set out a self-assessment exercise below, which introduces you to more of the dynamic issues involved when conducting action research. It is written in the form of dialogue and is entitled 'How *not* to do action research'. Please note that the dialogue is fictional but it is intended to be a vivid guide to the practical and ethical issues that could be encountered when doing action research.

Self-assessment exercise

How *not* to do action research

This is an exercise that you can do by yourself or you can do this as part of a class discussion. The following dialogue provides insight into a life-like scenario that could happen when running an action research project. While reading the dialogue, we would like you to think about some of the key considerations covered in this chapter and whether these things are appearing in this scenario too.

When you read the dialogue, answer the following question:

What are the major issues that were important in the researcher's attempts to manage and facilitate the action research project?

Action research mismanaged: Act I

Characters:

Geraldine Phillips	A nurse researcher working for Grantchester Hospitals NHS Trust on an action research project aimed at promoting dignity among patients on the Care of the Older Person wards in the hospitals.
Jamilla Akhtar	A nurse consultant, who is overseeing the running of the project.

Scene: Geraldine Phillips and Jamilla Akhtar are sitting at a desk in Jamilla's office. Jamilla sits at one end of the desk and Geraldine is seated at the other end. The atmosphere in the room between the colleagues is particularly frosty.

Geraldine: I am really sorry about how this is all turning out. But I don't think this is all entirely my fault. You only gave me 3 months to get this action research done and I've found that this is far too little time to do the job well. Our project plan should surely have included the time it took to get enough feedback from the staff and patients and we didn't even think about how long it would take to put together a plan for promoting dignity on the wards. I think if this project had been managed properly you'd have given me more time to do the things that matter, like making people think that their opinions were being valued and that we were going to act on what they said . . .

Jamilla: Have you finished?

Geraldine: Well . . . I guess so. I just don't want to be getting all the blame for the complaints that we've been getting.

Jamilla: Which complaints might they be? That you carried out some of the focus group interviews with staff within earshot of patients and relatives? For goodness sake,

---

Geraldine! What were you thinking?! I realise that the staff didn't want to be too far away from the patients in case of emergency, but doing the interviews in the staffroom. What kind of idea was that? At least choose a room with a closed door. And what about being very clear in the focus group with patients about what the project was all about? Some of the patients were talking about irrelevant things that didn't seem anything to do with preserving patient dignity!

Geraldine: But why did you have to sit in on that focus group? Now the patients daren't speak to me in case what they say gets back to you and you'll then make a big deal about it and make them feel uncomfortable. Why couldn't you just trust me to do the right thing?

Jamilla: Oh, like that other 'action' research that you did? There was absolutely no action coming out of that one with your feeble attempt to get patients to comply with their schedule of meds. What on earth did you think you were doing by asking the pharmacists to change the way they worked after more griping from patients and their relatives? It took a lot of work by me and some of the other senior nurses to repair the damage you created with Pharmacy after that piece of work. I think next time we're going to need a project done, we'll ask someone from Melchester Uni – they'll probably cost less than you and they'll do a much better job!

Geraldine: Maybe I should go and work there – at least my research would be treated with respect. Maybe you shouldn't have agreed to this project being done in the first place, as it's just opened up a big can of worms and you don't know how to put the lid back on again, do you? It's no wonder some of the nurses are neglecting their patients! They're so scared of you that they spend more time chasing shadows and looking busy to stay out of your way rather than actually listening to their patients.

Jamilla: Who told you that? Is this your rumour-mongering again or have you been talking to Pauline? She never really liked me after I got promoted instead of her and now she wants to have any excuse to moan about me. Don't listen to her. She spends too much time going off the hospital premises for a cigarette break and not enough time doing her job! I am merely saying that maybe we should bring in someone with more expertise when needing to do a highly skilled job or doing specific types of research in a collaborative way. Besides, I think you're much better at number-crunching rather than having to talk to patients. Some of the things they're saying to you are not the sorts of things I want spread around our team and I especially don't want the relatives hearing about it either!

Geraldine: But all I wanted to do was raise awareness of the issues among staff about what was going on and what the patient viewpoint on promoting their dignity was like. Also why did you stop me from talking to some of the patients' relatives? I know you wanted a quick and dirty action research project, but surely you could have given me a bit of latitude to talk to them as well?

Jamilla: And what good would that have done? We would have got these relatives even more worried than they already are.

Geraldine: This is probably why this project was doomed from the start. You probably just agreed to do it to look good with the Medical Director so that you're seen to be doing the right thing. I don't know why I went to all that trouble of writing the report on this action research if you were never going to do anything about it. You've held on to the report and let no one else see it. I wanted to write a brief newsletter too about all the positive things that can be done to promote patient dignity, but you didn't think it was a good idea. I wanted to put posters up on the walls to raise awareness of what we can all do but you're too hung up on the relatives being worried!

Jamilla: Okay, Geraldine, we can put up your precious posters if this'll make you happy. Will it? I think we should put an end to this meeting. You obviously have a different idea to me as to what action research should be about. I gave you a tightly prescribed agenda from the start remember? Our cash-strapped hospital can't afford to finance some of the weird and wonderful schemes that some of the patients are suggesting. I will take your report and show it to others but I will only give a shortened and adapted version of it to the Medical Director, as some of the things that are being suggested just aren't feasible. I'll put down some action points in the report that won't cost much and don't deviate too much from what we're already doing.

Geraldine: But . . . but is what you're saying you're going to do . . . is this ethical?

Jamilla: It's hospital politics, Geraldine. I don't expect you to understand it. Learn to live with it.

Geraldine: [gets up from her seat] Maybe I don't want to be in this job if this is how my work is going to be treated. I don't think I want to be here anymore. If you need me, I'll be in my office [exits].

We have provided some answers to this exercise in the Answers section at the end of the book that you could look at *after* you've had a go yourself. We have also provided below two more dialogues in the next section so you might further practise your analysis skills on your own or again with a group. Again, we have provided some answers to this exercise in the Answers section at the end of the book.

Additional self-assessment exercises

Action research mismanaged: Acts II and III

Two more dialogues

Main characters:

Lesley Ashworth	A patient in Grantchester Hospitals NHS Trust's Brickendonbury Ward.
Joyce Enwonwu	Another patient in Brickendonbury Ward.
Patience Enwonwu	Joyce's daughter.
Lee-Hai Ping	A health care assistant who works on Grantchester Hospitals NHS Trust's Care of the Older Person wards.
Brian Patterson	A staff grade nurse who works with Lee-Hai.

Act II:
Issues to consider when involving patients
and relatives/carers in action research

Scene: Lesley is sitting upright in her bed in Brickendonbury Ward. She is listening to the hospital's radio with a pair of headphones and is looking into the distance out of a nearby window. Joyce's bed is positioned opposite Lesley's bed. Joyce is sitting at the end of her bed and is trying to attract Lesley's attention.

Joyce: Lesley! Lesley! Can you hear me?

Lesley: Uh?

Joyce: Why don't you turn the sound down on those things? It makes you deaf, y'know?

Lesley: Okay, Joyce. [Lesley removes her headphones and places them on her bedside table] What did you want?

Joyce: Did you talk to that researcher? Y'know . . . Geraldine.

Lesley: I did have a word or two with her and I told her that we are all very well looked after and that this project of hers is just something to beat those hard-working nurses over their backs with a large stick. She seemed to want me to tell tales on the people I rely on every day and say that I'm not being treated with dignity. I said to her that she's badly mistaken if she thinks I'm going to say that. Did you talk to this researcher as well?

Joyce: Oh, yes! In a group with some of the other patients.

Lesley: And you told her everything's okay?

Joyce: Well . . . sort of. Towards the end of the session with Geraldine I got to thinking that we're not treated proper all of the time. Y'know that, don't you? When she mentioned about some examples like being left alone, it reminded me of the one time when the nurses took so long to help me when I really needed them. I felt so humiliated when I took too long to get to the toilet and I really should have had someone to help me. No one had noticed that I'd made a mess of myself as well for quite a while and I didn't feel like I had my self-respect after all that.

Lesley: How on earth can the nurses let things like that happen to you?

Joyce: Well, I told Geraldine about it when the group discussion had finished and we were making our way back to our beds from that so-called 'lounge' we have. I didn't really want to let anyone else know about it, but I thought that she should know. I had a quiet word with her because it's pretty embarrassing. I hope Geraldine can make sure we get enough staff on the ward so that I'm not put in such an awkward position again when it comes to making sure I'm not caught short. Geraldine seemed senior enough so maybe something will happen.

Lesley: Good for you, Joyce! Although I thought Geraldine was doing these group discussions with some of the patients quite a few days ago. At least that's when she was asking me to take part. Perhaps she can't really make any major changes because she doesn't have the authority.

Joyce: Well, anyways . . . it was good to talk to Geraldine about it. I felt really better when I did and I felt really listened to, but I do worry if anything like this will happen again, especially when the nurses have fed me with so much fluid that I'm bursting to go to toilet.

▶

Lesley: Well, Joyce, I think something should be done!

[Patience enters the ward and approaches the two women]

Patience: Do what, Lesley? Are you and my mother plotting on how to get this ward all spic-and-span again? [turning to her mother]. Hello, Mum. How are you feeling today? [kisses her mother].

Joyce: Hello, my darling. Don't worry about us, my sweetheart. It's just two women having a gossip about this fancy research that's being done and how we're hoping that what we said to the researcher will be used to tell the nurses what a splendid job they're doing and that we're grateful for all their help.

Patience: More research, Mum? I thought you had some medical researchers come to see you about the falls you've been having recently. They were doing some sort of investigation but they seemed really interested in how you keep falling over in the bathroom. I'm really worried about you, Mum. Why do you keep falling over? Surely you get help from one of the nurses to get to the bathroom and to get up and out of the bathroom too. I'm concerned that you're going to really hurt yourself if things carry on. Surely you should be a lot safer here? You're in a hospital, for goodness sake! Tell you what, Mum. Why don't I talk to this researcher you've just seen and I can tell them about the harm that might happen to you if these falls keep happening. After all, I've been with you for many years, especially when your health has got worse, and I think I can talk with authority about what could make you better, if you like.

Joyce: No, my love. I don't think it would be appropriate to talk to Geraldine. The sorts of things she was looking at are rather more private.

Patience: More private than my mother getting hurt by constantly falling? More private than the little 'accidents' you keep having and the staff don't seem to take a blind bit of notice about it? I have half a mind to complain to the hospital that your health's not getting any better since you've been here. If anything, it's got worse and I know whose fault it is.

Joyce: Please, dear, don't make a fuss about this. Your mother's health is just getting worse because I'm getting older. It's no one else's fault but my own. At least I'm keeping away from food that's liable to make me put on weight, especially as the doctor said I needed to lose a few pounds to make sure I have no more complications.

Patience: But that's the problem, Mum. If anything, you're getting thinner and thinner. What are they feeding you? I saw one time they were trying to feed you when you've just woken up and you were too drowsy to notice it was there. Did you eat your food later on or did it go to waste? It was probably stone cold by the time you ate it. I seem to remember also that there was another time when you didn't eat for virtually a whole day. Why was that? Were you sleeping again when the food trolley came around? I don't think they care if you eat properly at all.

Joyce: Don't be so hysterical. Of course I eat just fine. I'm just not hungry sometimes. The medication I'm on seems to affect my appetite sometimes. And don't go complaining to anyone about my food either. I'm doing just fine. Now can you please go and see if your brother has arrived yet. All your complaining is getting me all stressed out and I'd feel a lot better when both you and John are by my side. Go on! See if he's come . . . [Patience exits] and leave me be for a few minutes.

Question: Having read through this scenario, what are the main issues concerned with involving patients and carers in action research?

Act III:

Issues to consider when involving staff in action research

Scene: Lee-Hai Ping and Brian Patterson are in the staffroom that is adjacent to Brick-endonbury Ward. Lee-Hai is sitting on a lounge chair, sipping on her cup of coffee and reading a magazine, whilst Brian has only just entered the staffroom. He is pacing up and down and is occasionally looking outside of the staffroom's window.

Lee-Hai: [looks up from her magazine] Brian! Why are you so restless? If you keep doing that, you'll wear a hole in the carpet.

Brian: What's your problem? Am I disturbing you away from your trashy magazine?

Lee-Hai: Brian, there's no need to be so defensive. I'm just concerned about you. You've looked really worried and pale for quite a few days, you know. Have you been having problems at home?

Brian: Not that it's any of your business, but no. I haven't had these 'problems', as you call them. I'm just thinking about what that snooping Geraldine is after with her interviews.

Lee-Hai: Oh, you mean those focus groups that she's just been doing? I think she's after quite a lot of sensitive stuff, from the looks of things. She is expecting staff to admit to seeing patients who are not being treated with respect and dignity on the wards, but I think she might be a bit naïve in that respect.

Brian: It's not only the sensitivity of it, Lee-Hai. I'm concerned at what the agenda is to this action research and what they're going to do to staff as a result of it. Do you know that Geraldine seemed to be suggesting that leaving patients alone, if only for a little while, could affect their ability to preserve their dignity? I don't think this is realistic at all – she obviously doesn't see it from the staff perspective. For goodness sake, she's chattering on so much about being patient-focused that she's left out having any focus on the staff whatsoever. What about letting us have enough of a work–life balance so that we don't take work stresses with us when we go home? We're overloaded and short-staffed and can't do the sorts of things like being at the bedsides of all of our pa-tients all of the time. She's obviously never heard of the kind of emotional labour that we need to do day in and day out when we have to constantly be giving a 'pleasing' serv-ice to all of our customers. I don't know about you, Lee-Hai, but sometimes I just need to get away from the ward and keep away from this griping lot for just a little while. Whatever this Geraldine is doing seems to be promoting only the patients' interests and seems much too one-sided to me. I was tempted to tell her that in the focus group chat, but I then thought better of it because it's quite likely that any comments I make will fil-ter back to that ogre, Jamilla.

Lee-Hai: I know what you mean, Brian, about who is setting the agenda and suspect that, if Jamilla's had any part to play in this, there'll be actions that she's already decided on and this is all to pay lip-service to being more patient focused. If there were any serious problems that came out of the research, I'm sure that she'd sweep it under the carpet to make sure she didn't get poor PR but she'd also make our lives hell for anything bad get-ting filtered up to her.

Brian: You know what else I didn't like in that focus group? It looked like Geraldine had also got some clear ideas on what could already be done. She seemed to be suggesting that there might be some sort of training programme to get staff to give patients a good

▶

'customer' service and to make sure that our attitudes are 'proper' enough when it comes to treating them. She seems a right little do-gooder, but I don't know if she's thought it through properly as well. She mentioned about getting staff to attend regular refresher training days and I just can't see how she's going to be able to get the part-timers going along. And how on earth she thinks she can have any sort of influence on the agency staff who come and go and seem to be a law unto themselves . . . I don't know . . . She seemed to have little imagination and was always going on about these training days without thinking about alternative ways of promoting her do-gooding. Does she really think that going to these indoctrination sessions are going to make a difference to how we treat patients?

Lee-Hai: Well, it's not only that, Brian. I think it would have been better to have asked us more specific things that we'd like to see done. Many of the things that Geraldine was asking about were all quite general, you know? Did you also know that our focus group took nearly two hours in total? I was really tired out by then and I'm sure some of the staff were making up stories just to keep her satisfied. I must admit to feeling under pressure to tell her about anything that might please her and her agenda, especially as we've been told by Jamilla to co-operate with Geraldine as fully as possible. I don't think Geraldine was really listening to us and I personally don't think anything will come from this action research, certainly no 'actions' unless Jamilla wants these actions to happen.

Brian: Okay. You've set my mind at rest a little. It's just I can't stand thinking that some of these patients will be complaining to Geraldine and that this'll get back to Jamilla. Anyhow, we'd better get back to work or otherwise Jamilla's going to have plenty of reasons for making our lives hell.

Lee-Hai: Yes. We'd better go soon. You go first. I've got to finish this coffee and this so-called 'trashy' magazine. See you in a bit.

Brian: Fine. But don't go expecting me to see Mrs Enwonwu. She's really getting on my nerves. You can find me at the nurses' station if you want me. [Exits].

Question: Having read through this scenario, what are the main issues concerned with involving staff in action research?

Summary

In this chapter, we have introduced you to the general philosophy of action research and the main areas of focus that it sets out to achieve, namely an orientation to make meaningful and sustainable changes to practice. As a nurse, you will want to make sure that changes that are made to your practice are evidence-based and action research attempts to embrace many stakeholders' perspectives in gathering this evidence and implementing change accordingly. We have shown you that action research in nursing is very much like the stages of reflection that you would use as an effective, reflective practitioner. Action research can be an ongoing and exciting process and you have learned more about the four key stages to planning and conducting action research. You should also be well-equipped to identify the situations in health care that will be suited to an action research approach and you should also be more aware of some of the practical and ethical issues involved.

So far, we have shown you about how to blend quantitative and qualitative approaches when doing action research. Next, in the following chapter, we will be taking you through the 'nuts and bolts' of some of the tools that you could be using when doing quantitative research through the use of statistics.

Chapter 8

Quantitative analysis:
Using descriptive statistics

KEY THEMES

Descriptive statistics • Averages: mean, mode and median • Variability •
Range • Semi-interquartile range • Standard deviation • Bar charts •
Histograms • Pie charts • Box plots

LEARNING OUTCOMES

At the end of this chapter you will be able to:

● Be more aware of the role of variables in quantitative analysis when
conducting nursing research and be able to look for distinctions within
variables and between variables.

● Understand the different kinds of descriptive statistics that can be produced
in quantitative nursing research and the various ways of representing these
statistics.

● Be more knowledgeable of the role of frequency counts, averages, charts and
measures of variability within quantitative nursing research.

Introduction

IMAGINE THAT . . .

You are an occupational health nurse working for a hospital employing over 400 nurses. Over the past few weeks, you have had several nurses who have been referred to your department with chronic back pain. This is a problem as it is unlikely that some of these nurses will be able to return to work and there are the human costs to these nurses' well-being and their worries about ever being able to work as a nurse again. You wonder whether there are system-related issues about how nurses are moving and handling patients in the wards. Are some nurses failing to use slides or hoists when moving patients? Are some nurses susceptible to taking shortcuts when moving and handling? You want to see how common these practices could be within the hospital and so you and your colleagues have decided to survey a sample of nurses to find out their attitudes towards adopting shortcuts to moving and handling and whether some nurses admit to doing so. You want to see whether there are any patterns among the nursing staff that are cause for concern: is it one in five nurses who take shortcuts when moving and handling or is it as many as one in three? Have more than half of the nurses surveyed said that they experience moderate to severe back pain when moving and handling patients? All of these figures are what is known as descriptive statistics and can help guide your decisions in your clinical practice.

One well-known nurse who used descriptive statistics was Florence Nightingale. Although she is most renowned for being a pioneer of nursing and a reformer of hospital sanitation methods, her use of descriptive statistics played a part in such reforms. **Descriptive statistics** are techniques to collect, organise, interpret and make graphical displays of information. It was techniques such as this that allowed Florence Nightingale to outline the incidence of preventable deaths through unsanitary conditions in the army during the Crimean War and helped her to lead the way to sanitation reform.

In this chapter we will introduce you to descriptive statistics and, more specifically, frequency counts, averages, measures of variance and other measures of dispersion. We will also introduce you to graphical representations of data, such as bar charts, pie charts, histograms and box plots. Along the way we will also show you ways of noticing if there are interesting or peculiar things occurring within a data set. Here we will describe outliers, and distributions and skewness.

8.1 Practice in performing descriptive statistical analysis

Before you start, we are going to get your brain warmed up mathematically, and get you to carry out some simple calculations. These calculations are related to some of the concepts you will come across in the chapter.

For each set of numbers, add together the numbers.

4 3 2 1 5

3 2 1 2 5

For each set of numbers, rank the numbers in ascending (lowest to highest) order.

7 5 2 4 3 9 17

2 7 62 53 1 2

For each set of numbers, rank the numbers in descending (highest to lowest) order.

15 5 12 4 31 9 17

23 7 2 53 11 2

For each set of numbers, rank the numbers in ascending order. What is the middle number?

1 9 5 4 3 2 8

19 13 17 18 12 21 23

For each set of numbers, which is the most frequent number?

2 56 3 3 2 2 13 23

117 112 113 117 119

For each set of numbers, (i) add together the numbers in each set, and (ii) count how many numbers are in each set. Then divide your answer for (i) by your answer for (ii).

1 7 6 3 3 4

23 27 18 12 20

The above calculations actually refer to some of the statistics you are going to read about in this chapter.

8.2 Variables

Variables are integral to quantitative nursing research and in performing descriptive statistical analysis. In Chapter 1 we first introduced you to the concept of variables, and also how to identify variables in everyday literature as well as within academic titles and text. You may want to re-read this part of the chapter again to refresh your memory. However, unlike our discussion in Chapter 1, we are going to see how variables can be measured and analysed quantitatively.

From Exercise 8.1 (overleaf), you will see that there are many variables in which government scientists are interested. At one level it may seem that scientists are just interested in the levels of vCJD, and in how many people have died of vCJD. However, there are other variables that can be identified within this article, including:

● the year people have died in (to consider trends in the disease);

● changes in the frequency of vCJD, by looking at changes from one year to the next;

● the time period between which 'friends, relatives or doctors first noted the symptoms' and eventual death, which varies from 7 to 38 months;

EXERCISE 8.1

Identifying variables

Re-read the article by James Meikle (you will already have read this in Chapter 1). Again, see if you can spot different kinds of variables, i.e. things that might differ from person to person or from time to time.

Scientists warn of 30 per cent rise in human BSE

Government scientists yesterday warned of a sharply accelerating trend in the incidence of human BSE after studying the pattern of the disease so far. They said the number of reported cases may in fact be rising at between 20 per cent and 30 per cent a year despite the apparently varied annual death rates over the past five years. The prediction came as it was revealed that the death toll from the incurable condition officially known as vCJD had risen by a further two in the past fortnight to a total of 69, and 14 so far this year.

The scientists said that there was now a 'statistically significant rising trend' in the number of victims since the first casualties first displayed signs of the disease in 1994, although it was still too early to forecast the ultimate number of deaths caused by vCJD.

This year's toll is already equal to that for the whole of last year when the number dropped. A further seven people still alive are thought to be suffering from the condition. The scientists have come to their conclusion about the progress of the disease after analyses of monthly figures, including studying the dates at which friends, relatives or doctors first noted symptoms. The period between this and eventual death has varied between seven and 38 months, with an average of 14 months, although the incubation period before symptoms become evident is believed to be several years longer.

Stephen Churchill was the first known death from the disease in May 1995, although it was not formally identified or officially linked to the eating of beef in the late 1980s until March 1996. Three people died in 1995, 10 in 1996, 10 in 1997, 18 in 1998 and 14 last year.

Members of the government's spongiform encephalopathy advisory committee took the unusual step of publishing the figure immediately after their meeting in London yesterday because of the recent interest in a cluster of five cases around Queniborough in Leicestershire. These included three victims dying within a few of months in 1998, a fourth who died in May and another patient, still alive, who is thought to be suffering from the same disease. The scientists said this was 'unlikely to have occurred by chance but this cannot be completely ruled out' and they would be closely informed about local investigations. The Department of Health last night said it could not elaborate on the significance of the new analysis until ministers and officials had considered the scientists' new advice.

The figures came amid reports that sheep imported by the US from Europe were showing signs of a disease, which could be linked to BSE in cattle. Government scientists are to hold talks with their US counterparts after the US agriculture department ordered the destruction of three flocks of sheep, which were in quarantine in the state of Vermont.

Source: James Meikle, 'Scientists warn of 30 per cent rise in human BSE: What's wrong with our food?', *The Guardian*, 18 July 2000. © The Guardian Newspapers Limited, 2000, reproduced with permission.

- whether people have died of vCJD or another related disease;
- where the vCJD case occurred. Here, there is an emphasis on Queniborough in Leicestershire.

When using quantitative methods it is essential that you understand the central role of variables. One of the most important aspects in this area to understand is that distinctions can be made about different variables. These distinctions are made *within* and *between* variables.

Distinctions *within* variables

We need to understand that certain distinctions are made within variables. These distinctions are called levels of a variable, and are quite simply the different elements that exist within a variable. Therefore, all variables have a number of levels. Sex of a person has two levels: you are a man or a woman. Age has numerous levels ranging from birth to a probable maximum of 120 years old.

We have seen levels in all the examples we have used so far. Take, for example, the variables we identified in the vCJD article:

- *The year people have died*. The levels here are the years 1992, 1993, 1994 and so on.
- The time period between which 'friends, relatives or doctors first noted the symptoms' and eventual death, which varies from 7 to 38 months. The levels here are in months.
- *Whether people have died from vCJD or a related disease*. The levels here could be twofold. The first version might contain only two levels, those being (1) whether the person had died of vCJD, or (2) whether the person had died not of vCJD but of a related disease. A second version might contain levels that describe each related disease, leading to many more levels.
- *Where the vCJD case occurred*. Here there is an emphasis on Queniborough in Leicestershire. The levels here are different places, for example Leicestershire, Nottinghamshire, Derbyshire.

Distinctions *between* types of variable

You now know you can make distinctions within variables. We now need to expand on these distinctions and understand that researchers then go on to make distinctions *between* different types of variable. The main reason for these distinctions is that they underpin the choices that need to be made when using a statistical test. There are two common sets of distinctions that researchers make between variables and these rely on how researchers view the levels that exist within a variable.

Set 1: distinctions between nominal, ordinal, interval and ratio variables

In this set of variables, the first type of variable is called **nominal** and this entails merely placing levels into separate categories. The levels of this variable type (a nominal variable) are viewed as distinct from one another. For example, the sex of a person has two levels: male and female. As sex is biologically determined, individuals fall into one category or the other. There are other nominal variables such as classification of dressings (for example, multilayer versus short-stretch bandages) or variables taken from something like the ICD-10 classification system, which categorises medical conditions and treatments.

The next type of variable in this set is called **ordinal**, and this means that the levels of the variable can be placed into ranked ordered categories. However, the categories do not have a numerical value. A health care-related example is a pain rating score ranked from 0 to 3. One patient could have no pain (scored as 0), one could have mild pain (scored as 1), another could have moderate pain (scored as 2) and another patient could have extremely severe pain (scored as 3). We can see that although levels of pain go up with the scores given for each response, representing greater and greater pain, they do not represent equal differences between the categories that are suggested by the numbers. For example, there is a gap of 1 between mild pain (1) and moderate pain (2), but is this equal to the gap of 1 between moderate pain (2) and severe pain (3)? Therefore, the numbers that are assigned are arbitrary but are designed to give some indication of levels of pain.

The next types of variable are **interval** and **ratio**. The levels for both these variables are numerical, meaning that they comprise numerical values. These numbers do not represent something else, in the way that the numbers used above for the ordinal variable do, for rating pain. However, there is a distinction between interval and **ratio variables**. Ratio data have an absolute zero, in other words they can have an absence of the variable, whereas interval data do not have an absolute zero. So, for example, the number of children in a household is a ratio variable because a household can have no children.

Interval variables do not have an absolute zero. Common examples of interval variables are many concepts we use in everyday life, such as self-esteem. The measurement of self-esteem is not readily available to us (as opposed to simply counting the number of people in a family). Measurement of self-esteem in research will normally involve adding together the responses to a number of questions to produce a self-esteem scale. Consequently we refer to self-esteem in terms of low or high self-esteem, or relative terms, such as a person having higher, or lower, self-esteem than another person. Because of this type of measurement we can, at no point, establish that there is an absence of self-esteem (in other words that there is an absolute zero), so researchers treat many scales as interval data.

Set 2: distinctions between categorical, discrete and continuous variables

The other set of distinctions comprises those that are made between categorical, discrete and continuous variables. Categorical data are the same as nominal data. Yet in this set of distinctions, researchers make an important distinction between discrete and **continuous data**. Here, both these variables are numerical. However, continuous variables allow for decimal points (for example 10.5678 cm^2 of the total pressure sore area), whereas **discrete data** do not allow for decimal points (you can't get 3.5 patients waiting on trolleys in the ward).

Combining sets 1 and 2: categorical-type and continuous-type variables

As you can see from these two sets of distinctions between types of variables, there are different ways that researchers make distinctions between variables (and there are also a number of ways in which people merge these different sets of definitions and develop different understandings). Having different definitions can be terribly confusing for people starting out in statistics. This is sometimes particularly difficult, as teachers of statistics will adopt different definitions. If you are on a course you will probably, in time, come across different teachers who use different ways of defining variables.

To put it simply, one of the main sources of possible confusion is how teachers of statistics differ in the way they view the ordinal variable (set 1) and the discrete variable (set 2). There are two possible ways in which researchers perceive both types of variable. For many researchers, both ordinal and discrete variables are essentially ordered in a numerical way, and as such they believe that they should be viewed in the same way as continuous/interval/ratio variables.

However, for other researchers, ordinal and discrete variables represent separate, unique levels that do not represent numbers on a continuum. One example often cited, to support the latter point, is the distance represented *between* the levels of an ordinal variable. Unlike for numerical variables, in which the distance between levels is equal (the distance between 1 and 2, and 2 and 3, and 3 and 4, is the same, 1), for **ordinal data**, the distances between the levels are not the same (for example, in the example of the pain ratings above, the distances between severe, moderate and mild pain may not be of equal value). For simplicity's sake, it is easiest to treat variables as either **categorical-type** (variables that form separate categories), or **continuous-type** (numerically ordered and can be ordinal, interval or ratio).

However, you must always remember that different researchers treat ordinal and discrete variables differently. Some researchers insist that these variables are categorical and some insist that they are continuous. As such, there is no right or wrong view. Rather, you just have to be aware that this distinction occurs. This distinction has some implications for choosing which statistical test to use; we will return to this issue in Chapter 9 when an overall guide to the process of choosing which statistical test to use when testing hypotheses will be presented.

8.3 Descriptive statistics: describing variables

As a nurse, you are surrounded by statistics. For example, the BBC News health website (**www.bbc.co.uk/health**) and the *Nursing Times* website (**www.nursingtimes.net/**) list the following facts:

- Smoking is the single largest cause of preventable cancer deaths in the UK. On average, each year it causes 32,000 deaths from lung cancer and 11,000 deaths from other cancers.

- On average, nearly one in four British women dies as a result of heart disease. Women who have a heart attack are less likely than men to survive the initial event.

- Around 40 to 50 per cent of women diagnosed with ovarian cancer will still be alive five years later. When the disease is caught early, however, survival rates are much higher, although the particular type and severity of the cancer are also important factors.

- The Population Reference Bureau (2004) suggests that there will be a total of 10.5 million older people in the UK (16 per cent of the population) by 2050.

- It is estimated that there are about 338,000 new cases of angina pectoris (a common, disabling, chronic cardiac condition) per year in the UK (British Heart Foundation, 2004).

Nurses need to have an awareness of what these statistics might mean and how they have been calculated. In your profession, you will be continually presented with statistical descriptive data: mortality rates, average life expectancy, percentage recovery rate, average remission time. Most of your job, treatment strategies, policies that surround your job and all these facts described above are derived from the use of descriptive statistics.

All the statistics we mentioned above are ways of describing things: what mortality rates are, what effective treatment strategies are. Therefore, you wouldn't be surprised to find out that descriptive statistics are simply ways of describing data. There are many different types of descriptive statistics, but the aim of this chapter is to introduce you to some of the more frequently used statistics in nursing.

There are four main areas of descriptive statistics that we will cover. These are:

1. Frequencies
2. Averages
3. Charts
4. Variability.

Frequencies

The first aspect is frequencies of data. This information can be used to break down any variable and to tell the researcher how many respondents answered at each level of the variable. Consider an example where a hospital administrator is deciding whether to carry out an awareness scheme in his hospital of the causes of back pain in nurses while carrying out their daily duties (including heavy lifting, lifting patients correctly). He asked 100 nurses working in the hospital whether they had experienced any back pain in the past six months. Respondents were given three choices of answer: 1 = Severe, 2 = Minor and 3 = None. To examine the prevalence of back pain among nurses, the administrator adds up the number of responses to each of the possible answers, and presents them in a table in order to examine the frequency of answers to each possible response (see Table 8.1).

Table 8.1 Answers to the question 'Have you experienced back pain?'

Possible answer	Frequency of answer
Severe	7 respondents answered the question with this response
Minor	45 respondents answered the question with this response
None	48 respondents answered the question with this response

On this occasion, 7 respondents said they had experienced severe back pain, 45 respondents said they had experienced minor back pain and 48 respondents said they had experienced no back pain. As we can see, almost half of the nurses had suffered some sort of back pain, and as the occupational health nurse with responsibilities for back care in the hospital you may be concerned about this finding.

This type of breakdown of answers is how frequencies of information are determined. Frequencies refer to the number of times something is found. In statistics, frequencies are most often presented in the form of a **frequency table**, similar to Table 8.2.

This table refers to 24 people diagnosed as having learning difficulties, and this variable refers to the type of learning disability each person has. In this frequency table we can get two sets of information from the first two columns (ignore the other column for now). We are interested in the frequency of each level of the variable, and the percentage breakdown of each level. In this example we can see that the sample that has the highest frequency is for Down's syndrome (six reports), then Williams' syndrome and birth trauma (both three), and then brain damage and microcephaly (both two), and then for all the other diagnoses there is only one report.

This table also gives you a percentage breakdown. A percentage is the proportion of a variable falling within a certain value or category that is expressed in terms of 'out of 100'. Therefore, for example, if we said to you that 80 per cent of patients were

Table 8.2 Frequencies for diagnosis for learning disability

Diagnosis	Frequency	Percentage	Cumulative percent
Arrested hydrocephaly	1	4.2	4.2
Birth trauma	3	12.5	16.7
Brain damage	2	8.3	25.0
Brain damage RTA	1	4.2	29.2
Cerebral palsy	1	4.2	33.3
Chickenpox encephalitis	1	4.2	37.5
Congenital abnormality	1	4.2	41.7
Down's syndrome	6	25.0	66.7
Dysgenic features	1	4.2	70.8
Microcephaly	2	8.3	79.2
Multiple handicap at birth	1	4.2	83.3
Not recorded	1	4.2	87.5
Williams' syndrome	3	12.5	100.0
Total	24	100.0	

happy with the care they received in hospital, you would know that the majority of patients were happy about their standard of care. If we said to you 80 patients were happy with the care they received in hospital, your first question would be 'How many people did you ask?' (If we had asked 80, then great; but if we had asked 80,000, then perhaps not so great.) Therefore, percentages are descriptive statistics that allow us to quickly summarise and put some meaning behind our findings. In percentage terms, 25 per cent of our sample has been diagnosed with Down's syndrome.

Averages

Consider the following findings from published articles, noting when the term *average* is used.

Article 1

A study carried out by McEwen *et al.* (2005) to investigate the self-reported duties performed by sisters and charge nurses working on the wards reported the following findings: Sisters/charge nurses reported directly assessing on *average* 75 per cent of patients on their ward during a typical shift. Sisters/charge nurses were allocated patients for whom they had not planned to take primary responsibility in addition to being in charge of the ward a mean average of 2.5 shifts per week. On *average* they reported spending almost six hours a week outside of their contracted hours on ward business.

Article 2

Marshall *et al.* (2005) reported on a study which sought to reduce waiting times for a rapid-access chest pain clinic (RACPC). Between March and October 2003, patients referred to the RACPC waited an *average* of 34 days for an appointment. There was a high proportion of inappropriate referrals to the clinic. As part of a review of strategy, Marshall and her colleagues oversaw a service redesign, and a process-mapping session was conducted in which key players in the patient's journey informed each other of how their work was interrelated. As a result of the above changes, the team achieved, and sustained, a 14-day waiting target for the clinic, with the current *average* wait down to 8 days.

You have probably heard or read the phrase 'on average' a lot throughout your life, and probably many times during your time in nursing. Averages are ways in which researchers can summarise frequency data and find out what are the most common responses. Both the above articles use averages to describe a situation or event. Article 1 uses averages to indicate the amount of time spent by sisters and charge nurses on their duties. Article 2 uses averages to show falls in waiting times for a rapid-access chest pain clinic.

There are three types of average, known as the mean, the mode and the median.

- **Mean.** This is calculated by adding together all the values from each response to the variable, and dividing by the number of respondents.
- **Mode.** This is the value that occurs most often in the set of data.

Table 8.3 Answers to the question 'How long did you have to wait before being seen?'

Possible answer	Frequency of answer
10 minutes	3 patients
20 minutes	1 patient
30 minutes	
40 minutes	
50 minutes	
60 minutes	1 patient

- **Median.** This is calculated by putting all the values from responses to the variable in order, from the smallest value to the largest value, and selecting the value that appears in the middle.

Consider this example. A nurse consultant wants to assess quickly how long patients wait in the hospital's emergency ward before they are seen. The nurse consultant collates the information into frequencies, and displays the data in the form of a table (Table 8.3). The nurse consultant wishes to work out the mean, median and mode.

For the *mean* the nurse consultant adds all the responses, 10 + 10 + 10 + 20 + 60 (three patients had to wait 10 minutes, one patient had to wait 20 minutes, and one patient had to wait 60 minutes) and divides the total 110 (10 + 10 + 10 + 20 + 60 = 110) by the number of respondents asked. Here, five patients took part in the research, so 110 is divided by 5. Therefore, the mean equals 110 divided by 5, which is 22. Therefore, there is a mean of 22 minutes before people are seen.

For the *median*, you choose the middle number from all the numbers presented in numerical order. So, rank the numbers from the smallest to the highest, 10, 10, 10, 20, 60, and then select the middle number, which is 10. Therefore, there is a median of 10 minutes' waiting time. This is fairly straightforward when the researcher has an odd number of cases. When there is an even number, you select the middle two numbers and divide their sum by 2. So in the case of having four waiting times, say 10, 10, 20 and 60, you would add together 10 and 20 and divide by 2, giving 30 divided by 2 which equals 15. The median waiting time is 15 minutes.

For the *mode*, the most common number is selected. In the example, 10, 10, 10, 20, 60, the most common number is 10, so 10 is the mode. Therefore, there is a mode of 10 minutes' waiting time in the hospital.

Therefore, the researcher will report that among their sample the mean average waiting time for the five patients is 22 minutes, the median waiting time is 10 minutes and the mode waiting time is 10 minutes.

However, it is not common practice to report all three measures of average. Rather, the mean is the most commonly used, and as a rule the median and the mode tend to be used only when researchers suspect that reporting the mean may not represent a fair summary of the data. For example, in the case above, perhaps reporting a mean waiting time of 22 minutes would be unfair to the staff working in the ward. A much fairer assessment would be to use the median and mode because they seem to reflect more accurately the average of 10 minutes, particularly as all but one patient is seen in under 22 minutes.

In terms of statistics, it is sometimes best to use the mean and sometimes best to use the median. Throughout the rest of this book we will point out when (and why) it is best to use the mean and when (and why) it is best to use the median.

EXERCISE 8.2

Calculating averages

A researcher assessed probability of learning disability among five children. A score of '0' indicates nil likelihood of having a learning disability, whereas a score of '100' indicates profound and severe learning disability. A midpoint score of '50' would indicate moderately severe levels of learning disability.

Work out the mean, median and mode of the following values: 0, 25, 50, 25, 80, 80, 75, 10, 40, 90.

Charts: visual presentation of data

You can also provide graphical representations of variables. One advantage of descriptive statistics is that you can carry out a number of graphical representations. However, there is often a temptation to become over-involved with graphs. We are going to concentrate on the three simple graphs (the bar chart, the histogram and the pie chart), not only because they are frequently used but also because one of them (the histogram) will be used as an important building block in understanding further statistics in Chapter 9.

All of these charts are ways of presenting data graphically. Bar charts and pie charts tend to be used for categorical-type data, and histograms tend to be used for continuous-type data. We will, using the variables mentioned above (Type of Learning Disability [categorical-type] and Number of Consultations with the learning disability nurse [continuous-type]), show you how bar charts, pie charts and histograms are produced.

A **bar chart** is a chart with rectangular bars of lengths that represent the frequencies of each aspect and is mainly used for categorical-type data (data which is made up of different categories). We can show this for the type of learning disability variable in Table 8.2 (see Figure 8.1).

The variable levels (type of learning disability) are plotted along the bottom (this is called the x-axis) and the frequency of each level is plotted up the side (this is called the y-axis). Notice how the bars are separate; this indicates that the variable is categorical-type.

A **pie chart** is a circular chart divided into segments, illustrating the different frequencies, proportional to the size of the frequency to all the other frequencies (in much the same way as a percentage works). Florence Nightingale is credited with developing an early form of the pie chart and much of her work is credited to the fact that she was able to present her data in this way. Figure 8.2 shows a pie chart for the same variable – type of learning disability.

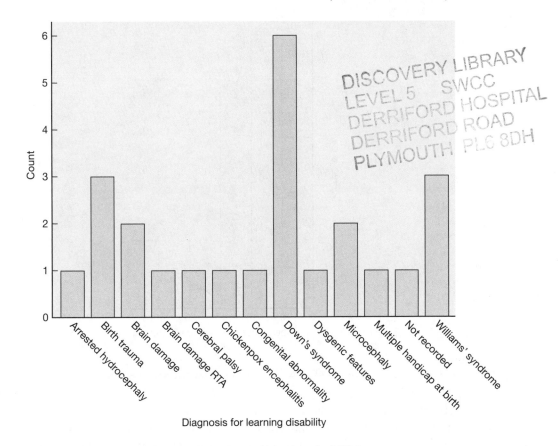

Figure 8.1 A bar chart for the variable 'type of learning disability'.

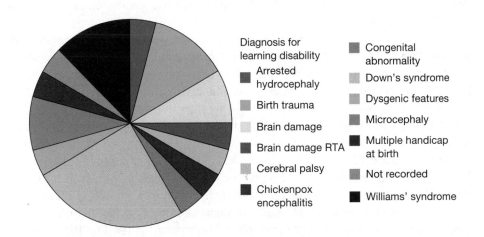

Figure 8.2 A pie chart of the variable 'type of learning disability'.

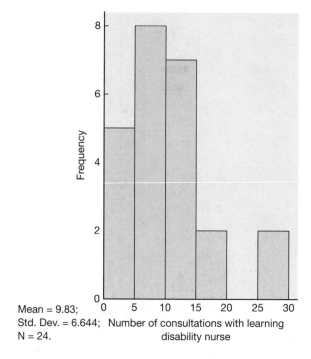

Mean = 9.83;
Std. Dev. = 6.644; Number of consultations with learning
N = 24. disability nurse

Figure 8.3 A histogram of the variable 'Number of Consultations' with learning disability nurse.

A **histogram** is a graphical display of the frequencies of a variable and is mainly used with continuous-type data (data comprising numbers in some numerical order). For this graph we are going to use the number of consultations the individual has had with the learning disability nurse (see Figure 8.3). The variable levels (possible scores) are plotted along the x-axis and the frequency of each level is plotted along the y-axis. Notice how the bars are together (unlike the bar chart), indicating that the variable is continuous-type.

Researchers have identified different types of distribution of a histogram. Histograms can be described as *skewed* (see Figure 8.4a), either negatively (where scores are concentrated to the right) or positively (where scores are concentrated to the left). An example of a **negatively skewed distribution** may occur when high scores on the variable are highly desirable. Therefore, if researchers develop a 'kindness' scale (in which higher scores indicate a higher level of kindness) containing items such as 'I am kind to other people' and 'I am a very kind person', we might expect most respondents to view themselves as being kind, as opposed to being unkind. Therefore, a negative skew would emerge as people respond with high 'kindness' scores. An example of a **positively skewed distribution** of a variable is often found with measures of depression. Measures of depression tend to identify greater and greater degrees of severity of depression, so researchers often find that most respondents score low on depression, as most people are not regularly depressed, and few people have high scores (as the highest scores indicate severe depression, and few respondents tend to be clinically depressed).

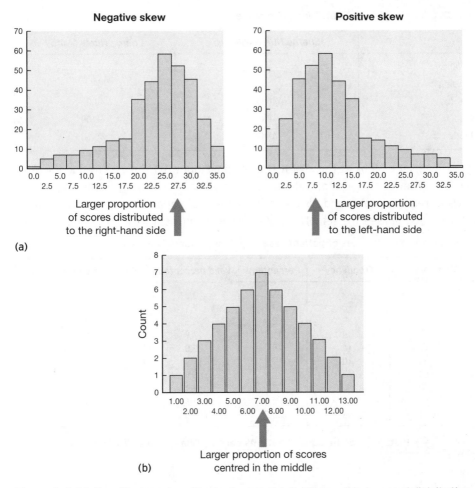

Figure 8.4 (a) Negatively and positively skewed distributions. (b) A normal distribution.

The final description is where the distribution of scores for a variable forms a **normal distribution**. This is where scores are distributed symmetrically in a curve, with the majority of scores in the centre, then spreading out, showing increasingly lower frequency of scores for the higher and lower values (Figure 8.4b).

Variability

So far we have looked at averages (mean, median and mode) and charts (bar charts, pie charts and histograms). However, let us put the following to you. In Table 8.4 we present you with the average statistics of the average age of two sets of patients assigned to two charge nurses in an Accident and Emergency unit: Charge Nurse Williams has 56 patients, and Charge Nurse Maltby also has 56 patients.

As you can see, the profile of the average statistics for the age of each set of patients (mean = 40, median = 40, mode = 40) suggests the two charge nurses are dealing with an identical set of patients (in terms of their age). Everything seems equitable.

Table 8.4 Mean age of patients by charge nurse

	Charge Nurse Williams	Charge Nurse Maltby
N Valid	56	56
Missing	0	0
Mean	40.00	40.00
Median	40.00	40.00
Mode	40.00	40.00

However, let us look at these statistics again. Figure 8.5 shows a frequency table and histogram of the age of patients seen by Charge Nurse Williams. Figure 8.6 shows a frequency table and histogram of the age of patients seen by Charge Nurse Maltby. As you can see, the actual ages of each set of patients *vary* for each charge nurse.

Frequency table of the ages of patients seen by Charge Nurse Williams

Years old	Frequency	Percentage	Valid percentage	Cumulative percentage
Valid <10	2	3.6	3.6	3.6
10	4	7.1	7.1	10.7
20	5	8.9	8.9	19.6
30	10	17.9	17.9	37.5
40	14	25.0	25.0	62.5
50	10	17.9	17.9	80.4
60	5	8.9	8.9	89.3
70	4	7.1	7.1	96.4
80	2	3.6	3.6	100.0
Total	56	100.0	100.0	

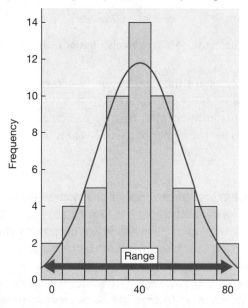

Histogram of the ages of patients seen by Charge Nurse Williams

Figure 8.5 Frequency table and histogram of the ages of patients seen by Charge Nurse Williams.

Frequency table of the ages of patients seen by Charge Nurse Maltby

	Years old	Frequency	Percentage	Valid percentage	Cumulative percentage
Valid	30	5	8.9	8.9	8.9
	35	13	23.2	23.2	32.1
	40	20	35.7	35.7	67.9
	45	13	23.2	23.2	91.1
	50	5	8.9	8.9	100.0
	Total	56	100.0	100.0	

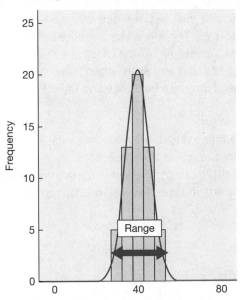

Histogram of the ages of patients seen by Charge Nurse Maltby

Figure 8.6 Frequency table and histogram of the ages of patients seen by
Charge Nurse Maltby.

Charge Nurse Williams sees patients ranging from newborn babies to those aged
80 years, whereas Charge Nurse Maltby sees patients ranging in age from 30 years
to 50 years. Therefore, their workload regarding the age range of the patients varies
greatly.

This is an example of variability, that is, the extent to which scores within a particular sample vary. What we will show you now are the three ways that statisticians
usually describe variability: through the use of (1) the range, (2) the semi-interquartile
range and (3) the **standard deviation.**

Range

The first way that we show variability is by reporting the range of scores. So, for
Charge Nurse Williams, his patients' ages range from 0 to 80, and therefore the range
of scores is 80 (worked out by subtracting the smaller number from the larger number). By contrast, the range of scores for Charge Nurse Maltby is 20 (= 50 − 30).

We can now see that although the average age of all their patients is similar, the ages of Charge Nurse Williams' patients have a much greater range (range = 80) than Charge Nurse Maltby's (range = 20).

Therefore, you can see how the use of averages might also be presented with some indication of the variability of scores. You will see, in research studies that use average statistics, that some mention of the variability of scores is made.

However, the range is sometimes considered a rather oversimplified way of showing variability. This is because sometimes it may over-emphasise extreme scores. Take, for example, another charge nurse, Charge Nurse Day, who has 100 patients; 99 of the patients are aged from 20 to 40 years, but there is one patient who is aged 80 years. With that patient included, the age range is 60. Without this one patient aged 80, the age range is 20. Therefore, the presence of this one 80-year-old patient has distorted the range. Consequently, the range is sometimes considered an unreliable measure of variability, and you will see two other measures of variability more commonly used: the semi-interquartile range and the standard deviation.

Semi-interquartile range

The **semi-interquartile range (SIQR)** is a descriptive statistic of variability that usually accompanies the use of the *median* average statistic (you will see why when we describe the semi-interquartile range). The semi-interquartile range is based on the idea that you can divide any distribution of scores into four equal parts (see Figure 8.7).

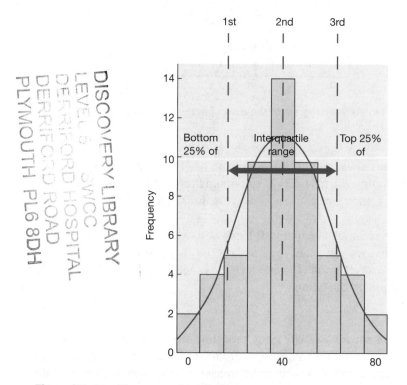

Figure 8.7 Quartile ranges of a set of scores.

Three cuts - **quartiles** - are made to create these four equal parts. They are:

- *First quartile* - this cuts off the lowest 25 per cent of scores (at the 25th **percentile**). It is also known as the *lower quartile* or Q1.
- *Second quartile* - this uses the median average (in other words, the 50th percentile score) to split the data in half. It is also known as Q2.
- *Third quartile* - this cuts off the highest 25 per cent of data, at the 75th percentile. It is also known as the *upper quartile* or Q3.

As you can see, we have four sections each representing 25 per cent of the scores (a quarter of the scores). You will have also seen that we have highlighted three sections, the bottom 25 per cent (those scores under the first quartile), the top 25 per cent (those scores over the third quartile) and the interquartile range, which are those scores between the first quartile (the bottom 25 per cent) and the third quartile (top 25 per cent). These are the basic ideas that underlie working out the semi-interquartile range.

To work out the semi-interquartile range, we first need to find out what the interquartile range is, and divide that into two (semi- means half, as in semi-detached, semiconscious, etc).

To use an example from practice, a district nursing team might want to measure the number of referrals it receives from the local Primary Care Trust's services and from the nearby hospital. They have recorded the number of referrals received over 11 days, which were 6, 2, 5, 6, 7, 4, 8, 5, 6, 3 and 4 patients. If the team wanted to find the semi-interquartile range for these referrals, they would treat this data as a set of 11 numbers, ordered from lowest to highest - 2, 3, 4, 4, 5, 5, 6, 6, 6, 7 and 8. They would then do the following:

- To work out the lower quartile, they would take the number of values (n, which stands for number of values in the sample of patients), which is 11, and add 1 (which is $n + 1$), this gives a value of 12.
- Then, to work out the lower quartile they would divide ($n + 1$) by 4; so here it is 12 divided by 4, which is 3. Therefore they would take the third value, which in this case is 5. So the lower quartile is 4.
- Then to work out the upper quartile they would multiply ($n + 1$) by 3 and then divide by 4. So this would be 12 multiplied by 3, and then divided by 4, which is 9. Therefore they would take the ninth value, which in this case is 6.
- Then to work out the interquartile range they would take away 4 (first quartile) from 6 (third quartile), which is 2. To work out the semi-interquartile range they would then divide this result by 2, which is 2 divided by 2, which is 1. Therefore for the set of numbers given above the semi-interquartile range is 1.

As with the median, if you find when working out what number value you should pick, the calculation says you should take, say, the 3.5th value, select the two numbers that surround this number in your list and divide by 2. The resulting number will be your quartile. So if, for example, your calculation of the lower quartile was 3.5, suggesting you choose the 3.5th value in the following set of number 1, 3, 5, 6, 7, 8, 5, . . . , you should take 5 and 6 (the 3rd and 4th numbers) and divide by 2, which is 11 divided by 2, which is 5.5.

In summary, the semi-interquartile range is another indicator of variability. This indicator of variability relies on splitting the sample; in other words, the second quartile division is based on a median split (i.e. the 50th percentile/halfway), in which you often find that when the median is used as an indicator of an average, the semi-interquartile range is used as an indicator of variability.

Standard deviation

Whereas the semi-interquartile range is a descriptive statistic of variability that accompanies the use of the median average statistic, the **standard deviation** is a descriptive statistic of variability that accompanies the use of the *mean* average statistic. Like the semi-interquartile range, the standard deviation provides the researcher with an indicator of how scores for variables are spread around the mean average (this is why it is sometimes referred to as a measure of dispersion).

Calculating the standard deviation is a little harder than calculating the semi-interquartile range. There are two formulae for working out the standard deviation. However, we are going to use the more common one. This is the standard deviation used with data from samples.

A nurse researcher has decided to examine how much a sample of five people with learning disabilities vary in the visits that they have from a learning disability nurse, Ms Kamal. The nurse researcher found out recently that with another learning disability nurse (Mr Smith), the mean visits required for a sample of clients was 3 and the standard deviation of visits was 2.34. From the sample the nurse researcher finds that the number of visits to the five clients by Ms Kamal over the past six months were 1, 3, 3, 4, 4 to the five clients respectively. To work out the standard deviation the nurse researcher would need to do the following:

Step 1: Work out the mean of the numbers.

Step 2: Subtract the mean average from each of the numbers to gain deviations.

Step 3: Square (times by itself) each of the deviations to get squared deviations.

Step 4: Add together all the squared deviations to get the sum of the squared deviations.

Step 5: Divide the sum of the squared deviations by the number of people in the sample minus 1 to find the variance.

Step 6: Find the square root of the variance to compute the standard deviation.

Calculating the standard deviation

Step 1: $1 + 3 + 3 + 4 + 4 = 15$, 15 divided by 5 = 3, mean = 3.

Score	Mean	Deviation (Step 2)	Squared deviation (Step 3)
1	3	$1 - 3 = -2$	$-2 \times -2 = 4$
3	3	$3 - 3 = 0$	$0 \times 0 = 0$
3	3	$3 - 3 = 0$	$0 \times 0 = 0$
4	3	$4 - 3 = 1$	$1 \times 1 = 1$
4	3	$4 - 3 = 1$	$1 \times 1 = 1$

Step 4: 4 + 0 + 0 + 1 + 1 = 6.

Step 5: 6 divided by (5 − 1), 6 divided by 4 = 1.5.

Step 6: Square root of 1.5 = 1.22. Standard deviation = 1.22.

Remember that the standard deviation value provides the nurse researcher with an indicator of how scores for variables are spread around the mean average. This finding suggests that though, on average, people tended to be visited by the two learning disability nurses at about the same number of times (mean = 3 with both learning disability nurses) there was less variability in visit frequency when comparing people visited by Ms Kamal (standard deviation = 1.22) versus those visited by Mr Smith (standard deviation = 2.34).

Sometimes it is hard to assess what all these measures of variability actually mean, but the higher the variability (that is, the higher the range, the semi-interquartile range or the standard deviation), the more scores are spread out around the mean. Therefore, a higher variability would be found for a set of five scores comprising 0, 15, 55, 78, 100 (the standard deviation here is 41.93), than for a set comprising 1, 2, 2, 3, 4 (here the standard deviation is 1.13). Though on its own a variability can often seem redundant, it is useful when you are comparing two sets of findings, because then you can also compare the dispersion of scores.

In the example above relating to the learning disability nurse visits, the standard deviation is helpful, because it tells us something additional about the data. It tells us that people's visits to the learning disability nurse are a lot more varied and that staff may wish to look into why this is: are some people not keeping appointments, while others are making too many, or does the administration of making appointments need to be looked at?

What is important is that it is good practice always to report the semi-interquartile range when reporting the median average statistic, and to report the standard deviation when reporting the mean average statistic.

8.4 Charts: visual presentation of variability with box plots

As with frequency tables and bar charts, pie charts and histograms, there is a way to graphically represent lower and upper percentiles and interquartile ranges. This is known as a box plot. A box plot is a way of showing five aspects of numerical data, the smallest value, the lower quartile (Q1), upper quartile (Q3), the median and the largest value.

Let us return to the district nursing team example from earlier in this chapter and the assessment of referrals made to the team over a period of 11 days. (i.e. 2, 3, 4, 4, 5, 5, 6, 6, 6, 7 and 8 patients during this time). Figure 8.8 shows a box plot of the data. Remember, we know from data analysis earlier in the chapter that the lower quartile is 4 and the upper quartile is 6. We also know that the highest value is 8 and the lowest value is 3. We also know with a quick scan of the data that the median is 5 as it is

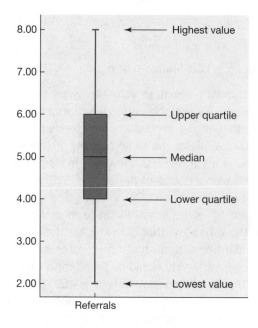

Figure 8.8 Box plot of the number of patients referred to the district nursing team (data taken over 11 days).

the 6th value, the middle value, in 11 numbers. You can see all these values outlined on the box plot. The box itself contains the middle 50 per cent of the data, i.e. that data between the lower quartile (Q1, 25th percentile) and the upper quartile (Q3, 75th percentile). The lower part of the box represents the lower quartile (placed at the value of 4) and the upper part of the box represents the upper quartile (placed at the value of 6). The line in the box indicates the median value of the data (here placed at the value of 5). The ends of the vertical lines at either end of the box represent the minimum and maximum values, here 2 and 8.

8.5 Beware of unusual data: outliers

Do you remember our example of waiting times, used earlier on in the chapter, to describe the mean, mode and median (look back at Table 8.3)?

In that table, we found the mean to be 22 minutes, the median to be 15 minutes and the mode to be 10 minutes. The mean is the most commonly used descriptive statistic and, as a rule, the median and the mode tend to be used only when there is a suspicion that the mean may not represent a fair summary of the data. In that example, we concluded reporting a mean waiting time of 22 minutes would be unfair to the staff working in the ward. A much fairer assessment would be to use the median and mode because they seem to reflect more accurately the average of 10 minutes, particularly as all but one patient is seen in less than 22 minutes.

Another term for the particular piece of data showing that one person had to wait 60 minutes is an outlier. An outlier is a piece of data (or pieces of data) that lies outside the rest of the data. So for example if you had 5 values in your data, 1, 2, 3, 3 and 71, 71 might be considered an outlier because it is very different from other data. We need to be wary of outliers in descriptive statistics because they can distort the assumptions we make after analysing the data.

Our demonstration of a box plot brings us to a final warning – be wary of outliers. A box plot also indicates any values that might be considered as 'outliers'. An outlier is a value that is numerically distant from the rest of the data and distorts the meaning of the data. So for example, if the hospital management had introduced a new initiative to improve average waiting times based on a mean calculation of the above data, the hospital management may be wasting its time, as the average (as calculated by the mode) is much more satisfactory; as a result, any future survey of average waiting times might not actually show improvements emerging from the initiative because they were already, in reality, quite low. The fact of the matter was that the data, and therefore the hospital management decision-making, was distorted by one outlier – so beware!

Usually, careful perusal of your data, by producing frequency tables, will allow you to identify outliers. However, a box plot is quite of a good way of identifying outliers. Take, for example, our example of the district nursing team and its record of referrals over an 11-day period (2, 3, 4, 4, 5, 5, 6, 6, 6, 7 and 8 patients). Let us imagine that the first piece of data was not 2, but actually 15 patients as a result of a mass of referrals from a hospital's bridging team to the district nursing team; let's also imagine that the last piece of data wasn't 8, but was in fact 20 patients who were referred to them after a spate of referrals from a nearby clinic. Now, 15 and 20 patients among that data set are clearly potential outliers. Let us see what it does to the box plot.

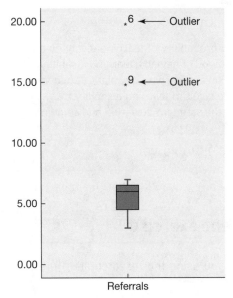

Figure 8.9 Box plot of the number of patients referred to the district nursing team (data taken over 11 days, with 2 data values altered).

You will see here that two points now appear on the graph (Figure 8.9). These are outliers, or at least suspected outliers. Therefore you will often see a box plot providing this information.

Now, what to do about outliers? Many people recommend deleting them. However, simply deleting outliers is controversial, and you need to think clearly about what you need to do. For example, we could easily have deleted the 60-minute waiting time listed in the above data that brought the mean up and didn't represent the overall picture in the data. However, that outlier did point to a problem with waiting times so examining what might have happened to make this patient wait longer than usual might be necessary. Likewise, with the example of referrals to the district nursing team, the presence of outliers could help us to get a better understanding of the demands placed upon them by knowing that referrals might be subject to massive variation due to unexpected referrals from certain hospital departments or community clinics.

This topic is perhaps too wide to consider here, however, we would suggest that if you have good reason for (or are confident of) deleting the outlier then do so. You might feel that a data point was inaccurate for some reason (someone giving an incorrect answer or was exaggerating) so perhaps there is reason to delete an outlier. Equally you may know that in your hospital on any given day no patient waits more than 30 minutes without being seen, in which case you may also wish to consider deleting this data. However, if you feel unsure about why the data might be an outlier then it might be best to leave the outlier in the data set.

EXERCISE 8.3

Calculating variability

A researcher assessed probability of learning disability among five children. A score of '0' indicates nil likelihood of having a learning disability, whereas a score of '100' indicates profound and severe learning disability. A midpoint score of '50' would indicate moderately severe levels of learning disability.

This time, work out the standard deviation and semi-interquartile range for the following values:

0, 25, 50, 25, 80, 80, 75, 10, 40, 90.

Self-assessment exercise

This exercise is to get you using the research literature to identify and understand descriptive statistics in research.

1. Your first task is to use either *Nursing Times* online or a library online database to find two research articles that include descriptive statistics.

2. Having found these two articles, in the boxes below write the reference for that article, what descriptive statistics are reported and what the descriptive statistics tell us about the topic studied.

Article 1

Reference for the article:

_____

_____

What descriptive statistics are reported?

_____

_____

_____

What do these descriptive statistics tell us about the topic studied?

_____

_____

Article 2

Reference for the article:

_____

_____

What descriptive statistics are reported?

_____

_____

_____

What do these descriptive statistics tell us about the topic studied?

_____

_____

Summary

In this chapter, we have introduced you to how descriptive statistics are used in quantitative nursing research. More specifically, we have looked at the importance of frequency counts, averages, measures of variance and other measures of dispersion, in getting a full picture of quantitative data. We have also covered the possibilities available in fully understanding quantitative data through the use of graphical representations, which include bar charts, pie charts, histograms and box plots. Finally, we have also warned you to be wary of what outliers might mean in a data set and how these could influence the interpretations that you undertake when analysing quantitative data. In the following chapter, we will introduce you to some of the types of statistical analyses that could be used when testing research hypotheses, and using inferential statistics to do so.

Chapter 9

Interpreting inferential statistics in quantitative research

KEY THEMES

Distributions • Probability • Statistical significance • Parametric and non-parametric statistical tests • Chi-square • Correlations • Pearson product–moment correlation coefficient • Spearman's rho correlation coefficient • Independent-samples t-test • Paired-samples t-test

LEARNING OUTCOMES

By the end of this chapter you will be able to:

● Understand what is meant by terms such as distribution, probability and statistical significance testing

● Understand the importance of probability values in determining statistical significance

● Undergo the decision-making processes informing the use of parametric and non-parametric statistical tests

● Determine a statistically significant result

● Interpret results from commonly used statistical tests including the chi-square statistical test, the Pearson product–moment correlation, the Spearman's rho correlation, the independent-samples t-test, and the paired-samples t-test.

Introduction

IMAGINE THAT ...

You are a busy leg ulcer nurse specialist and you need to find out at a glance whether one form of bandaging is better for effective leg ulcer healing than another type. You don't have time to mess around collecting data, putting the data into a computer, doing the analyses, and then coming to a conclusion about which form of bandaging is best. Instead, you want to look critically at studies that have compared the two types of bandaging. Many authors in the studies you have reviewed have used an inferential statistic called an **independent-samples** *t*-test. The authors have examined healing rates for one group of patients using the new form of bandaging compared to another group of patients who had the conventional form of bandaging. Can you trust the statistics that have been reported by these authors? Have the authors of these studies reported the means and the standard deviations, as well as other important statistics when comparing the healing rates?

Being able to answer these kinds of questions in this chapter will equip you with the skills you need for doing critical appraisal, which will be covered in more detail in the following chapter.

This chapter will help you decide whether some studies are more trustworthy than others; it will also introduce you to the concept of inferential statistics and how these statistics are different from the ones we introduced you to in the previous chapter. Inferential statistical tests (so called because they make inferences from data collected from a sample and generalise these trends to a population of people) are statistical tests that take data and provide answers to questions such as these – in fact any question you wish to devise. The only things you need in order to start using inferential statistics are two variables and some data collected relating to those two variables. After that, the statistical world is your oyster.

In the previous chapter, we introduced you to statistics and procedures that have described single variables by using frequency tables, mean scores and bar charts. However, the true usefulness of inferential statistics in nursing research is to take it one step further. Some of the main functions of inferential statistics include two things - exploring relationships between variables or finding differences between them. Have you ever wondered whether one type of anti-smoking campaign with your patients will be more effective than another type of anti-smoking campaign with another group of patients? Ever wondered whether senior nurses are more stressed out at work than their more junior counterparts? Or is it the other way around? Ever wondered whether stressed-out nurses will be more or less satisfied with their jobs? How about whether stress among nurses is related to the quality of the care they give to patients? Well, inferential statistics can help provide a more definitive answer.

In this chapter, we will introduce you to a series of commonly used inferential statistical tests. This chapter is designed to give you a brief overview of the rationale behind the use of inferential statistical tests and how to interpret the results from them. It will not go into a lot of statistical thinking and theory, as we feel this will put you off reading more, and over-complicate many of the things you need to know. Our main aim is to get you started with understanding how inferential statistics are used with nursing research that uses quantitative methods, so we are going to give you a simple and straightforward guide to the main ideas.

EXERCISE 9.1

Energiser activity

Before you start, we are going to get your brain warmed up mathematically and get you to carry out some simple calculations. These calculations are related to some of the concepts you will come across in the chapter.

Which of the two is the smaller number, 0.05 or 0.01?

Which of the two is the larger number, 0.05 or 0.001?

Is the number 0.10 larger or smaller than 0.05?

Is the number 0.50 larger or smaller than 0.01?

Between which two numbers does 0.02 fit in this series?

   0.50   0.30   0.10   0.05   0.01

Between which two numbers does 0.20 fit in this series?

   0.50   0.30   0.10   0.05   0.01

9.1 Distributions

In Chapter 8, you were shown a histogram (the distribution of scores for a continuous-type variable). Researchers have identified different types of distribution of a histogram to introduce an idea that is a cornerstone of inferential statistics. This idea is based on different ways of describing distributions. As we covered in the previous chapter, histograms can be skewed either negatively (i.e. scores are concentrated to the right) or positively (i.e. scores are concentrated to the left). The final description is where the distribution of scores for a variable forms a normal distribution. This is where scores are distributed symmetrically in a curve, with the majority of scores in the centre, then spreading out, showing increasingly lower frequency of scores for the higher and lower values.

Statisticians have noted that if scores on a variable (e.g. anxiety among the general population, with few people having high and low levels) show a normal distribution, then we have a potentially powerful statistical tool. This is because we can then begin to be certain about how scores will be distributed for any variable; that is, we can expect many people's scores to be concentrated in the middle and a few to be concentrated at either end of the scale. However, even if scores are not normally distributed, there are still ways and means of accommodating to this and we will explore this further when we look at the distinction between parametric and non-parametric statistics. By having an awareness of the role of normal or skewed distributions in quantitative studies, nurse researchers can be more confident in comparing differences in samples of patients or looking at relationships between a type of treatment and health outcomes. This confidence has come through being able to examine the data collected and analysed through inferential statistics by having a full understanding of the concept of probability.

9.2 Probability

With the advent of the National Lottery in the United Kingdom, the use of the word 'probability' has increased in society. The chances of winning the National Lottery jackpot are thought to be about 14 million to 1, meaning that there is a very small probability that you will win. We can make a number of assertions about life based on probability. It is 100 per cent probable, if you are reading this sentence, that you have been born; there is a 50 per cent probability (1 in 2) that a tossed coin will turn up heads (50 per cent probability that it will turn up tails), 16.66 per cent probability (1 in 6) that a roll of a dice will show a 6.

Some of the ideas about uses of probability in statistics have come from recognising that scores are often normally distributed. With normal distribution we are able to talk about how individual scores might be distributed. An example of this would be for a variable in which scores are normally distributed between 0 and 10. We would then expect most scores (the most probable) to be around 5, slightly fewer scores around 6 and 4, slightly fewer scores again around 7 and 3, and so on (8 and 2; 9 and 1), until the least expected scores (the least probable) are 0 and 10.

These expectations lead us to the key issue emerging from probability: the idea of confidence. Researchers use probability to establish confidence in their findings. The reason why researchers are concerned with establishing confidence in their findings is a consequence of their using data that are collected from samples. Owing to constraints of time, money or accessibility to possible respondents, researchers always use sample data to generalise, or make **statistical inferences** (hence the generic name of *inferential* statistics for the tests we will use in the next few chapters), about a population. This means that there is always a chance that researchers will make an error, because they never have access to the whole population, and therefore can never be certain of how every possible respondent would have scored on a variable. However, because researchers find that variables often form a normal distribution, they can use samples to generalise about populations with confidence. Researchers try to establish confidence by talking about their findings with regard to probability. An example of how they do this can be seen in the horse racing form card in Table 9.1.

At the bottom of this form is the betting forecast. As you can see, 'Nursing sister' is the favourite, at evens, with 'Call bell' being the least favourite, at 33/1. In a similar

Table 9.1 Racing form card for the Fantasy Health Care Horse Novices' Hurdle

3.40 p.m. Fantasy Horse Novices' Hurdle (Class D) (4 y.o. +) 11 run Winner £2,260		2 m 7 ½ 2 fl Going: Good	
No.	*Horse*	*Weight*	*Jockey*
1	Nursing sister	10-12	C. Barton
2	Physical assessment	10-12	L.M. Alcott
3	Antibiotic	10-12	E. Church
4	Case management	10-12	E. Cavell
5	Clinical protocols	10-14	D.L. Dix
6	Person-centred care	10-12	M.E. Mahoney
7	Stats for nurses	10-12	E. Robson
8	Multidisciplinary team	10-12	J. Delano
9	Interprofessional care	10-12	E. Kelly
10	Health promotion	10-12	M.E. Zakrzewska
11	Call bell	10-7	F. Nightingale

Betting forecast: Evens, Nursing sister; 2/1 Physical assessment; 7/2 Antibiotic; 6/1 Case management; 10/1 Clinical protocols; 14/1 Person-centred care; 16/1 Stats for nurses; 18/1 Multidisciplinary team; 16/1 Interprofessional care; 25/1 Health promotion; 33/1 Call bell.

way to that in which bookmakers suggest that it is probable that 'Nursing sister' will win and that 'Call bell' will probably not win, researchers use probability to grade findings as more or less probable. However, unlike bookmakers, researchers use criteria to decide whether something is probable or not probable. The way this is done is through significance testing.

9.3 Significance testing

Significance testing is a criterion, based on probability, that researchers use to decide whether two variables are related. Remember, because researchers always use samples, and because of the possible error, significance testing is used to decide whether the relationships observed are real.

Researchers are then able to use a criterion (significance testing) to decide whether their findings are probable (confident of their findings) or not probable (not confident of their findings). This criterion is expressed in terms of percentages and their relationship to probability values. If we accept that we can never be 100 per cent sure of our findings, we have to set a criterion of how certain we want to be of our findings. Traditionally, two criteria are used. The first is that we are 95 per cent confident of our findings; the second is that we are 99 per cent confident of our findings. This is often expressed in another way. Rather, there is only 5 per cent (95 per cent confidence) or 1 per cent (99 per cent confidence) probability that we have made an error. In terms of significance testing these two criteria are often termed as the 0.05 (5 per cent) and 0.01 (1 per cent) significance levels.

In this chapter, you will be interpreting tests to determine whether there is a **statistically significant** association or relationship between two variables or there is a significant difference between two groups/conditions. These tests always provide a probability statistic in the form of a value, for example 0.75, 0.40, 0.15, 0.04, 0.03, 0.002. Here, the notion of significance testing is essential. This probability statistic is compared against the criteria of 0.05 and 0.01 to decide whether our findings are statistically significant. If the **probability value** (p) is less than 0.05 ($p < 0.05$) or less than 0.01 ($p < 0.01$) then we conclude that the finding is statistically significant.* If the probability value is more than 0.05 ($p > 0.05$) then we conclude that our finding is not statistically significant. Therefore, we can use this information in relation to our research idea and we can determine whether our variables are statistically significantly related. To summarise for the probability value stated above:

> The probability values of 0.75, 0.40 and 0.15 are greater than 0.05 (>0.05) and these probability values are not statistically significant at the 0.05 level ($p > 0.05$).

> The probability values of 0.04 and 0.03 are less than 0.05 (<0.05) but not less than 0.01, so these probability values are statistically significant at the 0.05 level ($p < 0.05$).

> The probability value of 0.002 is less than 0.01 (<0.01)); therefore this probability value is statistically significant at the 0.01 level ($p < 0.01$).

An analogy of significance testing to research is the use of expert witness with evidence in court cases. In a court case, an expert witness is asked to comment on a piece of evidence to help the jury draw a conclusion about the accused. In the same way, the researcher uses significance testing (the expert witness) to help to determine whether the finding (evidence) is significant (the jury conclusion).

EXERCISE 9.2

Deciding on statistical significance through probability

Using the following probability values, decide whether the statistic is statistically significant or not statistically significant. Then decide, if the result is statistically significant, which level of significance the statistic is at (0.05 or 0.01).

0.060   0.030   0.500   0.002   0.978

So, we now know we can do amazing things with numbers. They are not just numbers: things happen with them. The normal distribution allows us to make statements about where scores are likely to happen in a population. Probability introduces us to ideas of things being likely to happen or not happen. What these ideas in statistics do is lead us to the idea of **inferential statistical** tests.

---

*Note that if the probability statistic is below 0.01 (say, 0.002) then we don't need to bother mentioning that it is below 0.05 as well - we already have greater (99 per cent) confidence in our finding.

9.4 Inferential statistical tests

We are now on to the really exciting stuff. Whereas descriptive statistics were exciting in their own right with their ability to describe single variables, inferential statistics can be used to provide answers to our naturally inquisitive minds. As a nurse you are always asking investigatory questions:

- Does the length of waiting lists have an effect on patients' health?
- Does atypical anti-psychotic medication have fewer side effects than typical anti-psychotic medication?
- Are the attitudes of parents to the measles, mumps and rubella (MMR) jab related to parents' anxieties over the general health of their children?

However, to test any of these questions, the first problem is that there are many statistical tests to choose from – which one to use? We will cover five in this chapter as a bit of a 'taster'. The type of statistical test that is chosen depends on:

- The types of variable being used, in other words whether they are categorical-type or continuous-type (see Chapter 8 for a reminder);
- If they are continuous-type variables, whether they should be used in parametric or **non-parametric statistical tests.**

The distinction between parametric and non-parametric statistical tests was mentioned earlier in this chapter so let's go into this area in more depth.

The importance of the parametric and non-parametric distinction

What do we mean by parametric and non-parametric? Remember that earlier in this chapter we said that if data form a normal distribution then they are very powerful because they allow us to be *certain* about how scores will be distributed in a variable. This certainty then led to the development of a number of statistical tests that allowed us to be confident in looking at relationships between variables. These tests were called parametric statistical tests, which are based on the normal distribution curve.

However, statisticians, in their wisdom, wondered what would happen if we had data that didn't form a normal distribution. Rather than give up and go home, they also developed a series of tests that were to be used when the data did not form a normal distribution and, therefore, were less certain about how scores were distributed within a variable; this is a back-up plan for us all to use. These tests became known as non-parametric statistical tests.

So, within statistics, a major distinction is drawn between parametric tests and non-parametric tests. An important idea you must understand is that, with continuous-type data, the nurse researcher must always decide whether the test used to verify them should be a parametric or non-parametric statistical test. The central

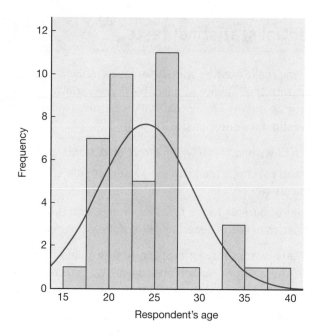

Figure 9.1 Histogram of mothers' ages.

criterion to help them decide on the type of test is whether or not the data form a normal distribution. If their continuous-type data form a normal distribution, then they should be used in a parametric statistical test; if they do not form a normal distribution, then they should be used in a non-parametric statistical test.

The next question is, how do you tell whether your continuous-type data are parametric or non-parametric? There are two ways to do this. The first is to create a histogram of the data and see whether they form a normal distribution. The second is to see whether your data are skewed, that is, do not form a normal distribution.

Take the examples shown in Figures 9.1 and 9.2, which represent data from a maternity hospital where researchers have recorded the mother's age and time spent in labour. You can see from both graphs that the distribution of scores is *compared* against the black line, which is a normal distribution curve. You can see that the amount of time spent in labour forms a normal distribution, but the age variable seems to be skewed towards the lower end (positively skewed). This is perhaps not surprising given that mothers will tend to have babies earlier on in life.

However, you may see that there are problems with making this judgement. More often than not it is not easy to tell whether a variable is normally distributed. For example, the time in labour variable does seems to have properties of a normal distribution: it has a high middle, among other things. However, it is not always easy to tell whether your data form a normal distribution. Another approach to this is through the skewness statistic (see box on the opposite page).

Therefore we suggest that the main guideline to use when deciding whether your continuous-type data are suitable for parametric or non-parametric tests is whether

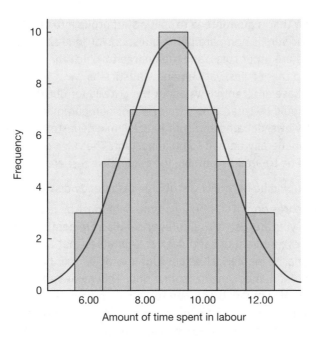

Figure 9.2 Histogram of mothers' time spent in labour.

the data are skewed. If they are not skewed, then they probably are suitable for use in parametric tests. If they are skewed, then you might wish to use them in non-parametric tests instead.

> **THINGS TO CONSIDER**
>
> ### The skewness statistic
>
> Now you will not come across this in the book, but sometimes there may be information about the extent of skew and therefore it will be useful for you to be aware of this. The skewness statistics can either be positive or negative, indicating in which direction the skewness may lie. There is a test to decide whether your skewness statistic means you have a skewed distribution, but this is vulnerable to the number of people you have in your sample. Most researchers use a general criterion that any statistic above 1.00 (either + or −) means your distribution is skewed.

Complications with the parametric and non-parametric distinction

So far, the criterion to decide whether data should be treated as parametric or non-parametric seems simple. Do the data form a **normal distribution** or not? Unfortunately, it is not always that simple in practice. Before we say why, it is as well to know that the question of what constitutes parametric is one that is hotly debated in statistical teaching. Your lecturers may look as if they are all friendly with each other, but if there is one thing that is guaranteed to split a staff group into factions it is their views on the parametric versus non-parametric question. Intrigued? Read on.

You see, there are other rules, and the degree to which they apply, and the importance attached to these rules, vary among statisticians.

Many people have different views about the criteria for deciding whether continuous-type data should be treated as parametric or non-parametric. Our consideration of the different views, debates and split in academic departments begins with three rules, which are generally agreed to be important. The rules of whether continuous-type data should be treated as suitable for parametric test are:

- **Rule 1:** Data should be normally distributed (as already discussed).

- **Rule 2:** The scores on any continuous-type data must be interval or ratio data (or continuous if you are using the categorical/discrete/continuous distinctions between variables); interval or ratio data are variables that are numerical, meaning that they comprise numerical values (for example, age, hours spent in labour), where the actual number means something. This means that the levels of these variables are real numbers that mean something numerically. Therefore, data such as ordinal data, which are of a continuous type but represented by artificial numbers, do not count. For example, a measure of pain where no pain is scored as 0, mild pain is scored as 1, moderate pain is scored as 2, and extremely severe pain is scored as 3 is not a variable of real numbers; instead it comprises numbers we've assigned to understand the amount of pain.

- **Rule 3:** If two continuous-type variables are being used or compared, they must have similar standard deviations. The standard deviation provides the researcher with an indicator of how scores for variables are spread around the mean average (this is why it is sometimes referred to as a measure of dispersion). The higher the standard deviation, the more the scores are spread out (the scores 0, 1, 2, 2, 0 will have a low standard deviation, whereas the scores, 0, 50, 100, 200, 500 will have a much higher standard deviation).

These are all rules for determining whether your data are parametric. They can be used to determine whether your data are suitable for use in a parametric statistical test.

Furthermore, if your continuous-type data do *not* follow these rules, you do *not* use a parametric statistical test; instead you use a non-parametric test. So, for Rule 2, if your data are not interval or ratio data, then you should use a non-parametric test. For example, consider an ordinal variable which asks the respondent how their anxiety might be scored: 1 = Not at all, 2 = Sometimes, 3 = Often, 4 = Always. It is sometimes argued that this scoring does not reflect numerical properties, as the score of 4, for instance, given for responding 'Always' to the question, does not represent a behaviour that is twice as much as the score of 2, given for 'Sometimes' ('Always' is not twice as much as 'Sometimes'). Similar principles apply for Rules 1 and 3. If your continuous-type data are *not* normally distributed (Rule 1) or if two sets of continuous-type scores are being used or compared and they do *not* have similar standard deviations (Rule 3) then a non-parametric test should be used.

But, and this is a big *but*, people don't always use these three rules. Or, they will vary in the application of these rules. Even when the data do not comply with the rules, researchers may treat data as parametric that look more suited to being treated as non-parametric. They may do this for a number of good reasons, including the following:

- The statistics test has been previously used by other researchers to look at the same variable. This is sometimes done to provide consistency in the research literature.

- Although some continuous-type variables may not comprise real numbers (such as ordinal data which ranks the data), we can make the assumption that they *are* real numbers because researchers are assigning these values to responses.

- Sometimes, researchers will assume their continuous-type data are normally distributed because they have collected data with adequate sampling techniques and, therefore, have data that are in general representative of a variable which would be expected to be normally distributed in a larger population. For example, if you do a study of 40 people then the data will not likely form a normal distribution because you haven't got enough cases.

- The scale used to measure the continuous-type variable is a well-established, reliable and valid measure of that variable and has been shown by previous research (among larger samples) to demonstrate a normal distribution of scores.

- Because their lecturer/teacher has told them so. Lecturers and teachers may suggest you use a certain version of the test because of wider learning reasons or for reasons of being consistent with the literature.

What you need to be aware of most is that researchers do vary in practice and people do not always agree with each other's approaches. People will be very definite about their way of doing things and insist that their way is correct. This is often a source of confusion for students of statistics, and the best strategy you can employ is just to be aware that researchers do vary in practice. Usually, there is little point in adopting one position only, because often you will work with colleagues, complete reports for employers/teachers/lecturers, or submit papers to academic journals that will insist you adopt a different tactic. Ideally, you should be aware that different valid practices exist and be able to employ and engage with these different practices when needed.

It is best to use these various rules and practices as guidelines to decide whether to use parametric or non-parametric versions of tests. However, overall, you should remember that this decision shouldn't be viewed as a big problem. The purpose is not that you should develop a concept of parametric versus non-parametric tests. Rather, you should appreciate that statisticians have provided us with different ways of solving problems. Therefore, there is nothing to worry about if you find that the continuous-type variables you have measured do not show parametric properties: you simply use non-parametric tests as an alternative.

What we suggest you do at this stage, to keep things as simple as possible, is to use the normal distribution criterion and the skewness statistics as ways of determining the parametric versus non-parametric question when it is needed. Then, as you become more experienced with statistics (or as you come across them), you could begin to consider the other rules.

Moving forward

In moving forward to the next stage, you need to remember two things before being introduced to the world of statistical tests, namely that:

- variables can be generally defined as two types: categorical-type or continuous-type (we have covered this throughout the book so far);
- when using continuous-type variables, a distinction is made between whether the data should be used in parametric or non-parametric statistical tests, and this choice rests on whether your data form a normal distribution.

9.5 Statistical tests and the decision-making table

Let us introduce you to all the statistical tests you will use in the book and the context for using these tests. Remember, the aim of any inferential statistical test is to answer your question of whether there is something happening between two variables. Although there are a number of statistical tests, you use only one statistical test with any one question. *The problem is that you have to use the right one*. How do you ensure you use the right one? Let us introduce you to our decision-making chart (see Table 9.2).

Table 9.2 Decision-making table for choosing statistical tests

Question 1: *What combination of variables have you got?*	*Which statistical test to use?*	*Question 2:* *Should your continuous-type data be used with parametric tests or non-parametric tests?*	*Which statistical test to use?*
Two categorical-type variables	Chi-square		
Two separate/independent continuous-type variables	Go to Question 2	Parametric	Pearson correlation
		Non-parametric	Spearman correlation
Two continuous-type variables which is the same variable administered twice	Go to Question 2	Parametric	Paired-samples *t*-test
		Non-parametric	Wilcoxon sign-ranks
One categorical-type and one continuous-type variables	Go to Question 2	Parametric	Independent-samples *t*-test
		Non-parametric	Mann-Whitney *U*

In our decision-making chart you will notice a number of blocks with terms such as **chi-square**, **Pearson correlation**, **Spearman correlation** (to name just a few) written in them. Of these tests, we will cover only a few to give you a taster on how the results of inferential statistics are interpreted and reported. For further information about other statistics for nurses, you can read *Statistics for Nurses* (Maltby, Day and Williams, 2007), which gives an in-depth overview of each of the tests covered in the decision-making chart and how to calculate these statistics by hand or with a computer.

The aim of the decision-making process is to reach one of these end points in Table 9.2. To reach each end point, what you must do is to answer *two* questions in each of the columns in turn, choosing your response from the rows below. What you must then do is continue along each row until you reach an end point. Then, when you reach this end point, you should know which type of statistical test you should use.

The two questions are:

- What types of variable are being used, and in what combination?
- Should the continuous-type variables be used in parametric or non-parametric statistical tests (remember, your answer to this question rests on whether your data form a normal distribution)?

If you are able to answer both of these questions successfully then you will always choose the right statistical test to be used.

To illustrate this process let us use an example. Hospital staff are interested in examining recent findings that women who have an epidural to ease the pain of childbirth are more likely to need medical help to have their baby (BBC News, 2005a). One important aspect to this study is that women opting for an epidural were more likely to experience a longer second stage of labour. The staff members want to see whether this is occurring in their hospital. The researchers have decided to measure the following variables:

- Whether or not the mother has had an epidural during childbirth (i.e. this is categorical-type variable with two categories, or levels).
- The length of the second stage of labour. This continuous-type variable has been found to have a normal distribution.

In terms of moving forward, we have to choose which statistical test to use. In answer to the two questions in our decision-making table:

- we have one categorical-type variable and one continuous-type variable;
- the continuous-type variable has a normal distribution, and therefore it is suitable for use in a parametric test.

Therefore, we would choose an independent-samples *t*-test.

Now, we know you have no idea what an independent-samples *t*-test does, but you can see that you can already find your way through different statistical tests. And that skill is an important aspect of statistics. Have a go yourself in the next section.

EXERCISE 9.3

Choosing an inferential statistical test

Following efforts by NHS Lothian to combat the MRSA hospital superbug via information packs, leaflets and posters (BBC News, 2005b), your local health authority has decided to see whether hospitals under its control could benefit from such a drive. Research staff at the local health authority have then surveyed each of the authority's hospitals on two issues:

● Whether there have been any special initiatives within the hospital, such as information packs on infection control and prevention given to staff, or posters and leaflets aimed at patients and visitors to raise awareness of the problem. Responses are either 'yes' or 'no'.

● Whether the hospital has been given a clean bill of health in terms of there not being a reported case of the MRSA superbug in the hospital. Responses are either 'yes' or 'no'.

To help you, the research staff have decided that both variables are categorical-type data and Figure 9.3 shows the data obtained in this study.

Initiative *Free of MRSA Cross-tabulation

Count

		Free of MRSA		Total
		No	Yes	
Initiative	No	15	6	21
	Yes	6	13	19
Total		21	19	40

← Frequency counts

Figure 9.3 Example of cross-tabulated frequencies for a chi-square test.

What statistical test should the researcher use?

You would be right if you chose chi-square.

9.6 Making sense of inferential statistics: chi-square

By now we can tell that you are itching to find out about these inferential statistical tests. In this section we introduce you to your first inferential statistical test: the chi-square.

Table 9.3 Breakdown of 100 respondents by sex and type of work

	Full-time work	Part-time work
Males	40 (25)	10 (25)
Females	10 (25)	40 (25)

As you know from the last exercise, the chi-square test provides a test for use when a researcher wants to examine the relationship between two categorical-type variables. For example, if we had two variables, Sex of respondent and Type of work performed by the respondent (full- or part-time work), we would be able to examine whether the two variables are associated. Often, people think that men tend to have full-time jobs and women tend to have part-time jobs. This type of thinking might be a research question. That is, is there a relationship between the variables? Does the sex of the respondent tend to determine what sort of work they undertake?

The key idea underlying the chi-square test is that we examine two sets of frequencies: observed and expected. To illustrate this, let us take the everyday example of males and females in full-time or part-time work. Table 9.3 sets out these two aspects: observed and expected frequencies (in brackets). The researcher, interested in whether the sex of a person influences the type of work they engage in, has asked 100 respondents their sex and whether they were employed in full-time or part-time work. The chi-square test analyses a matrix (often referred to as cross-tabulations) made up of cells representing each of the possible combinations of the levels of each categorical-type variable, in this case males and full-time work, females and full-time work, males and part-time work, and females and part-time work. As you can see from the table, there are two possible sets of frequencies.

The first set of numbers is the **observed frequencies**. These are an example of a set of frequencies the researcher might have found having gone out and collected the data from 100 people (Males and full-time work = 40, Females and full-time work = 10, Males and part-time work = 10, and Females and part-time work = 40).

The second set of numbers (in brackets) is the **expected frequencies**. These are the frequencies the researcher would expect to emerge from 100 people if everything was equal and, therefore, there was no association between the two variables. These frequencies are spread evenly across the possible combination of levels for each of the categorical-type variables (Males and full-time work = 25, Females and full-time work = 25, Males and part-time work = 25, and Females and part-time work = 25).

The chi-square test uses significance testing to examine whether two variables are independent (sometimes the chi-square test is referred to as the test of independence). What this means is that if the two variables are independent of each other, that is, are not related, then the *observed* frequencies would be split pretty evenly across the different rows and columns of the cross-tabulation (much like the expected frequencies are). Using our example, if the two variables are independent of each other, that is, if sex has no bearing on the type of work a person does, then you would expect to find that the observed frequencies are evenly split across the matrix.

However, if the observed frequencies are not even across the matrix, and if certain levels of one variable went together with other aspects of the other variable more so than would be expected, then we might begin to think that the two variables are linked in some way.

This is what appears to be happening with the observed frequencies in our example of sex of respondent and type of work. In terms of frequencies, 40 males are in full-time work (whereas only 10 males are in part-time work), and 40 females are in part-time work (whereas only 10 females are in full-time work). Therefore, what we can see in these data is a tendency for men to be employed in full-time work and women to be employed in part-time work. This suggests that the two variables might not be independent of each other and may be related. This possible relationship within a chi-square is often referred to as an association (which is why you will also sometimes find the chi-square referred to as a test of association as well as a test of independence; don't worry though – just remember, if the variables are related then they are 'associated'; if they are not related they are 'independent'). The chi-square statistic allows us to determine whether there is a statistically significant association (relationship) between two variables.

A research example to which this type of test could be applied is that by Powell *et al.* (2004). Their study looked at different staff perceptions of community learning disability nurses' roles. One of the things that the researchers were interested in was whether health care staff or social care staff were more likely to see assessment as part of the community learning disability nurses' role. Therefore, the study has two categorical-type variables with two categories for each of these variables:

- The type of staff member (health care staff versus social care staff) and
- Whether the respondent believes that it is the community learning disability nurses' role to carry out assessment (yes or no).

Seeing a chi-square test in action

A chi-square analysis here could help us find out whether there is an association between the type of staff (health or social) and their view on whether it is the community learning disability nurses' role to carry out assessment (or whether these two variables were independent of each other, that is, whether the type of staff had no bearing on their views of the learning disability nurses' role to carry out assessment).

This must then be incorporated into a text, to help the reader understand and conceptualise your findings. In writing about the chi-square statistic, the researcher needs to do the following:

- Remind the reader of the two variables you are examining.
- Describe the relationship between the two variables in terms of the cell counts (and percentages).

- Tell the reader whether the finding is significant or not.
- You can use all the information above to write a fairly simple paragraph, which conveys your findings succinctly but effectively. However, you will also need to include a table.

Therefore, a typical report of the chi-square test results might be as follows:

The following table shows a breakdown of the distribution of respondents by area of residence and heart disease. The frequency of respondents in each cell was distributed such that the highest counts were for when the case lived in Glasgow and had heart disease, and when the case lived in Edinburgh and did not have heart disease. A chi-square test was used to determine whether there was a statistically significant association between the two variables. A statistically significant association was found between the area of residence and heart disease ($\chi^2(1) = 9.19$, $p < 0.05$).

You might find different ways in which chi-square statistic results are written up, both in your own reports and in those of other authors, but you will tend to find in each write-up all the information you need but it might vary in the order that it is presented. Read the following boxes for further points to consider when using chi-square.

THINGS TO CONSIDER

What are degrees of freedom?

Whenever you use a statistical test you will always be asked to report your degrees of freedom. It is sometimes considered more a matter of convention than essential, but it is good practice to do it. This is always very straightforward and easy to do. Many authors rightly shy away from explaining what degrees of freedom are. However, one of the best explanations of how to conceptualise degrees of freedom is presented by Clegg (1982).

Clegg suggests you imagine two pots, one of coffee and one of tea, but neither is labelled. Clegg asks the question, 'How many tastes do you require before you know what is in each pot?' The answer is one, because once you have tasted one, you not only know what is in that pot, but also what is in the other. Similarly, if you had three pots, coffee, tea and orange juice, you would need two tastes before you could conclude what was in all three pots. What is important here is that you *do not* need to taste all of the pots before you are certain about what is contained in each pot.

These ideas are used in the measuring of variables. In both examples, all the pots represent your sample, and your tasting represents your sampling. Each pot-tasting represents another procedure to establish certainty for your findings. Further, your number of attempts will be one less than the total number of pots. Degrees of freedom can be visualised in the same way. Overall, degrees of freedom are important, as you use them to decide whether your result is statistically significant.

THINGS TO CONSIDER

Writing up a statistically non-significant result for the chi-square test

Researchers at the local health authority have surveyed each of their hospitals on two issues:

1. Have there been any special initiatives within the hospital, such as information packs on infection control and prevention given to staff, or posters aimed at patients and visitors distributed to raise awareness of the problem? Responses are either Yes or No.

2. Whether the hospital has been given a clean bill of health in terms of there not being a reported case of the MRSA hospital superbug in the hospital. Responses are either Yes or No.

A table was compiled, which showed the breakdown of respondents by each of the table cells. The frequencies of respondents in each cell were distributed evenly across the categories. A chi-square test was used to determine whether there was a statistically significant association between the two variables. No statistically significant association was found between the presence of initiatives and the hospital being given a clean bill of health with regard to the MRSA superbug ($\chi^2(1) = 1.05$, $p = 0.78$). The present findings suggest that there is no association between initiatives to combat the MRSA superbug in hospitals and a hospital's reporting cases of MRSA in it, and that the two variables are independent of each other.

THINGS TO CONSIDER

Further information on the chi-square test

There are two conditions under which it is not advisable to do a chi-square test:

1. When you have a chi-square that comprises two rows by two columns and any of the expected frequencies is less than 5.

2. When you have a chi-square that comprises more than two rows by two columns and any of the expected frequencies is less than 1, or more than 20 per cent of the expected frequencies are less than 5.

9.7 Pearson and Spearman correlation statistics

What we intend to do now is to build on your knowledge by introducing you to two more tests. Cast your mind back to the decision-making table presented in Table 9.2. The Pearson and Spearman statistics are two statistics that you use when you want to examine the relationship between two separate continuous-type variables. The

Pearson correlation statistical test is a parametric statistical test (you remember, when your data show a normal distribution and are not skewed). The Spearman correlation statistical test is a non-parametric statistical test (when your data are not normally distributed or you find evidence of their being skewed). We will next introduce you to the thinking that lies behind these two statistical tests.

What is a correlation?

The aim of both the **Pearson** and **Spearman correlation coefficients** is to determine whether there is a relationship between two separate continuous-type variables.

Imagine two variables: amount of chocolate eaten and weight. It is thought that chocolate contains a lot of fat, and that eating a lot of fat will increase your weight. Therefore, it could be expected that people who eat a lot of chocolate would also weigh a lot. If this were true then the amount of chocolate you eat and your weight would be positively correlated. The more chocolate you eat, the more you weigh. The less chocolate you eat, the less you weigh. This is a correlation, but this is a positive correlation, because when the scores are high on one continuous-type variable, they are high on the other continuous-type variable (and low scores on one are accompanied by low scores on the other). This is visualised in Figure 9.4(a), with the plotted points moving from the lower left-hand corner up and across to the upper right-hand corner of the chart.

Conversely, a negative correlation between two variables is the opposite of that: a high negative correlation would mean that while scores on one variable rise, scores on the other variable decrease. An example of this would be the amount of exercise taken and weight. It is thought that taking exercise will usually lead to a decrease in weight. If this were true then the amount of exercise you take and your weight would be negatively correlated. The more exercise you take, the less you weigh. The less exercise you take, the more you weigh. This is visualised in Figure 9.4(b), with the plotted points moving from the upper left-hand corner down and across to the lower right-hand corner of the chart.

Finally, some variables might not be expected to show any level of correlation with each other. For example, the number of hot meals you have eaten and the number of times you have visited the zoo. Usually, we expect that there would be no logical reason why eating hot meals and zoo visiting would be related, so that eating more hot meals would mean you would visit the zoo more, or less (or vice versa). Therefore, you would expect the number of hot meals you have eaten and the number of times you have visited the zoo not to show any correlation. This is visualised in 9.4(c) by a random scatter of plots; the plots show no clear direction, going neither up nor down.

One nursing research example of a correlation was carried out by Cherri Hobgood and her colleagues (2005). The researchers were interested in the relationship between emergency department volume and the impact this had on nurse time at the bedside in an emergency department. Therefore, they measured the volume of people in the emergency department and compared this against the amount of time nurses spent at the patients' bedsides. They found a negative correlation between these two variables, suggesting the greater the volume of people in the emergency ward, the less amount of time nurses were able to spend at the bedside of patients.

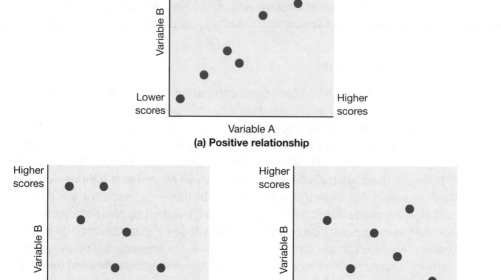

Figure 9.4 Examples of positive, negative and no relationships between two variables.

The correlation statistic

We now know what a correlation generally is, and the description of the relationship, but so far we have vague information. However, the Pearson and Spearman correlation statistics can give us much more information. The correlation coefficient provides a statistic that tells us the direction, the strength and the significance of the relationship between two variables.

What do we mean by direction and strength? Well, both the Pearson and Spearman correlation statistics use the number of the data and present a final figure that indicates the direction and strength of the relationship. This final figure is always known as the correlation coefficient and is represented by *r* (Pearson) or rho (Spearman). The correlation coefficient will always be a value ranging from +1.00 through 0.00 to −1.00.

- A correlation of +1.00 would be a 'perfect' positive relationship.
- A correlation of −1.00 would be a 'perfect' negative relationship.
- A correlation of 0.00 would be no relationship (no single straight line can sum up the almost random distribution of points).

All correlations, then, will range from −1.00 to +1.00. So a correlation statistic could be −0.43 (a negative relationship) or 0.53 (a positive relationship). It could be 0.01, close to no relationship. This figure can then be used with significance testing, such as the chi-square, to see whether the relationship between the two variables is statistically significant. Let us show you how one of these correlation statistics works.

Pearson product–moment correlation

Remember from Table 9.2 that the Pearson product-moment correlation is a test used with parametric data, and is used when you have two continuous-type variables that you believe should be used in a parametric test (for example, it shows a normal distribution, or rather that the data are not skewed). Remember, too, that the key idea of the correlation statistical test is to determine whether there is a relationship between the two variables. The following example reflects a study that tried to examine the relationship between physical functioning and general health. The study used two validated questionnaire scales among a non-clinical sample of five respondents - one scale to measure physical functioning and one to measure general health. The aim of the study was to see whether poorer levels of physical functioning were equated with lower levels of general health. A high score on physical functioning would mean that a person could do plenty of physical things like climb stairs, walk a mile without needing to take a break, etc., and a high score on general health would mean that the person had high-quality health in many spheres of their lives. By contrast, low scores on the two scales meant poor physical functioning and low general health.

Interpreting and reporting Pearson product–moment correlations

From the output that you would get from a statistical program, you will need to consider the following things:

1. The statistical test statistic. It is important to note whether the statistic is positive or negative. This indicates whether the relationship between the two variables is positive (positive number, which is often without a '+' sign in front of it in journal articles) or negative (represented by a '−' sign).
2. Whether the relationship between the two variables is statistically significant. Remember, if this figure is below the $p = 0.05$ or $p = 0.01$ criteria, then the finding is statistically significant. If this figure is above 0.05, then the findings are not statistically significant.

Let us say that we got a Pearson's r statistic of 0.45 and the significance level was 0.002. The Pearson's r statistic tells us that there is a positive relationship between the two variables. The thing we need to remember is how the scales are scored; the lower the scores on both questionnaire scales, the poorer the physical functioning and lower the general health, and vice versa. If the relationship was a negative one, the statistic would have a minus sign in front of it. The significance level is $p = 0.002$, which is below the level of $p = 0.05$ or $p = 0.01$, so we can decide that the relationship we have found is not likely to have occurred by chance. Therefore, we can conclude that there is a statistically significant positive relationship between physical functioning and general heath.

The next stage is to report these statistics. There is a formal way of reporting the Pearson product-moment correlation coefficient, which comprises two elements. The first element is that a formal statement of your statistics must include the following:

- *The test statistic.* Each test has a symbol for its statistic. The Pearson product-moment correlation has the symbol *r*. Therefore, in writing your results you must include what *r* is equal to. In the example, $r = 0.45$.
- *The degrees of freedom.* This is a figure that is traditionally reported (though it is worth noting that it is not always reported). For the Pearson product-moment correlation coefficient, the degrees of freedom equal the size of your sample minus 2. The minus 2 represents minus 1 for each set of scores (the set of scores for the physical functioning scale and the set of scores for the general health scale). The figure is placed between the *r* and the equals sign and is written in brackets. Here, the degrees of freedom are 3 (size of sample = 5, minus 2 = 3). Therefore, $r(3) = 0.45$.

  Traditionally, this was done in relation to whether your probability value was below 0.05 or 0.01 (statistically significant) or above 0.05 (not statistically significant). Here, you use less than (<) or greater than (>) the criteria levels. You state these criteria by reporting whether $p < 0.05$ (statistically significant), $p < 0.01$ (statistically significant) or $p > 0.05$ (not statistically significant). In the example above, $p < 0.01$ and place this after the reporting of the *r* value. Therefore, with our findings, $r(3) = 0.45$, $p < 0.01$.

The second element is the incorporation of these statistics into the text, to help the reader understand and interpret your findings. In writing the text, use the 'describe and decide' rule to inform the reader of your findings:

- Remind the reader of the two variables you are examining.
- Describe the relationship between the two variables as positive or negative.
- Tell the reader whether the finding is statistically significant or not.
- Give some indication of what this means.

You can use all the information above to write a fairly simple paragraph which conveys your findings succinctly but effectively. Therefore, using the findings above, we might report:

A Pearson product-moment correlation coefficient was used to examine the relationship between physical functioning and general health using the subscales from the SF-36 Health Survey. A statistically significant positive correlation was found between physical functioning and general health (r(3) = 0.45, p < 0.01), suggesting that poorer physical functioning and general health are statistically significantly related to one another.

You will come across different ways of writing up the Pearson product-moment correlation coefficient, both in your own writing and in that of other authors, but you will find all the information included above in any write-up. Read the next two boxes for further things to consider when using a Pearson product-moment correlation.

THINGS TO CONSIDER

Significance testing with one- and two-tailed hypotheses

One-tailed and two-tailed tests involve making statements regarding the expected direction of the relationship between the two variables you are measuring. With a one-tailed hypothesis the researcher would make a statement regarding the specific direction of the relationship. With a two-tailed statement, prediction is not made regarding the direction of the expected relationship. We can illustrate this with the present example because we believe there is going to be a statistically significant *positive* (this is the expected direction of the relationship) relationship between physical functioning and bodily pain. A two-tailed hypothesis may be that we might expect a significant relationship, but we are unsure of the final direction of the relationship (here, the researcher would state that there is an expected statistically significant relationship between the two variables). As we can see from the present example, by making a specific prediction about the direction of the relationship between these aspects of physical health these ideas are incorporated into statistical significance testing and we would use a one-tailed test.

In reality you are more likely to get a statistically significant result using a one-tailed test because the way the significance testing is set up allows you more leeway because you have made a prediction. This increases your chances of a statistically significant finding; it also increases your chances of making an error by suggesting there is a statistically significant relationship between two variables when in fact there is no such relationship (this is known as a **Type I error**). In nursing, it is crucial to avoid making this sort of mistake. You don't want to say a drug has a statistically significant effect when it doesn't. Therefore, many researchers don't make this distinction any more and tend to use two-tailed tests regardless of a-priori predictions. Therefore, in future you might be best advised always to perform the correlations using the two-tailed test.

THINGS TO CONSIDER

Writing up a statistically non-significant result for the Pearson product-moment correlation

Knowing how to write a statistically significant result is of little use if, in your research, you have a statistically non-significant finding. Therefore, whenever we suggest how you might report test results, we will also give you the alternative way of writing up your results. Here, let us imagine that we found no statistically significant relationship between physical functioning and bodily pain, i.e. $r = 0.032$ and $p = 0.76$ (therefore $p > 0.05$ and is statistically non-significant). A Pearson product-moment correlation coefficient was used to examine the relationship between physical functioning and general health using the subscales from the SF-36 Health Survey. No statistically significant correlation was found between physical functioning and general heath ($r(72) = 0.032$, $p > 0.05$), suggesting no statistically significant relationship between physical functioning and general health.

Spearman's rho correlation

The Spearman correlation is the non-parametric version of the parametric test the Pearson product-moment correlation. Whereas the Pearson product-moment correlation is used to examine whether a statistically significant relationship occurs between two continuous variables, which demonstrate properties suitable for use in parametric tests, the Spearman rho correlation is used to examine whether a statistically significant relationship occurs between two continuous variables, which demonstrate properties suitable for use in non-parametric tests. Apart from this, the Spearman rho correlation works in exactly the same way, but with a rho value between −1.00 and +1.00 being generated (though some people just use r). As with the Pearson correlation, significance testing is then used to determine whether a statistically significant relationship occurs between two variables.

Some further things to know about correlations

So there we are. That is how you perform correlations. However, before we finish we just need to tell you three things about correlations. These are particularly useful things to consider when you are discussing your findings, which include the points that:

● Correlation does not represent causation;
● Issues of association;
● The size of correlation.

Correlation does not represent causation

It is important to remember, when reporting any sort of correlation, not to infer that one variable causes another. Therefore, in the example above we could not conclude that role limitations due to physical health problems necessarily cause bodily pain, as it may be that worse bodily pain causes role limitations due to physical health problems. It is more likely that the two variables influence each other and/or work together. Remember to reflect this in your wording and always to talk about relationships, associations or correlations between two variables. Do not say that one variable causes another, unless you have a very good reason for thinking so.

Issues of association

You will often find authors reporting the association between the two variables in a Pearson product-moment correlation coefficient, and this is thought to represent the shared variance between two variables. In theory, two variables can share a maximum of 100 per cent of the variance (identical) and a minimum of 0 per cent of variance (not related at all), and the association can be used to indicate the importance of a statistically significant relationship between two variables. The association is found by squaring (i.e. multiplying by itself) the *r* value, and reporting it as a percentage. For example, if the correlation between role limitations due to physical health problems and bodily pain is 0.356 we would work out the association in the following way: calculate $0.356 \times 0.356 = 0.126736$, and report it as a percentage by multiplying the number by 100, so 12.6736 per cent, or 12.67 per cent (to two decimal places). You often find researchers reporting the variance as part of their discussion, sometimes used as an indicator of importance of the findings (or lack of importance of findings – as the smaller the percentage, the less important any relationship between the two variables).

Effect size: size of the correlation

The consideration of the importance of findings is now common practice in statistics. This importance of findings has become what is known as **effect size**. The consideration of effect size is an important addition to statistical testing through significance. Why? Well, significance levels depend on sample size. The larger the sample size, the lower the criterion is for finding a statistically significant result. For example, while a correlation of 0.2 is not statistically significant among a sample of 50 participants, a correlation of 0.2 will be statistically significant among a sample of 1,000 participants. This has led to an interesting dilemma for researchers. Imagine two drug trials, one with drug A and one with drug B, both designed to help one particular illness.

In the trial with drug A, among 50 participants, the correlation between drug A and improvement with patients was $r = 0.32$. The probability value was $p = 0.10$, not a statistically significant result.

In the trial with drug B, among 1,000 participants, the correlation between drug B and improvement with patients was $r = 0.22$. The probability value was $p = 0.01$, a statistically significant result (though the correlation statistic is smaller than in the first study). Therefore, if we studied these two drug trials separately we would come to different conclusions about the relationship between the two drugs and patient improvement. We would, based on significance testing, be likely to recommend drug B because there was a statistically significant relationship between the drug and patient improvement, even though drug A had a stronger association with patient improvement.

This has led to a general rethink about reporting statistics, and the notion of considering effect size when reporting statistics. Effect size just refers to the strength of the relationship, and you will now commonly find a reference to the effect size of any finding in the literature.

Luckily, the criteria introduced by American statistician Jacob Cohen (1988) to label the effect size are used across the majority of the statistics mentioned (though it won't surprise you that practice varies, but to a lesser extent than in other areas of statistics). Cohen suggested that effect sizes of 0.2 to 0.5 should be regarded as 'small', 0.5 to 0.8 as 'moderate' and those above 0.8 as 'large'. Even luckier for us at this stage, when it comes to correlation statistics the *r* value is considered the indicator of effect size. So correlation statistics of:

0.1 represent a *small* effect size

0.3 represent a *medium* (or moderate) effect size

0.5 represent a *large* effect size.

It is best to see these criteria in tabular form, as set out in Table 9.4. Remember, these are used as indicators of your findings to help you in your consideration. If you have a statistically significant correlation of 0.25, it is important not to conclude that this is a strong relationship. More importantly, if you have found a number of statistically significant correlations in your study, Cohen's criteria can be used to determine which correlations represent more important findings, and which are less important.

Let us consider effect size with some data in a fictionalised study into the number of falls among older people in care of the older person wards. Table 9.5 sets out the correlation between three variables: (1) the age of the patients, (2) the number of falls they've had and (3) the number of other reported accidents.

Let us show you how to interpret the correlation matrix in Table 9.5. There are five columns and four rows and this whole table shows you how all of the variables are related to each other. All of the variables are listed in the rows and also in the columns too. If you look at the 2nd row and the 3rd column, in this cell there is a value of 1. This is correct as the 2nd row and 3rd column is age correlated with age (i.e. the same variable correlated with itself will always equal 1). Let us look at another cell in this correlation matrix. In the 4th row and the 3rd column we can see that, although there is a positive correlation between number of other reported accidents (the 4th row) and age (the 3rd column) which has a correlation of $r = 0.239$; we also know that the correlation is statistically significant as there is a value

Table 9.4 Cohen's effect size criteria

Criteria: effect size	r
	0.65 0.60 0.55
Large	0.50 0.45 0.40 0.35
Medium/moderate	0.30 0.25 0.20 0.15
Small	0.10 0.05 0.0

Table 9.5 A correlation matrix showing age of patient, number of falls and the number of other accidents (apart from falls)

		Age	Number of falls	Number of other accidents reported (apart from falls)
Age	Pearson correlation	1	0.613*	0.239[†]
	Sig. (2-tailed)		0.000	0.040
	N	74	74	74
Number of falls	Pearson correlation	0.613*	1	0.355*
	Sig. (2-tailed)	0.000		0.002
	N	74	74	74
Number of other accidents reported (apart from falls)	Pearson correlation	0.239[†]	0.355*	1
	Sig. (2-tailed)	0.040	0.002	
	N	74	74	74

*Correlation is significant at the 0.01 level (2-tailed).
[†]Correlation is significant at the 0.05 level (2-tailed).

directly underneath the correlation, which is 0.040. This value is less than 0.05 and is therefore significant. Overall, the trend that we have found from this cell in the correlation matrix means that the older the patients are, the more often they have other accidents beyond falls. However, this correlation would be considered small.

A much more important correlation to consider can be found in the 3rd row and the 3rd column, which shows a statistically significant positive correlation between age and number of falls ($r = 0.613$, $p < 0.01$), meaning that the older the patients are, the more falls that they have (and vice versa). The effect size of this correlation is large, and therefore in any writing-up of the results we would emphasise this finding when compared to the other result as being a more noteworthy trend.

THINGS TO CONSIDER

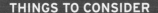

Small effect sizes

There is one point to consider from a nursing perspective of small effect sizes. Robert Rosenthal (1991) has pointed out that the importance of effect sizes may depend on the sort of question we are investigating. For example, finding a small correlation between emergency ward volume and time spent at patients' bedsides might suggest that there isn't an important effect on emergency ward volume and the amount of bedside care. However, when it comes to aspects such as medication, if there is a small effect size between a new drug and its ability to save lives suggesting that it saves 4 out of 100 lives, if we translated that figure to a population of 100,000, that would mean 4,000 lives and the finding is certainly an important one regardless of the effect size. Therefore we might, in nursing, have to consider what we are studying before drawing final conclusions.

9.8 Comparing average scores: statistics for all sorts of groups and occasions

Earlier in this chapter, we looked at correlation statistics, which are statistics that find out whether there is a relationship between two continuous-type variables (such as age and wage earning). However, there are other statistics that are used for measuring variables before and after an intervention (such as the support group scheme for carers) or for assessing group differences in a variable (for example, comparing participants in the support group scheme with non-participants).

In this section, we are going to look at these tests. You are going to use again terms such as significance testing and scores, but you will also learn more about why certain tests are used to examine differences between groups, and you will learn how to interpret results from these tests.

The common theme between these tests that we will look at is that they are comparing how people score on average (see the previous chapter on descriptive statistics and averages).

The two tests that we are going to examine in more detail will focus primarily on the average scores. The first group of tests will involve looking at average scores between two groups (e.g. a control group and an experimental group). These two tests are:

- **Independent-samples *t*-test** - used when you have one categorical-type variable with two levels, and one continuous-type variable that you have decided can be used in a parametric test.
- **Mann-Whitney *U* test** - used when you have one categorical-type variable with two levels, and one continuous-type variable that you have decided to use in a non-parametric test.

The second group of tests will entail examining average scores over time (e.g. Time 1 versus Time 2). These two tests are:

- **Paired-samples *t*-test** - used when you have the *same* continuous-type variable, administered on two occasions, and you have decided the data are suitable for use in a parametric test.
- **Wilcoxon sign-ranks test** - used when the *same* continuous-type variable has been administered on two occasions but you have decided to use the variables in a non-parametric test.

Tests that compare two groups of people on a continuous-type variable

These tests compare two groups of data on a continuous-type variable. A simple example of this would be male and female nurses (these are two groups: male nurses and female nurses) might be compared on their average wages to find out whether there are equal pay structures in the profession.

An example from the research literature of the way this type of test is used is provided in the study by Maureen Smith (2005). Smith wanted to examine whether encouragement and praise during an eye acuity test (a test for sharpness and clearness of eyesight) improved patients' performance. Therefore, she compared two groups of people who underwent eye examinations: one group received encouragement from the nurse (for example, 'Well done' and 'That was good, see if you can read any further') and the other group received no such encouragement. A group type of *t*-test would be used to compare the two groups on how well they did on the eye acuity test, with the expectation that the 'encouragement' group would have done better.

The two tests that fall into this group are:

- the independent-samples *t*-test – this is the parametric version within this group of tests;
- the Mann-Whitney *U* test – this is a non-parametric version within this group of tests.

A term that is used to sum up these types of tests is that they are tests dealing with independent groups/samples of data. In other words, whether your continuous variable is parametric or non-parametric, you, as researcher in this situation, are comparing two *independent* (or unrelated) groups of cases on the same variable (in our example, people who were encouraged by the nurse in the eye acuity tests and those that were not encouraged by the nurse in the eye acuity tests).

The independent samples *t*-test

The independent-samples *t*-test (see the box below for other names for this test) is used to compare mean scores for a continuous-type variable (that you want to treat as usable in a parametric test) across two levels of a categorical-type variable.

THINGS TO CONSIDER

Different names for the same independent-samples *t*-test

The independent-samples *t*-test is known by a number of names. These include unmatched *t*-test, *t*-test for two independent means, independent *t*-test, *t*-test for unrelated samples, and Student's *t*-test. Do not concern yourself; they all refer to the same test.

What the independent-samples *t*-test does is work out for each group the mean score on the continuous variable by each group and then calculate whether there is a difference between the group, by means of the *t* statistic (which looks at the scores, and the spread of scores) and significance testing (that is, working out whether any differences observed between the groups are not likely to have occurred by chance and we can be confident of our results). Let us work through an example with data in a table on how male and female patients have rated how well they can mobilise when

Table 9.6 Mean self-rated mobility scores according to patient's sex

Patients	Mean mobility ratings (and standard deviations in brackets)
Males (*N* = 14)	3.8 (1.3)
Females (*N* = 10)	3.6 (1.1)

NB *N* = the number of patients who rated themselves.
$t(22) = 0.2581, p = 0.343$.

using a new walking frame. These patients were able to rate themselves on a validated mobility scale from 1 ('Not at all') to 5 ('Very well') and therefore a higher score indicates high levels of mobility using the walking frame. Table 9.6 illustrates the mean scores for the male and female patients, along with the standard deviations for these mean scores.

Using 'describe and decide' to interpret the independent-samples *t*-test

Mean scores and standard deviations. These are the basis of our description. We note both the mean scores (with the standard deviation, which is a statistic that indicates the spread of scores) and which mean score is higher.

The *t value*. The statistical test statistic. Unlike correlation statistics, it is not important to note whether the *t* statistic is positive or minus. The *Sig. (2-tailed)*. The significance level. This is the probability level given to the current findings. The significance level found in the table above (Table 9.6) tells the researcher whether the difference noted between the means is significant. Remember, if this figure is below the $p = 0.05$ or $p = 0.01$ criterion then the finding is statistically significant. If this figure is above 0.05 then the findings are not statistically significant.

Therefore, the average mean score for males in terms of their mobility is 3.8 (with a standard deviation of 1.3). The mean score for females in terms of their mobility is 3.6 (with a standard deviation of 1.1). Next is the *t* value. The *t* value for the independent-samples *t*-test is 0.2581. This tells us very little at this stage. However, the significance level is 0.343, and therefore $p > 0.05$. Therefore, we conclude that there *is* no statistically significant difference between males and females for the number for their mobility.

Using 'describe and decide' to report the independent-samples *t*-test

The next stage is to report these statistics. There is a formal way of reporting the independent-samples *t*-test, which comprises two elements. First there is a formal statement of your statistics, which must include the following:

- *The test statistic*. Each test has a symbol for its statistic. The independent-samples *t*-test uses the symbol *t*. Your write-up must include what *t* is equal to. In the example above, $t = 0.2581$; however, we would abbreviate this to two decimal places, therefore $t = 0.26$.

- *The degrees of freedom*. For the independent-samples *t*-test, the degrees of freedom equal the size of your sample minus 2. Here, the minus 2 represents minus 1 for each sample, because you have asked only two sets of respondents (males and females). The figure is placed between the *t* and the equals sign and is written in brackets. Here the degrees of freedom are 22 (size of sample = 24, minus 2 = 22). Therefore, $t(22) = 0.26$.

The traditional way is to report whether your probability value is below 0.05 or 0.01 (statistically significant) or above 0.05 (not statistically significant). Here, you use less than ($<$) or greater than ($>$) the criteria levels. You state these criteria by reporting whether $p < 0.05$ (statistically significant), $p < 0.01$ (statistically significant) or $p > 0.05$ (not statistically significant). So in the example above, $p > 0.05$ and place this after the reporting of the *t* value. Therefore, with our findings, $t(22) = 0.26$, $p > 0.05$.

You can use all the information above to write a fairly simple paragraph which conveys your findings succinctly but effectively. Therefore, using the findings above, we might report:

> *An independent-samples t-test was used to examine statistically significant differences between males and females in terms of their mobility. Males (mean = 3.8, SD = 1.3) and females (mean = 3.6, SD = 1.1) did not score statistically significantly differently (t(22) = 0.26, p > 0.05) in terms of their mobility. This finding suggests that males and females in our sample did not differ significantly in their mobility.*

The Mann-Whitney *U* test

The Mann-Whitney *U* test is the non-parametric alternative to the independent-samples *t*-test. The Mann-Whitney *U* test is used to examine for statistically significant differences between two levels of a categorical variable on a continuous variable that is described as *non-parametric* data. When reporting the Mann-Whitney *U* test the procedure is much the same as the independent-samples *t*-test, but unlike its parametric counterpart, there are two differences. The first is the test statistic. The test statistic symbol is a *U*, rather than a *t*, but it works in much the same way.

The second difference is that, unlike the independent-samples *t*-test which reports the mean and standard deviations, here the descriptive statistics are mean ranks, which aren't as familiar or as informative to people. Therefore, some people prefer to give the median score along with the semi-interquartile range as an indicator of variability, as this is more informative. (We outlined the median and the semi-interquartile range in Chapter 8.) It is a temptation not to give the median score but rather the mean when performing the Mann-Whitney *U* test. Nonetheless, we would recommend that you consider providing this median and the semi-interquartile range instead of the mean rank scores as these are well-recognised indicators of average and variability (remember, we stressed the importance of providing variability statistics alongside average statistics in Chapter 8).

Tests that compare the same subjects on a continuous-type variable on two occasions

The two tests that fall under this category are the:

- **Paired-samples *t*-test** – used when you have the *same* continuous-type variable, administered on two occasions, and you have decided the data are suitable for use in a parametric test.
- **Wilcoxon sign-ranks test** – used when the *same* continuous-type variable has been administered on two occasions but you have decided to use the variables in a non-parametric test.

The paired-samples *t*-test

A paired-samples *t*-test is one test in which two sets of data on the same continuous variable are compared on two separate occasions (see the box below for the different names of this test). A simple example of using the paired-samples *t*-test would be when comparing the average ratings of patients of their pain (scored on a scale of 1 = No pain at all to 10 = A lot of pain) before, and after, taking a new drug designed to decrease pain.

THINGS TO CONSIDER

Different names for the paired-samples *t*-test

The paired-samples *t*-test goes under a number of different names. Sometimes the test is referred to as the related *t*-test, related samples *t*-test, paired test, dependent groups *t*-test, *t*-test for related measures, correlated *t*-test, matched-groups *t*-test and, most importantly for our needs, the paired-samples *t*-test. Don't worry. These are just different terms for the same test.

However, one point to note is that the matched-groups *t*-test is so named because the test is sometimes used under other circumstances. Sometimes researchers cannot administer the same measure twice to the same sample, and instead have to use two samples. Here, researchers will try to match their sample in as many ways as possible (it may be by variables such as sex, age, educational attainment, length in treatment, and so forth) to simulate using the same sample. On these occasions you will find researchers using a related *t*-test, referring to it as a matched-groups sample.

An example from the research literature, where this test might be used, was demonstrated by Christopher Hodgkins and his colleagues (Hodgkins *et al.*, 2005). Stress has been identified as an important issue among residential carers looking after individuals with learning disabilities. Staff were asked by Hodgkins and his co-workers to assess themselves on a measure of stress. The staff then underwent an intervention programme according to their needs in which it was ensured that they had support, such as appropriate training, regular staff meetings, reviews of internal procedures and guidance in counselling skills and how to respond to stressful situations. Three months later, staff assessed themselves again on the same measure of stress. This type of *t*-test would be used to compare the two occasions in term of people's scores, with the expectation that stress would be lower after the three-month period.

A term that is used to sum up these types of tests is that they are tests that are dealing with dependent groups of data. In other words, whether your continuous variable is parametric or non-parametric, you, as researcher in this situation, are comparing two dependent (or related) groups of cases on the same variable (in our example, the same group of carers *before* and *after* a clinical intervention).

To illustrate the paired-samples *t*-test, we will use the data from a fictitious clinical trial for patients with mental health problems. In this trial, 40 patients with schizophrenic disorders were given the antipsychotic medication, Olanzapine. Researchers are interested in finding out whether Olanzapine will make a difference to the level of psychotic symptoms that patients experienced. Researchers have devised a checklist to assess the patients' symptoms in four areas: paranoia, hallucinations, delusions of grandeur and disorders of streams of thought. Each part of the checklist is scored on a four-point scale ranging from 0 = Non-existent, 1 = Mild, 2 = Moderate to 3 = Severe. Responses are then totalled to provide an overall checklist score, with higher scores indicating a greater level of psychotic symptoms (with possible scores ranging from 0 to 12). Researchers want to test whether Olanzapine will decrease patients' psychotic symptoms scores (and please forgive the lack of a control group, for now we are only looking at the data for the people who were administered the drug). Therefore, they used the Psychotic Symptom Checklist with the 40 patients before Olanzapine was received, and then one day after they had received the medication to see what had happened to psychotic symptoms.

Using 'describe and decide' to interpret the paired-samples *t*-test

From the findings, you will need to consider three things:

1. *Mean scores and standard deviations.* These are the basis of our description. We note both the mean scores (with the standard deviation) and which mean score is higher; in this case, we want to know whether the psychotic symptoms are higher or lower when comparing before and after the administration of Olanzapine.

2. *The t value.* The test statistic.

3. *The significance level.* This is the probability level given to the current findings. The significance level tells the researcher whether the difference between the means is significant. Remember, if this figure is below the $p = 0.05$ or $p = 0.01$ criterion, then the finding is statistically significant. If this figure is above 0.05, then the finding is not statistically significant.

We can see from Table 9.7 that the mean score on the first administration of the psychotic symptoms checklist before the use of Olanzapine is 6.6 (with a standard deviation of 1.1) and the average mean score on the psychotic symptoms checklist after the use of Olanzapine on the second administration is 2.00 (with a standard deviation of 0.7) (note that all these figures are rounded to two decimal places). It

Table 9.7 Mean scores on Psychotic Symptoms Checklist when comparing before and after administration of Olanzapine

Phase of study trial	Mean psychotic symptoms checklist scores (and standard deviations)
Before	6.6 (1.1)
After	2.00 (0.7)

$t(39) = 2.104, p = 0.003.$

looks as if the psychotic symptoms checklist scores for the second phase are lower than for the first administration. The t value for the statistic is 2.104. This tells us very little at this stage. However, the significance level is $p < 0.05$. Therefore, we conclude that a statistically significant difference for mean scores exists between the two administrations of the psychotic symptoms checklist. This suggests that the dosage of Olanzapine had a statistically significant effect on lowering psychotic symptoms among the present sample.

Using 'describe and decide' to report the paired-samples t-test

The next stage is to report these statistics. There is a formal way of reporting the paired-samples t-test, which should include the following:

- *The test statistic.* Each test has a symbol for its statistic. The paired-samples t-test has the symbol t. Therefore, in your write-up you must include what t is equal to. In the example, $t = 2.104$.

- *The degrees of freedom.* For the paired-samples t-test, the degrees of freedom equal the size of your sample (which is 40) -1. Here, the minus 1 represents minus 1 for the sample, because you have asked only one set of respondents. This figure is placed between the t and the equals sign and is written in brackets. Here, the degrees of freedom are 39 (size of sample = 40, minus 1 = 39). Therefore, $t(39) = 2.104$.

- *The significance level.* You also need to use the traditional way of indicating whether the trend you have found is statistically significant in relation to whether your probability value is below 0.05 or 0.01 (statistically significant) or above 0.05 (not statistically significant). Here, you use less than ($<$) or greater than ($>$) the criteria levels. You state these criteria by reporting whether $p < 0.05$ (statistically significant), $p < 0.01$ (statistically significant) or $p > 0.05$ (not statistically significant). In the example above, as $p = 0.003$, we would write $p < 0.01$ and place this after the reporting of the t value. Therefore, with our findings, $t(39) = 2.104., p < 0.01.$

In writing up the report use the 'describe and decide' rule to inform the reader of your findings:

- Remind the reader of the two variables you are examining.
- Say which mean score is the higher.
- Tell the reader whether the finding is statistically significant or not.

You can use all the information above to write a fairly simple paragraph which conveys your findings succinctly but effectively. Therefore, using the findings above, we might report the following:

> *A paired-samples t-test was used to examine whether Olanzapine had a statistically significant effect on psychotic symptoms. A statistically significant difference (t(39) = 2.10, p < 0.05) was found for mean scores on a psychotic symptoms checklist, with mean scores for psychotic symptoms being statistically significantly lower for the second administration of the psychotic symptoms checklist (mean = 6.60, SD = 1.1) than for the first administration of the psychotic symptoms checklist (mean = 2.00, SD = 0.7). The current findings suggest that Olanzapine reduces psychotic symptoms.*

Wilcoxon sign-ranks test (non-parametric test)

The Wilcoxon sign-ranks test is the non-parametric alternative to the paired-samples *t*-test. It is used when you have measured the same continuous variable on two occasions among the same respondents and you do not wish to treat your continuous data as parametric. Whereas the paired-samples *t*-test was based on examining whether statistically significant differences occur between mean scores (with standard deviations), the Wilcoxon sign-ranks test, because the data are ranked, is based on examining statistically significant differences between average ranks. There is little other difference aside from the test statistic for the Wilcoxon sign-ranks test is a W (and not a *t* for the *t* test) and also, unlike its parametric counterpart, the paired-samples *t*-test which reports the mean and standard deviations, here the descriptive statistics include mean ranks, which aren't as familiar or as informative to people. Therefore, some people prefer to give the median score along with the semi-interquartile range as an indicator of variability, as this is more informative. It is a temptation not to give the median score but rather the mean when performing the test because sometimes it seems more meaningful. Nonetheless, we would recommend that you consider providing this median and the semi-interquartile range instead of the mean rank scores as these are well-recognised indicators of average and variability, and we stressed the importance of providing variability statistics alongside average statistics in Chapter 8.

Effect sizes for tests of differences

You may remember earlier in this chapter, we talked about effect sizes with correlations. Effect sizes can be used to estimate the magnitude or the importance, rather than just relying on significance. One handy thing you may want to know is that effect size can be calculated for tests of difference. The criteria are slightly different for tests of differences mentioned here. Cohen suggested that effect sizes of 0.2 to 0.5 should be regarded as 'small', 0.5 to 0.8 as 'moderate' and those above 0.8 as 'large'. To calculate the effect size for differences between two sets of scores, subtract the mean of one set of scores from the mean of the other set of scores, and then divide it by the standard deviation statistic for the total scores. This will give you your effect size.

Let us use an example of two means. The mean for group 1 = 2.9762 and the mean for group 2 = 2.1563, with an overall standard deviation for both groups of 1.24639.

Now we have all the information we need. So, we first subtract the mean of one group from the mean of the other (it doesn't matter which way round), but let us take the smallest from the largest, so 2.9762 − 2.1563 = 0.8199, then we divide that number by the overall standard deviation, 1.24639.

So 0.8199 divided by 1.24639 = 0.66 (rounded up to the nearest two decimal places). This means we have an effect size of 0.66, which is medium to large. When reporting it, you call it d. So here $d = 0.66$. So we know that the effect size for these means are medium (or moderate). Easy. You can also do this with the paired-samples t-test (although you may have to do some rearranging of data as they wouldn't all be in the same column). Nonetheless, you now know that if you do a series of t-tests, you can calculate the effect size to determine which is the most important finding.

Self-assessment exercise

This exercise is to get you using the research literature to identify and understand inferential statistics in research.

1. Your first task is to use either *Nursing Times* online or a library online database to find two research articles that include inferential statistics.

2. Having found these two articles, in the boxes below write the reference for that article, what inferential statistics are reported and what the inferential statistics tell us about the topic studied.

Article 1

Reference for the article:

_____

_____

What inferential statistics are reported?

_____

_____

_____

What do these inferential statistics tell us about the topic studied?

_____

_____

_____

Article 2

Reference for the article:

_____

_____

What inferential statistics are reported?

_____

_____

_____

What do these inferential statistics tell us about the topic studied?

_____

_____

_____

Summary

In this chapter you have been introduced to probability, significance, inferential statistics and the decision-making for choosing a specific statistical test. You should hopefully be better able to understand what is meant by terms such as distribution, probability and statistical significance testing; you should be able to understand the importance of probability values in determining statistical significance; you should be more aware about how to decide whether the use of a parametric or a non-parametric statistical test is needed and you should be able to determine whether a result is statistically significant or not. In this chapter you have also learnt the rationale for five statistical tests and how to interpret the results from these tests. These tests were: chi-square, Pearson product–moment correlation, Spearman's rho correlation, independent-samples t-test and paired-samples t-test.

In the next chapter, we will take you through how to critique studies that have used quantitative methods and we will show you what to look out for when critiquing a qualitative study, which we covered in Chapters 6 and 7.

Chapter 10

Critical appraisal of quantitative and qualitative research

KEY THEMES

Evaluation • Methodological rigour • Quantitative data • Qualitative data • Critical appraisal frameworks

LEARNING OUTCOMES

At the end of this chapter you will be able to:

- Understand that qualitative and quantitative studies are meant to answer different types of research questions and are thus judged by different standards.

- Apply critical appraisal criteria to evaluate qualitative research and quantitative studies that analyse relationships between variables that are naturally occurring (i.e. correlational data) or studies with an experimental/intervention design.

- Decide whether a study has met acceptable 'best practice' standards by using appropriate research design and analysis strategies.

Introduction

IMAGINE THAT . . .
You are a mental health nurse who is working with a service user who has chronic depression and is worried about the recent bad publicity on the medication that he is taking. The service user has heard that Seroxat (paroxetine) has been found to have side effects that are worrying him, especially in terms of feeling suicidal. How would you be able to draw on the 'best' evidence to reassure him or to give him choices on any other possible evidence-based medications to use for his depression?

Critical appraisal is a process of looking at a study, or groups of studies (e.g. systematic reviews of the literature) in a rigorous and methodical way. In this chapter, we will only be guiding you through the process of doing a critical appraisal with one study at a time, rather than doing an evaluation of how well systematic reviews have been done. Centrally, it involves a questioning element by systematically working through a series of questions (i.e. a critical appraisal framework) to weigh up a piece of evidence and assess its 'quality' by examining the strengths and limitations of the methods used and the reported findings within a particular context or setting. Importantly, it also allows you to evaluate whether the methods that have been used in a study or review are appropriate for the research question or proposed area of enquiry. One thing to bear in mind is that not all questions that are created for doing critical appraisal are created equally. For instance, you will soon be looking at whether a study has stuck to good principles of research design but, if the researchers have not followed accepted ethical practice, some of the findings might have to be treated with caution.

Although critical appraisal involves a distinct process the use of terminology may be confusing, implying for example that the process should be negative. This is not the case. With critical appraisal, you should not only be looking for the potential flaws in a study but rather should be examining the limitations *and* strengths of each study that you appraise. Critical appraisal may be more fruitfully viewed as casting a *critical eye*, by examining the evidence presented in an objective way, rather than accepting it at face value. All of this process enables you to interpret the evidence in a systematic way in terms of its overall quality and allows to you to judge the relevance of this evidence to your area of nursing practice.

In this chapter, we provide you with the fundamentals and equip you with the essential groundwork that you need to cover when evaluating different types of research evidence. For an in-depth treatment of how to do critical appraisal, you may want to read Greenhalgh (2001), which looks at a wide range of various types of studies or systematic reviews that a clinician can critically appraise.

10.1 Why should you use critical appraisal?

In an era of evidence-based practice, and the accompanying plethora of published materials, it is important that all nurses are aware of, *and* undertake, critical appraisal as a recognised part of their practice. It is important in terms of informing your nursing practice by accurately identifying and acting on up-to-date, relevant and clinically sound sources of information. It is also important in terms of developing dialogue amongst your colleagues to develop clinical practices and challenge the status quo in a health care team.

There are a variety of reasons for wanting to use critical appraisal techniques and these methods are important for you to be an effective nurse in dealing with patient enquiries and in ensuring that your clinical practice is based on the best evidence available. But how do you know that the evidence that you look at in a journal article is the best evidence? What makes it the 'best'? Some of you may think that the use of a bit of jargon like needing to implement 'best practice' is a useful concept and every nurse know what is meant when you, or other nurses, use this phrase. There's 'really bad' practice, 'okay' practice and 'best' practice, but which criteria do you use to tell the difference? Let's consider the following situations that you might encounter in which you'll need to be able to judge a research study and maybe use this as the basis for changing your own nursing practice or for recommending changes to practice amongst your colleagues.

Being posed difficult questions when working in clinical practice

As you can see, there are a variety of patient/service user queries that you may face as a nurse. For instance, as a health visitor, you may be advising parents to let their children have the all-in-one measles, mumps and rubella vaccine, but these parents could be very concerned about media coverage of the potential problems with doing this. Some of the parents may have heard about the debate on the safety of this triple vaccine (e.g. Wakefield *et al.,* 2004) and may be worried that their children could be at risk of getting autism or inflammatory bowel disorders. There are other instances, in which you could be dealing with service users who don't want to adopt a certain health-related behaviour because of a range of reasons, including social pressures, the healthier behaviour 'doesn't feel right' or is hard to maintain, etc., etc. . . For instance, as a health visitor, you are working with other health visitors and with midwives to promote breastfeeding among mothers. A mother may say the following to you,

> *How do you know that breastfeeding is best for my child? What evidence do you have to support this claim? Is all of the evidence supporting my use of breastfeeding? I know of mothers who don't breastfeed their children and their kids are still healthy!*

If the mother wanted you to show them a balanced perspective, some studies show-ing that breastfeeding can be beneficial versus those that show breastfeeding has a negligible effect on a baby's development compared to formula bottle feeding, would you know which studies to choose and how to evaluate these studies in a clear and concise way so that the mother understands the evidence in a balanced way? The mother is right in some senses, by looking at things that she has experienced or has been told about by other mothers. In some ways, you may also learn from experi-ences that you and your colleagues have had and these experiences could affect what you do in your everyday clinical practice. However, it would be dangerous for you to rely solely on personal experience or the experiences of other health profes-sionals, as you need to make sure you're acting on the best possible evidence to en-sure your practice is safe. This is why you need to be able to look at evidence that has been collected by expert researchers in the field so that you can compare their find-ings to your current ways of working. In this chapter, we will be showing you how to use a systematic method to do this evaluation (known as 'critical appraisal') with a range of studies.

Being clinically and professionally competent

As well as needing to respond to difficult patient/user queries, critical appraisal can be used to justify your nursing practice to your patients/service users and to your colleagues. If you can critically appraise research evidence, then you are well on your way to meeting professional standards of competence, such as those put forward by the Nursing and Midwifery Council (NMC, 2008); this is why critical appraisal is treated as so important as a skill within pre-registration and post-registration train-ing courses for nurses. By using critical appraisal, you can evaluate whether you have the best evidence available to you through examining the pros and cons of orig-inal research, literature reviews, sensationalised headlines or reports in the mass media, clinical guidelines, new treatments that have been commissioned by an NHS Trust or recommended by the National Institute for Health and Clinical Excellence (NICE). All of these things can be looked at by posing a series of questions in a sys-tematic manner.

Looking at better use of health care resources

Critical appraisal is a powerful tool because you can use it to argue for more re-sources to bring about more effective ways of treating patients or for working more efficiently and safely in your health care team. Perhaps you are an infection control nurse who is aiming to cut down on the number of hospital-acquired infections that are spread throughout the wards and you are trying to convince colleagues in the hospital to use alcohol-based hand-cleansing solutions - what is the evidence that these methods are as good as using soap and water? To have a bigger picture of the available evidence you may need to make sure you look further than asking 'does it work?'. You may need to ensure that you look at qualitative studies into the acceptability of alcohol-based hand-cleansers, because poor subjective experiences among patients or relatives or amongst the staff members themselves may make it difficult to implement a change in infection control as a result. For example, some Muslim health care staff and patients may not wish to come into any contact with alcohol and could view it as a practice that goes against the tenets of their religion (Ahmed *et al.*, 2006). This shows that, as nurses, you face unique challenges by needing to look at how widely applicable a certain health care practice can be; you may be able to find the best clinical evidence to support this practice, but the very important human elements, including cultural differences, may make it difficult for this practice to work in all settings and with all types of patients and service users.

Being able to judge studies as being credible

When critically appraising a piece of research, you will probably need to gauge how credible it might be. For instance, you could be asking whether the authors are sufficiently qualified and experienced in the area of interest (e.g. is there a leg ulcer specialist nurse who is part of the research team conducting a study into leg ulcer treatment?). You could also evaluate the credibility of a study by looking at how the project has been designed. By using the expertise that you will have gained from previous chapters, you should be able to spot whether the quantitative study has a case-control, or a cohort, or a cross-sectional or a randomised controlled trial design. You can query if researchers in a quantitative study have tried to remove any possible bias in how the data are collected, how participants responded when data were collected from them, and how the data are analysed. You should be able to decide whether the sample of participants in a quantitative study is large enough to come up with meaningful statistically or clinically significant findings. You should be looking out for whether there is a noticeable drop-out rate by participants in an experimental study or that there is a high enough response rate in a survey, for instance. You should be asking questions about how the researchers have come up with their conclusions and recommendations and whether these are linked to their findings in a clear and transparent way. Or does it look like the researchers have decided what they're going to recommend before they've even started collecting the data in the study? You should be able to appraise the credibility of a study by asking critical questions about which clinical settings the results can be applied to and considering about the types of patients with whom the same types of results would still be found. In other words, you could be asking questions about how reliable the research is.

We will cover more on the concept of reliability later in this chapter and show you how being reliable has many different parts to it, if you are evaluating research relevant to you as a nurse. We will also be looking at a related concept – validity – later in this chapter too. We will be seeing how validity and reliability are very important in nursing research and that different types of validity and reliability become more prominent depending on whether you are evaluating a qualitative or a quantitative study.

10.2 How do you *do* critical appraisal?

Initially, you need to make sure that you're doing critical appraisal with a quantitative or a qualitative study as they are judged by different criteria in terms of what makes up a rigorous and acceptable piece of research. From looking at earlier chapters in this book, you will know that different standards are used to judge the way that research is conducted and that different research questions will be addressed as well. When you wish to evaluate a study you will need to stick to the proper set of criteria in your critique. Of course, some studies may involve using quantitative and qualitative data analyses (known as 'mixed methods' designs, which we will look at later on in the book). As a result, you may need to use both sets of criteria for assessing different parts of this type of mixed methods study. First, we will look at the sorts of things that you should be looking for when critically appraising a quantitative piece of research.

Critical appraisal of quantitative studies

The general philosophy of quantitative research

Quantitative research in nursing involves looking at probabilities by looking at whether research findings are due to a chance result or because they are due to some real-life mechanisms that are at work. These real-life mechanisms are the sorts of 'laws' or 'principles' that a quantitative researcher is looking for. Questions are asked about whether the results would apply in all or most situations and with all, or most, people who are given the same intervention/treatment. This is really important in nursing because you would want to have some confidence that a specific treatment, like a dressing for a leg ulcer, will work for patients with a leg ulcer at a certain stage of healing. It is looking at these findings and seeing them occur consistently that should make you feel more certain next time you have a patient needing a similar dressing for a certain type of leg ulcer. In order to have confidence in the findings, you will also need to be reassured that there is a minimal chance of external factors having a biasing influence on the results. The importance of minimising bias in quantitative research was emphasised earlier in this book and it is vital that this is kept to a minimum, especially if you are interested in knowing whether a clinical intervention has had a substantial impact on people's health.

Putting numbers to your patient's/service user's experiences

Quantitative research is also underpinned by another set of assumptions, namely that the subject of study can be analysed as quantities through the use of statistics. In this way, a nurse researcher using a quantitative approach would often use 'how' to precede many of the research questions posed, such as the following:

- 'How long should a mother breastfeed for the infant to reap the physical (or psychological) benefits when compared to using bottle feeding?'
- 'How many side effects are found among patients who are treated with Haloperidol and experiencing acute psychotic episodes?'

- 'How severe is the pain experienced after an operation when a patient is given "I'm chilled out" (patent pending) pain relief when compared to "Ow-it hurts!" pain relief?'

- 'How likely is it that a 20-a-day smoker will give up smoking when using cognitive behavioural therapy when compared to the use of nicotine patches or willpower alone?'

- 'How often, and for how long, should a patient exercise when recuperating from an acute episode of myocardial infarction?'

As can be seen from the examples above, these sorts of questions are very different to the kinds of things that a qualitative nurse researcher would ask; whilst a quantitative study would involve asking how often or how severe something occurs, a qualitative study might entail looking at the human element of why people refuse to take certain medications, their perceptions of their health care, the meanings that they derive from having a specific illness or the motivations for undertaking a health-related behaviour like overeating. Quantitative studies would also require looking for differences or relationships between phenomena that vary (i.e. variables). When you're critically appraising quantitative studies, look to see whether the statistical tests are appropriate for the research questions being posed. As we covered earlier when discussing the use of inferential statistics, there are certain kinds of tests that should be done on specific types of data and in line with a certain kind of question. For example, studies that look for *differences* between various patient groups (e.g. one group that has had treatment X versus one group that has had a placebo) might use an independent-samples *t*-test. Likewise, other research focusing on comparing differences over time could entail using the related *t*-test that we covered in the chapter on inferential statistics. Overall, it is crucial to look out for what questions the researchers are analysing – are they looking for differences or relationships? In other studies using quantitative methods, relationships between variables might be analysed with tests like chi-square statistics, correlations (e.g. Spearman's rho or Pearson's *r*), or other similar statistics.

Validity

Validity is defined simply as 'measuring what you're intending to measure'. However, there is more to validity than just this. From a nursing researcher's perspective, it should be recognised that there are many different types of validity and these ways of looking at validity may have an impact on how much credibility you give to a particular study. Some of the various kinds of validity that researchers look for include:

- **External validity:** this is also called **ecological validity** and refers to the degree with which the findings can be generalised to other groups of people and how representative the sample in a current study might be.

- **Construct validity:** this can sometimes be found when researchers use a statistical technique like factor analysis to look at the underlying concepts relating to a specific phenomenon, such as the experience of burn-out among nurses; for example, researchers (Maslach and Jackson, 1986) used this technique of factor analysis with data from those in the helping professions to find that there are three main components to these people being burned out – (1) emotional exhaustion (i.e. feeling drained and emotionally numb), (2) depersonalisation of service users (i.e. not seeing the service users as human beings after a while) and (3) feelings of not achieving much at all.

- **Criterion validity:** this can be found when using a new measurement tool and judging how effectively it matches up to a well-established measure, such as by comparing a new measure designed to look at depression among older adults with something like the Beck Depression Inventory (BDI; Beck, *et al.*, 1996).
- **Face validity:** this is sometimes also called 'acceptability', but is probably the least acceptable form of validity because it is often not subjected to any form of statistical analyses to enable people to differentiate between various levels of this type of validity. Instead, with face validity, a tool is shown to people who have a stake in studying the phenomenon and these people give their views on how well they believe this tool seems to measure the phenomenon, on the face of it.

Validity is not necessarily to do with an instrument and way of measuring; it's also to do with whether the instrument is making valid assessments with different groups of people.

Reliability

Reliability is also important in nursing research for a number of reasons. First, if you're using an instrument in a study, you need to have the confidence that it will produce the same, or very similar, results time and time again. Second, you will also be interested in getting the same, or very similar, findings if someone else used the same instrument with the same participants. The first type of reliability that we have just mentioned is known as test-retest reliability. If we assume that a patient's temperature has not changed in the time that you first tested her, we should expect the same results the next time we test this person. However, if the instrument has poor test-retest reliability, this would mean wildly different results when doing the measuring, even when the participant's state has not changed. With the second type of reliability, this is known as inter-rater reliability, which means that two people who are doing the testing of the same research participant with the same instrument should get very similar findings. In both cases of these two types of reliability, there is a correlation that is calculated. This correlation is analysed between the first time of testing and the second time (i.e. test-retest) and the first person in relation to the second person doing the testing (i.e. inter-rater); the higher the correlation, the more reliable the test.

Another concept to bear in mind with quantitative studies is the need to do a partial replication of a study's research findings, but in another setting or with a similar group of participants (see the box below on problems with publishing identical replications of the same study in different journals). An example of a partial replication of a study would be to see whether the Edinburgh Postnatal Depression Scale (EPDS) (Cox *et al.*, 1987) is sufficiently sensitive to pick up risk of postnatal depression in teenage mothers and also among mothers from ethnic minorities.

THINGS TO CONSIDER

Publication biases with replication studies

When it comes to replicating a study, you need to recognise that journal editors rarely publish an article that just reproduces exactly the same study that has already been done and published with the same type of research participants. Instead, journal editors are often looking for something that is a bit more original so you will often see partial replications of studies that have been done before, rather than exact replications. An example of a partial replication of a study would be when researchers are trying out the same study design but with the addition of some variables that were not examined in the previous study.

Overall, we can see that there are potential pitfalls to address when doing a quantitative study, particularly in terms of threats to validity and reliability. Let us now introduce you to a critical appraisal framework (i.e. a set of questions) to use systematically when going through an article that describes using an intervention or experiment.

10.3 Top ten issues to consider with quantitative studies using an intervention

When doing a critical appraisal with an experimental/intervention-type study, we need to make sure that we are asking questions relating to keeping many things in the study as consistent as possible. It is important to minimise any intrusion from other variables that might influence how much of an effect an intervention has on a health-related outcome. By using the critical appraisal framework in Table 10.1, you should be able to gauge how good the study has been in minimising bias and other threats to how valid and reliable the study might be.

We will now expand on the issues that are raised in the framework in Table 10.1 so you can be sure about what things you need to look out for.

1. *Removing bias.* Are the people collecting the data and the participants 'blind' to the study hypotheses and the experimental conditions, or is it likely that either data collectors or participants can guess the purpose of the study? Are participants randomly allocated into the different groups or is there a possibility of them being able to select which group they go into (i.e. self-selection bias)?

2. *Having a benchmark.* Is there a control (or comparison) group so that you can see how the intervention compares with a treatment standard and/or no treatment at all? Is it possible that there may be a placebo effect (Harrington, 1997) in which treatment of any form will have a beneficial effect on the participants?

Table 10.1 Critical appraisal of a quantitative intervention study

Issue to address	Questions to answer	Where to look
1. Bias	Is it a single-blind (i.e. participants are unaware of the hypothesis) or double-blind (i.e. participants and persons collecting the data are unaware of the hypothesis) design?	Method
2. Benchmarks	Is there a control group? Is there a way of comparing participants before and after they have received the intervention?	Method
3. Sampling and sample size	Is there a large enough sample to find a statistically significant effect? Are there enough participants to detect a clinically significant effect?	Method
4. Use of objective indicators	Have objective indicators of a person's health been taken, if appropriate?	Method
5. Analyses appropriate	Are differences being analysed (e.g. before versus after *or* control group versus the group with the intervention)?	Method and results
6. Transparency	Was the procedure clear and replicable?	Method
7. Variables	Have the researchers openly excluded certain people from taking part (e.g. those with heart problems)? Have some variables been statistically controlled (e.g. looking out for personality factors that might affect how people respond to a treatment)? Have the people in the control group and experimental (intervention) groups been matched according to their demographic background?	Method and results
8. Psychometrics (validity/reliability)	How valid and reliable are the instruments/measures that have been used in the study?	Method
9. Effects: long-lasting	Have the researchers looked at the long-lasting effects of the intervention by tracking changes in the participants over a meaningful and substantial period of time?	Results and discussion
10. Effects: knock-on	Have the researchers used counterbalancing when interventions follow a certain sequence (e.g. therapy A then therapy B)?	Results and discussion

3. *Sample size.* Does it look like the researchers have collected data from a large enough sample to find a clinically significant effect? (See Chapter 10 of Maltby *et al.*, 2007 for how you can calculate this.)

4. *Objective indicator variables.* Have the researchers obtained information about the physiological status of a patient/service user (e.g. heart rate), as well as measuring something a bit more subjective (e.g. pain ratings), or do the researchers

rely solely on subjective data? Other very acceptable objective indicators could include measures of blood pressure, size of pressure sore, body temperature.

5. *Appropriate analyses.* Does it look like the researchers are looking at relationships between variables when they should be looking at *differences* between conditions (e.g. treatment vs. placebo, health before treatment vs. health after treatment)?

6. *Transparency.* Was the procedure for conducting the study very clear and easy to reproduce with another set of participants?

7. *Variables included/excluded.* Have the researchers been open about the criteria for deciding on which people to include in, or exclude from, the study? Has there been any statistical control for any variables that might have a biasing effect? For example, maybe people with high levels of a personality trait (e.g. high levels of anxiety-proneness) will react less well in response to a drug intended to calm a patient's nerves. Have the researchers measured all, or most, of the variables that could affect how well the intervention works out? Has there been a process of matching people in a control group and the experimental group in terms of their demographic variables (e.g. age, sex, amount of time with a certain health condition, etc.)?

8. *Validity/reliability of variables measured.* Have there been prior studies into how valid a specific scale of measurement has been or has the instrument been relatively untested? Has the instrument been tested with various populations (i.e. the general population or with clinical or subclinical groups)?

9. *How long-lasting is the intervention and its effects?* Does it take a series of treatments before the intervention's benefits take hold or are there some short-term effects as well? For example, if studying how effective having postnatal 'listening visits' are with women at risk of postnatal depression, it might be wise to ensure that data are collected at a range of time points to pick up short-term, medium-term and longer-term effects of the intervention on the well-being of these women.

10. *Knock-on effects.* In a similar vein, you may need to consider whether the order in which a certain intervention is administered could have an effect on the outcome of the study. For example, if a group of mental health care users with a generalised anxiety disorder are given initially some medication to enable them to relax more effectively and then systematic de-sensitisation therapy to target their anxieties, it might be useful to counterbalance this design so that half of the participants in this group receive the therapy first and the medication afterwards.

10.4 Top ten issues to consider with quantitative studies using correlational data

When doing critical appraisal of a study in which data are correlated with each other, we need to bear in mind that there is no experimental manipulation of people being allocated into different groups and that the researchers are mainly just looking at variables as they naturally occur with each other. In Table 10.2 we provide you with a

Table 10.2 Critical appraisal of a quantitative correlational study

Issue to address	Questions to answer	Where to look
1. Rationale for research questions	Can the researchers justify why they are looking for a certain type of correlation between variables?	Introduction
2. Differences vs. relationships	Are the researchers looking for relationships or differences between variables?	Introduction and results
3. Psychometrics (validity/reliability)	Is the study being used to look at the validity or reliability of a measure?	Introduction and results
4. Not considering a third variable	Are the researchers assuming that the relationship between two variables is meaningful or have they looked for a possible third variable?	Results and discussion
5. Common method variance	Have the researchers only used one method of measurement (e.g. just using a self-report questionnaire)?	Method
6. Multicollinearity	Do some of the variables correlate really highly?	Results
7. Doing too many correlations	Have the researchers correlated variables together on the basis of a solid theoretical background?	Method and results
8. Causality vs. causation	Is correlation being interpreted as causality?	Results and discussion
9. Wrong variables types for a correlation	Have the researchers tried to do a correlation between inappropriate types of variables (e.g. nominal variables related to variables measured on an interval or ratio scale)?	Method and results
10. Too sensitive a measure	Have some of the variables been measured with too sensitive a scale (e.g. looking at a patient's pain on a 100-point scale)?	Method

checklist of the sorts of issues that need to be addressed in this kind of study and the sorts of questions you might ask.

We will explore the issues/questions to consider when using this critical appraisal framework in more detail below:

1. *Not having a rationale behind formulating a one-tailed hypothesis for a correlation* (e.g. expecting patient condition to *improve* with treatment X, rather than being open to the possibility that treatment condition could deteriorate as well).

2. *Are the researchers looking at relationships and not differences?*

3. *Is research being used to assess the validity or reliability of a measure?* If wishing to look at test-retest reliability of a tool, it will be important to have more than one time point for measuring the participants, there should be a sufficient time gap so that the previous attempt at measurement does not affect the next period of measurement, and also there should be no anticipated changes in the participant's status regarding the specific concept being measured in the interim period between measurements; we can ask various other questions about the ways in which the researchers have been looking for validity or reliability of the

measurements being taken. These measurements often involve analysing the relationships between variables.

4. *Not taking into account the presence of a third variable.* Is there any consideration of a third variable that could account for the relationship between two variables? For example, if a research team was to come to the conclusion that improvements to the eyesight among older patients was able to decrease the number of falls they had, this might be missing out other crucial variables, like how easily each patient can mobilise. Another instance of falling into the trap of assuming a link between two variables might be in assuming that increased treatments for cancer of chemotherapy can lead to an increase in survival rates when this link might miss out the vital variables of type of cancer or how severe the malignancy of the cancer has been.

5. *Common method variance.* This occurs when there are several variables correlated together and they are all obtained via the same measure (e.g. a self-report questionnaire); this is a problem because the measure itself may have an influence on how people respond when participating in a study, so there is usually a need for other objective measurements (e.g. physiological indicators of blood pressure or of heart health through saliva samples) or other supplementary subjective measures to be taken, so that people's responses are not solely affected by the common method being used.

6. *Multicollinearity.* This is more of a statistical point, but is important because you might have two variables that correlate very highly such as with a correlation of 0.80 or higher (Bryman and Cramer, 1997). If the two variables are that strongly correlated, it might not make much sense to treat the variables as two separate entities.

7. *Doing too many correlations.* This occurs when doing so many correlation analyses that some significant relationships are bound to be detected; if anything, there needs to be some form of theoretical rationale for looking at relationships between certain variables, rather than going for a fishing expedition when doing the analysis and being happy with whatever you catch!

8. *Is correlation being interpreted as causality?* It should be noted that the variables might be measured at the same time so we might not necessarily be able to infer that one variable causes the other variable to change.

9. *Using the wrong kinds of data combinations.* For example, using nominal data (e.g. categories) and correlating these data with scale data (e.g. interval or ratio units of measurement). This sort of correlation isn't particularly meaningful; if researchers were to correlate a nominal variable with three categories (e.g. whether a person is an inpatient, an outpatient, or not receiving any treatment) and any other variable such as pain levels, this would not make much sense. Instead, it would probably be better to look at **differences** in pain levels with this particular variable of patient type.

10. *Having a too sensitive scale of measurement that picks up significant relationships with virtually everything.* For example, measuring pain or a scale of 1-100 may pickup very minor changes, while using a scale 1-5 may not be sensitive enough to changes.

10.5 Critical appraisal of qualitative studies

As we mentioned previously, there are distinct differences between qualitative and quantitative research and this is experienced through the methods that are utilised and arguably more centrally through the particular 'lens' or way that the researcher views the social world. Unlike positivist approaches, in which it is assumed that there is an objective reality that is visible, measurable, and can be repeated in a variety of settings, qualitative researchers are likely to argue against the use of quantitative methods with human beings. These researchers would argue that the quantitative methods of the natural sciences are not entirely appropriate for studying individual experiences and their perspectives of their own worlds.

At first glance, critical appraisal of qualitative studies may appear to be less clearly defined than its quantitative counterpart. For example, there is an absence of percentages and numbers, and researchers appear more concerned with the 'richness' of the data collected rather than the generalisability and replicability of a study. As we will discuss in the course of this section, these concepts are not redundant but rather are interpreted and applied in a different way. You are unlikely to find control groups or randomisation but rather descriptions of participants and purposive sampling. However, this does not mean that qualitative studies are less rigorous. The rigour and reliability of qualitative studies still needs to be transparent and open to scrutiny; however the criteria for establishing academic and practice rigour will be different. Therefore, while critical appraisal of qualitative evidence will share some of the facets with quantitative work, there are also clear differences.

In a similar vein to critical appraisal of quantitative literature there needs to be a systematic approach to the appraisal process. Unlike quantitative studies, where research design issues of avoiding bias might appear more black and white, qualitative researchers have a more difficult task to justify the methods they have used. Qualitative research has been based on a number of different philosophical approaches to seeing, measuring and interpreting people's social worlds. Despite this diversity of approaches in qualitative research, there still needs to be some form of clarity when reporting the ongoing processes of data description, analysis, synthesis, and theory-generation; this is what you should seek to become more clear about when doing critical appraisal of such studies.

A critical appraisal framework for evaluating qualitative research

The following framework will help you to systematically consider the quality of qualitative studies. In Table 10.3, you can see the main issues that you need to address, the questions to be answered, and the typical sections in a research report or article where you might find answers to the critical appraisal questions.

A more in-depth overview of the issues raised in this critical appraisal framework is presented after Table 10.3.

Table 10.3 Critical appraisal of a qualitative study

Issue to address	Questions to answer	Where to look
1. Authors	Who are the authors and what is their background? Have they published work elsewhere in this field?	Near the title or at the end of the paper
2. Aims	Has the aim of the study been clearly defined? Are the aims justified with reference to the supporting literature and presented succinctly within the opening 'background' section?	Introduction/ end of literature review
3. Background	Does the background literature provide a clear rationale and/or links to the development of the present study?	Introduction or literature review
4. Design	Do the research methods chosen support the research question, i.e. is a qualitative approach appropriate in this instance?	Method/ methods/ methodology
5. Ethics	Have the general and particular ethical issues arising from the study been identified and adequately addressed?	Method/ methods/ methodology
6. Sample and sampling	Where was the sample (the participants) sited and do the authors explain why a particular site was chosen? Who was selected and how were they selected to take part in the study? How was the final sample size chosen?	Method/ methods/ methodology
7. Data collection and analysis	Is the overall process involved in data collection clear or 'transparent' for the reader? Does data collection address the original research question or field of exploration? How was data analysis undertaken and what methodologies informed this process? How rigorous was the data analysis process? Does it just look like the themes that have 'emerged' are just a result of the types of questions asked? Do the authors address issues of transferability and trustworthiness?	Methods and findings
8. Data presentation	Are sufficient data, including the full range of responses, presented to support the findings as stated by the authors?	Findings (maybe discussion if merged with findings)
9. Findings placed in context	Do the authors contextualise their findings within the existing literature?	Discussion
10. Role of researcher/s	What is the relationship of the researcher to the people being researched?	Methods or discussion

1. Authors

Who are the authors and what is their background? Have they published work elsewhere in this field? Both of these questions will help to establish the past experience and particular standpoint or academic perspective of the authors. However, this is not crucial, as there are many first time and novice authors who publish material of an extremely high quality, for example the findings of research dissertations and theses.

2. The aim of the study

Has the aim of the study been clearly defined by the authors? The aim of the study should be clearly defined through the title, abstract and where included keywords, which will also indicate for example the subject area and methodology. However, if you have conducted a literature search by using electronic databases like CINAHL or PubMed, you will have experienced the phenomenon whereby the title may sometimes not truly reflect the study or topic under consideration.

Although this may seem to be common sense, it is important to consider the aim of the study, that is, what the paper seeks to explain or illuminate should also be clearly stated in the 'aims' section of the paper. This is important later on when you consider the data and discussion as you will need to consider if the study as a whole has met the aims as stated at the beginning.

Are the aims of the study justified with reference to the supporting literature and presented succinctly within the opening 'background' section? This is important for several reasons. First, it will help the reader to contextualise the work, for example, even if you are unfamiliar with the area under study you should be able to understand the key theories and arguments being discussed in the Introduction/Literature review section. This, in turn, should help you to understand the way in which the authors have developed their thinking and led to the generation of research questions, in light of the existing literature by identifying links and gaps for further exploration.

3. Background literature

Does the background literature provide a clear rationale and/or links to the development of the present study? The background literature section also provides the forum for the authors to provide an account of the development of their work, for example, comparing the data collected with prior research and theory and being able to establish whether new ground is being covered in the study. There is an ongoing process from study design to write-up of engaging with the literature in terms of going from description to interpretation. The literature review will also enable the reader to see how the researchers have developed their own work in light of the existing literature. For example, in a study that explored the experiences of older informal carers, McGarry and Arthur (2001) used the existing literature regarding informal caregiving as a whole to develop their work while considering the particular situation of older people.

4. Study design

Do the research methods chosen support the research question, i.e. is a qualitative approach appropriate in this instance? While traditionally qualitative and quantitative research methodologies were seen as being at opposing ends of the research spectrum, within contemporary frameworks it is now widely acknowledged that different methods are appropriate for different kinds of investigation rather than issues of credibility *per se*. As such, researchers will need to justify their choice of methodology within the context of the phenomena under study. In contrast to quantitative studies, qualitative studies do not generally encompass issues relating to quantification or number in the same way. However, irrespective of the underpinning methodology a good qualitative study design will enable the reader to make clear links between the research question and the choice of research method or approach. As you will already know from previous chapters, qualitative methods are concerned with using an 'interpretative approach' which is about understanding the meanings that people attach to particular phenomena within their social worlds, for example beliefs regarding illness or ageing.

5. Ethical issues

Have the general and particular ethical issues arising from the study been identified and adequately addressed? Similar ethical considerations will need to be addressed irrespective of the methodology and research methods utilised and these should be clearly stated within the paper, for example, ethical approval, informed consent and confidentiality. However, in addition, any particular issues arising from the specific methods utilised within the study should also be addressed within this section. For example, the nature of fieldwork within the sphere of qualitative research, the relationship between the researcher and the researched (a point we will return to later) and the potentially sensitive nature of the data collected through personal disclosure or observation will need to be considered.

6. Sampling

Where was the sample (the participants) sited and do the authors explain why a particular site was chosen? Sampling in qualitative studies encompasses both the study site and the participants. As we mentioned earlier, sampling in qualitative research is a central issue, but unlike its quantitative counterpart does not usually involve the same issues, for example randomisation. Sampling within qualitative research is more concerned with selecting individuals who are likely to be able to inform the development of the study, while ensuring that the sample includes a representative group of the phenomena under study.

Who was selected and how were they selected to take part in the study? There are a number of ways in which potential participants may be selected to take part in qualitative research and this will be dependent upon a number of issues, for example, accessibility and time and resources available. You may come across a number of terms when reading papers and studies and we have included a few of the main terms:

- *Purposive sampling:* participants are specifically chosen because they share commonalities which the researcher wishes to explore in-depth, for example, socio-economic characteristics or particular experiences, such as being informal caregivers.

- *Snowball sampling:* existing participants are asked to identify further potential participants who 'fit' the particular study criteria.

- *Convenience sampling:* is as it sounds and is based on ease of access to potential participants.

All of these approaches have their merits and shortfalls and the authors will need to clearly explain the thinking behind their choice of sampling strategy.

How was the final sample size chosen? Irrespective of the sampling strategy, researchers will still need to justify their final choice of sample and size. Qualitative researchers refer to 'saturation' of data to describe the point at which they do not uncover any new insights from the data. However, researchers may also be restricted by time and resources. This does not necessarily mean that the study is not credible, but as before will need to explain the thinking behind the decision for the approach.

7. Data collection and analysis

Is the overall process involved in data collection clear or 'transparent' for the reader? The overall process of data collection should be clearly defined for the reader. Specific areas, for example the setting, the type of data collected and how it was managed all need to be explained adequately. This will include the consideration of how data were collected, for example did researchers use a field journal? Were data recorded and transcribed?

Does data collection address the original research question or field of exploration? As the research unfolds it is also important that the researchers are able to show that they have remained focused towards the original research question or area of exploration.

How was data analysis undertaken and what methodologies informed this process? Within the tradition of qualitative research, data collection and analysis do not comprise distinct facets of the research process but rather 'inform' each other in terms of the direction of the developing research. For example, issues may come to light during data collection which the researcher would like to pursue further with other participants or through the research. You may come across the term 'iterative' and this is often used to describe the interrelated processes of data collection and analysis.

How rigorous was the data analysis process? It isn't enough for researchers to state that the findings simply 'emerged' from the data and while qualitative researchers remain 'true' to the original data, there is still an element of interpretation within the process. As such, the authors should be able to explain to the reader how the analysis was undertaken and what type of framework or theoretical model informed this process.

Do the authors address issues of transferability and trustworthiness? This is a central issue when assessing the quality of the paper as a whole. Within qualitative research the term 'transferability' is often used to describe the extent to which the findings of the study may be 'transferred' to other populations or the wider population from which the sample has been drawn, quantitative researchers may refer to this as 'generalisation'. However, transferability has to be treated with a certain amount of caution as qualitative research is largely context-specific and therefore cannot be applied broadly without careful thought.

In quantitative research you will have come across the terms reliability and validity, within qualitative research these terms have been called into question with researchers preferring other terms, for example, 'trustworthiness'.

8. Presentation of the findings

Are sufficient data, including the full range of responses, presented to support the findings as stated by the authors? In presenting the findings the authors should include a range of responses, including any differences of perspectives, therefore ensuring that the data as a whole are representative of the perspectives of the participants as a whole.

9. Discussion and conclusion

Do the authors contextualise their findings within the existing literature? Do the authors highlight the limitations of the study and possible developments arising from the findings? It is important that the authors engage with the literature in order to look at similarities with previous findings, and where the study has contributed to the knowledge base in a particular topic or field of study.

10. The role of the researcher

What is the relationship of the researcher to the people being researched? With qualitative studies, some of the ways that we can test out whether these criteria can be met are through looking at issues through reflexivity. Reflexivity means taking a step back, reflecting, and considering one's position in relation to the people being researched and choice of research topic. A good qualitative study will involve this process of being reflective and the researchers should consider some of the following (see McGarry, 2007b):

- *Motivations:* what motivated the researchers to study this area? Is it because they have experienced this phenomenon in clinical practice? Is it the concerns of their patients/service users that have led to the researchers being interested in this area? Do the researchers have an emotionally rooted basis for doing the study (e.g. being upset at the number of men who leave it very late to seek help with possible testicular cancer)?

- *Production of data:* what might motivate participants to take part in the study? How does the participant view the researchers? Do participants see this as an opportunity to spread their world-view to others (e.g. some parents may feel driven to share their experiences with others and explain why they don't wish to give their children the MMR vaccine)? Might the participants view the researchers with an air of caution, particularly if the qualitative study involved observation of clinical practices being employed by nurses? Some nurses being observed may be anxious about whether their practice is being judged as unsafe or not sufficiently evidence-based. If this were the case, the researchers may need to reflect on how they are positioned in relation to the participants and how the participants may be reacting as a response to this positioning.

- *The social context of the study:* what is the significance of the geographical space and the era within which the study has been conducted? For example, within the UK it may be perfectly normal to wish to examine people's views concerning the ban on smoking in enclosed, public spaces, whereas this may be looked upon with some amusement in countries where such a ban is not being debated or even considered!

Self-assessment exercise

Using the critical appraisal framework with a qualitative study

An excerpt from the following brief fictionalised article is meant to reflect the kind of issues to look out for when doing critical appraisal with a qualitative study. The excerpt is deliberately in need of some improvement and we have highlighted with **CA** (critical appraisal) where there might be issues that need addressing or where the article looks to have met some of the criteria in the critical appraisal framework. It is purposefully brief (method and findings section included only) so that you can have a quick skim through and try to spot some of the main points covered in the critical appraisal framework. Have a go at using the framework for qualitative research from Table 10.3 with this article. Our suggested answers are in the answers section at the end of the book.

Fictionalised article

Postnatal depression among fathers – a grounded theory analysis

End of Introduction section:

The aims **[CA1]** of the study were to:

- Explore **[CA2]** the particular experiences of first-time fathers
- Describe the issues that impact on the ways that new fathers perceive their role within the family
- Discuss the implications for health care professionals in terms of recognising the key issues and supporting new fathers

---

Methods

Participants

Eight men were interviewed during the first six months of fatherhood. They were recruited among a population of 50 men who had reported feelings of depression to the health visitor or general practitioner. The services provided by the local Primary Care Trust were used as a means for recruiting possible participants. [CA3] Participants were selected by using purposive sampling. Firstly, they needed to be first-time fathers; secondly, their experiences of depression was not supposed to be acute and severe in nature; thirdly, they were only supposed to be on medication for their depression and should not have received any psychotherapy prior to participation in case the psychotherapy interfered with their perceptions of the depression; fourthly, and finally, the potential participants needed to have identified their depression as being linked to the event of becoming a father for the first time. [CA4] Only eight participants were needed in this study, as we reached a state of data saturation in which the fathers were providing very similar accounts of their experiences and no new insights were emerging.

Procedure

Before the study could commence, ethical approval [CA5] needed to be obtained from the Trust's Local Research Ethics Committee. Safeguards were put in place to protect the well-being of the participants so that they had a confidential helpline to use at any time after being contacted about participation. Participants were debriefed at the end of the study so that their well-being was checked and they were still comfortable with the interview data being used for this project. They were given the option to withdraw their data from consideration at various stages up until the write-up of the project findings. The interviews were carried out within the participants' homes [CA6] and would follow a semi-structured format by using an interview schedule with questions touching on the cognitive, affective (i.e. emotional), and behavioural effects of postnatal depression on each participant's well-being. Interviews took an average of 15 minutes to conduct, [CA7] with the longest interview being 30 minutes and the shortest one being 10 minutes. By cognitive effects of depression, we asked about how being a parent has adversely affected the way in which the participant views the world. In terms of affective and behavioural symptoms of postnatal depression, we asked the participants about how they felt and how they acted when they were depressed as a consequence of parenthood.

Analyses

The data were recorded verbatim on a dictaphone and were analysed using a recognised analytical framework. A grounded theory approach was used for the analysis. This meant that we needed to focus primarily on producing an account of these participants' experiences and perceptions based purely on *their* perceptions rather than on our own perspectives of the phenomenon of postnatal depression among fathers. [CA8]

Findings

Three main themes emerged from the grounded theory analysis – cognitive, affective and behavioural symptoms [CA9] of postnatal depression. In the following excerpts, we report illustrative quotes that were taken from the interviews and epitomised each of the themes.

▶

Cognitive symptoms

Several fathers reported feelings of self-doubt and their perceptions of the world had changed in an adverse way too. Typical concerns involved the following comments including, 'My world had changed for the worse. I didn't know what my role was in the family any more' (Participant #2, lines 18-20) and '. . . when my child was crying, I no longer saw the world as one that I could control' (Participant #3, line 99) and 'I don't think I'm doing things right. Everything seems so confusing' (Participant #5, lines 5-6).

Affective symptoms

Postnatal depression manifested itself with emotional components too. Some participants reported feelings of worthlessness, generalised anxiety and psychosomatic symptoms such as experiencing migraine attacks and irritable bowel problems. A comment from one participant typified the affective component of his postnatal depression:

> 'I just felt anxious all of a sudden and was sweating buckets! My heart was pounding really fast and I couldn't really focus on any one thing. I felt like such a worthless wimp and didn't feel like a man anymore' (Participant #1, lines 31-35).

Behavioural symptoms

The behavioural symptoms of postnatal depression among these men took many different forms and related to these men doing things that they wouldn't ordinarily do. Sometimes these men would begin crying openly when they had some time to be alone. They would also display some behavioural problems, such as avoiding going home and also consuming more alcohol and smoking more tobacco than they usually would do. One participant reported some of the following dysfunctional ways of behaving in response to become a father:

> 'I spend more time at work, you know? I make excuses with her so that I can stay on at work. I don't like to let my wife know that I'm feeling down and I often try to avoid getting intimate with her any more. If this is what it's like with one child then heaven help us if we have any more! When I tried to hold this child one time, it started crying so much, that I wouldn't want to hold it for a good few days after that . . .' (Participant #8, lines 56-60).

Summary

In this chapter we have introduced you to the concept of critical appraisal and why this process is vitally important for you to make sure your practice is evidence-based and that you have assessed research according to appropriate standards. Through showing you three different critical appraisal frameworks, you should have a template of questions or issues to raise when critiquing at least three different types of research studies. We have given you critical appraisal frameworks for studies that (1) use an experiment or intervention, (2) that analyse naturally occurring data (i.e. correlational study) and (3) that use qualitative methods. We will now move on to further issues relating to the communication of research findings but in the following chapter we will equip you with the skills you will need when communicating your research to others at conferences or in other published formats.

Chapter 11

Presenting your work to others

KEY THEMES
Dissemination • Research report writing • Journal article writing •
Oral presentations • Poster presentations

LEARNING OUTCOMES
By the end of this chapter you will be able to:

- Write a research report of a quantitative or qualitative study by following a recommended structure

- Know about how to write the key sections of a research report, which comprises the abstract/summary, introduction, methodology/method, results/findings and discussion

- Be aware of what one should expect from a research report

- Understand the key principles of making an effective oral presentation of your research

- Apply key principles for effective design of a research poster.

Introduction

IMAGINE THAT . . .

You are a research nurse who has completed a project into the most effective method of leg ulcer care; you have designed the study, collected the data and analysed the data; you have obtained findings that point to using a specific type of compression bandaging to help the healing rate of patient leg ulcers. You might think that the hard work has been done (in a sense, much of it has) but you still need to convince other nurses that your research is credible and your findings need to be implemented in leg ulcer care. Who do you approach to tell them about your findings and how do you tell them? Do you submit it to a professional nursing publication like *Journal of Community Nursing*? Do you present your results at a professional conference, for example one organised by the Royal College of Nursing? In this chapter, we will take you through a number of options to choose when presenting your research work and the decisions to make when presenting your study in a text form or an oral form.

One way to build knowledge in nursing and to share best practice is to let other people know about your research findings. It is most likely during your nursing course that you will be asked to write up or present the findings of a piece of work, for example the evidence base surrounding a particular intervention. You may also, at some time either during your nursing course or after you have qualified, undertake a research study. In all research situations the most common ways of letting other people know about your research (known as dissemination) is through research reports, oral presentation and poster presentations. In this chapter we're going to take you through how to present your research when:

- Writing a report about a quantitative or qualitative study, perhaps as an article in an academic journal or maybe in a professional publication, such as *Nursing Times*.
- Making an oral presentation to colleagues at a forum like a journal club or conference.
- Presenting a poster, usually at a conference.

11.1 Writing a quantitative or qualitative research report

When presenting a report, be it quantitative or qualitative, there are a number of key sections that most reports need to have. These are the following:

- *An abstract or summary.* This is a short paragraph which summarises the main ideas and findings of the research.
- *An introduction.* With quantitative studies, this would often mean outlining the theoretical context to the research and a summary of the main research literature

in the area that provides the background to the research. It

jectives and aims of the research. With qualitative resear

that much prior theory or research into a specific area;

shorter than if it were a quantitative study because the aim

could be to build up theory rather than give an overview of

in qualitative studies it is important to cover some literature

periences that have influenced the decision to conduct such

to expose to the readers why you have chosen to use a quali

covering some of the studies that have been done in a cert... ....,

your introduction might outline that there have been many quantitative studies into the quality of life among people with neurofibromatosis type 1 by using a number of questionnaire scales, but there may be very little in-depth exploration of the perceptions of people who have such a disease; this could act as the rationale for you choosing a qualitative approach.

- *Methodology or method.* This section outlines the method or the overriding paradigm within which the research was conducted. Often 'methodology' and 'method' are used interchangeably in a research report but do remember from previous chapters that 'methodology' relates to the underlying philosophy that is being applied when approaching the research problem (e.g. an ethnographic methodology) whereas 'method' mainly deals with techniques used to carry out the research (e.g. details on questionnaire administration, the use of a behavioural checklist, development of an interview schedule or analysis methods like discourse analysis). This section contains information on who took part in the study and details surrounding the collection of the data.

- *Results/findings.* This section seeks to summarise the main findings of your analysis. Whether it is a quantitative or qualitative analysis, this section outlines the key patterns obtained from your analysis. With a quantitative study, descriptive statistics should be reported first and then inferential statistics, which test hypotheses, are reported afterwards. In reports of qualitative studies, this section is often called 'findings' rather than 'results'; sometimes due to the tendencies of some qualitative researchers to emphasise the differences between qualitative and quantitative studies. With quantitative studies reporting 'results', this seems to suggest trends that are objective and akin to the types of sections that someone might find in a physical science lab report. By contrast, 'findings' is preferred by some qualitative researchers, as it emphasises more about the fluid nature of the data and that the findings can be interpreted in a variety of ways; the qualitative researcher is making every effort to report the best interpretation of the findings at that time but is also aware of the potentially various ways that the data could also be interpreted. As a result, qualitative researchers might often treat any themes or categories that have emerged from the analysis with an air of caution.

- *Discussion.* This section outlines the interpretation of your results and what they mean in terms of your research objectives and aims, and the wider research literature and practice. In qualitative studies, sometimes the findings and discussion s are merged so that the researcher is able to flit from reporting a theme has arisen from the analysis to ideas in the literature and developing theory, and then back to other themes obtained from the analysis.

In the following section we are going to outline each of these sections and details of how to write up each of the sections. Accompanying each section we will be using a small sample paper to illustrate each section. The fictional paper we've used before in this book deals with falls among older people and is referred to as follows: Ward, F., Williams, G.A., Maltby, J. and Day, L. (2008) Assessment of nutritional problems and risk of falling in hospital-based older person care: Brief research report. *Optimal Nursing Research, 25 (3)*, 25-29. It should be noted that this is a small paper and won't fully cover the actual length and in-depth nature of some research reports. For the purposes of this chapter it will still illustrate specific points to look out for when writing your research report.

Abstract or summary

An abstract or summary is usually between 150-250 words and provides a short paragraph that summarises the main ideas and findings of the research.

Abstracts are useful to other researchers because they can use the abstract/summary to gauge whether they will want to read the research paper - does it have information that is important or useful to them? Consequently, online research databases contain an abstract so researchers can work through many of them quickly to carry out a literature review. Clearly the abstract/summary can be useful in attracting readers to your research.

In essence you have to quickly convey four main points: *problem*, *approach*, *answer* and *conclusion*. Think of four key questions linked to each of the sections in an abstract/summary:

1. Why do the study?
2. How did you do the study?
3. What did you find?
4. What are the implications of your study for further research, theory and health care practice?

These questions are reflected in the following four main points:

- What was the *problem* the study tried to address? The first part of the abstract should outline the problem that is examined in the study. There is a reason why the researcher carried out the study, and mainly it will be due to trying to advance the nursing literature in some way. Therefore there should be one or two sentences outlining the problem to be solved.

- What *approach* did the study adopt to solve this problem? Here you should outline the main method that was used in the research to investigate the problem. The researcher would also include some details on the sample, the variables measures and the exact design used.

- What *answer* did your approach produce? Here the researcher reveals their main finding(s). The researcher may have many findings, but the results should outline the main findings that were most pertinent to the problem being examined.

- What *conclusion* did your answer produce? Finally, the abstract/summary will outline the main implications of the finding. What does your result mean, how does it add to the literature, i.e. what is the main thing the research has taught us or identified as new?

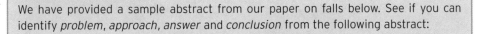

EXERCISE 11.1

We have provided a sample abstract from our paper on falls below. See if you can identify *problem*, *approach*, *answer* and *conclusion* from the following abstract:

Abstract:
Falls among older people are problematic in the hospital environment and a cause for concern among administrators, patients, relatives and health professionals alike. In the current study, the views of 31 nurses on falls' risk assessment were obtained from a randomly selected sample of 50 nursing staff working in three Care of the Older Person wards. We focused on nurses' consideration of poor nutrition among patients as being a major factor for making falls more likely and hypothesised that there would be a relationship between the type of ward that a nurse was based on and acknowledging nutritional problems as being implicated with falls. No significant link was found between ward type and nurses looking at nutrition. We outline the implications for staff training with needing to ensure that more nurses see nutrition as a falls' risk factor. It is also recommended that this education does not need to be targeted to those working in only one type of Care of the Older Person ward.

Introduction

The introduction is your first main section. It provides a context and general review of the area being investigated and sets out the objectives of your research. Overall the introduction to your research paper should represent an overview of the 'state of play' of the literature and the problem to be investigated.

In the main the introduction generally comprises three sections:

- A general literature and background
- A more specific literature and background
- A rationale for the study and a statement of research aims/objectives.

Ideally you should retain in your mind where you are going. That is, your introduction should always be moving to research questions or aims (or a hypothesis). A way of visualising this is depicted in Figure 11.1 in which you move from general aspects of the current state of the research to an eventual statement of your research aims and objectives. You would not subtitle your introduction like this; rather it should be an overall narrative with these elements moving seamlessly from one to another.

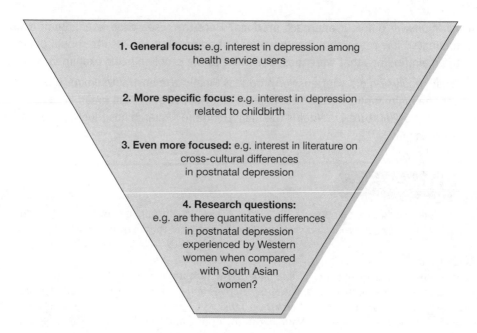

Figure 11.1 Creating a 'funnel' from the general to the more specific for your Introduction.

Let us now illustrate each of the main features of an introduction.

A general literature and background

An introduction must include a quick idea of the topic of the paper, identify the central theme and hint at the organisational pattern of the literature to be covered. One early statement might centre on the current situation or problem and should provide a context for all the literature that is to be covered. There should also be an introduction to the general perspective or ideas, and most certainly an indication of the general areas the paper is likely to draw upon, whether it be theoretical, policy-driven or methodological. There is no need to cover a large range of sources here (that is for later in the introduction), but rather identify recent sources (or most recent sources) and begin to lay the foundations of the areas to be covered in the introduction and that is a potential area for study.

A more specific literature and background

The next part provides a more comprehensive view of the literature and is likely to comprise the larger body of your introduction. In this section you would identify areas of theory and research that clearly need to be considered, known or understood by the reader before reading about your research. That is, you should only include theory, research and methodological ideas that inform, or are used to directly address your research. So what theory, research and methodological issues inform your research? For example what theory is debated in the area? What research evidence is there in the area? What methods and problems have been identified in the area that impact on the research you have done?

There are no hard and fast rules about how to structure this part of your introduction, but what you must try to do is present an organised and relevant analysis that covers all relevant aspects to your research, and only your research. There are a number of different ways to organise this section and the choice will depend on the nature of the theory, research and methodological issues that you need to cover. So before you write your introduction, think about whether you could order the introduction in either of the following ways:

- *Chronological.* Chronological means by date. What might be appropriate is to order the literature to outline the way it has developed over the years. Therefore you would look to order the literature, or ideas, mostly by year of publication.

- *Themes.* Here your review would be organised around particular topics or issues, rather than the date of publication. Therefore this section will identify major aspects of the research, which may or may not be related, but that you may feel come together and inform your research. Within themes you might want to still order the ideas by date, but here you are focusing on the dominant ideas that inform your research.

A rationale for the study and a statement of research aims/objectives

The final part of the introduction entails bringing together all these ideas and making a statement about what your research is aiming to achieve. At the beginning of this section there should be a summary statement and rationale that brings together all the ideas and justifies the need for the research. Then what follows is a formal statement regarding what the aim of the research is. Sometimes this is simply written in terms of the aims of the research or the study objectives. This statement should say clearly what you hope to achieve or examine in the current study. However, there is one formal statement that is worth dwelling on, and that is the use of hypothesis statements to outline the aims of a study.

Quantitative analysis is thought to be of better scientific quality if it has explicit statements of predicted relationships between variables or differences between participant groups in the form of a hypothesis. Likewise, it will be useful to know what the researchers have set as an acceptable level of statistical significance to gauge whether such relationships or differences can be put down to chance or a real statistical effect. Using hypotheses is the same as using questions. However, there is some formal terminology associated with using hypotheses to describe the type of research question proposed.

You won't tend to see hypothesis statements in qualitative research, and in fact many quantitative papers won't make formal statements. However, they are used most in experimental reports. One good clue to whether or not you should include them is whether the literature you have been looking at tends to use them. Regardless of this decision, at the end of the introduction there will be a formal statement of what the research aims to achieve.

EXERCISE 11.2

We have provided a sample introduction from our paper on falls below. See if you can identify the different sections (general literature, specific literature and statement of research aims) from this introduction. Also see if you can identify the problem we have set out and to what extent we have identified theory, previous research and methodological debates. Given that this is a rather short introduction (due to the space allowed in the book) is there any more information that you would look for that we haven't provided here?

Introduction:

Falls among older people contribute greatly to mortality and morbidity throughout this country and the government (Department of Health and Health Care, 2003) has been implementing action plans to target this growing problem. The Dietetic Society (2007) has claimed that one of the major risk factors for falls among older people is that many of them are undernourished, thus leading to dizziness when older people are mobilising. In the hospital environment, there should be less chance of older patients not having sufficient nourishment, as there should be more control over what food is administered to them. However, there is evidence that the older patient has problems with diet and feeling hungry due to polypharmacy (i.e. needing to take a cocktail of prescribed drugs throughout the day) (Jefferies and Dealer, 2006). In the current study, we were aiming to see whether nurses involved with care of the older patient were taking poor diet/malnourishment into account when considering a patient's risk of falling. This study focused on the reported falls' risk assessment practices of a sample of registered general nurses working at three Care of the Older Person wards in a community hospital based in a city within the New Pleasant state. We also sought to explore whether there was a relationship between the type of ward that the nurses worked on and the reported assessment practices. It was hypothesised that there would be a link between ward and assessment of diet when examining risk of falling. This hypothesis was grounded in observations by the research team that one of the wards (Spongebury) appeared to have patients with higher dependencies than in the other two wards, which dealt mainly with rehabilitation, and that staff would thus have less time to consider nutrition as an issue.

Method

In this section you should state what you did to carry out the research. Did you carry out an experiment, interviews or use a survey? How did you collect your data and from whom? What variables did you try to measure and what variables did you measure? When writing the method part of the report the golden rule is that you should provide enough information so anyone wishing to carry out your study again has enough information to do so.

It may not surprise you to find that there are differences between how quantitative and qualitative reports are typically written up and we will now distinguish between the two types of quantitative method sections; one for experimental and one for survey; and a qualitative method section.

Quantitative experimental studies

In an experimental report you will tend to see a number of headings, usually four: Sample, Design, Materials and Procedure. We will go on to explain each of these in turn.

Sample

Here some detail could be provided on how the sample was recruited and the constitution of samples, i.e. how many people were there, what were their ages, sex and ethnicity.

Design

In the design section you describe the type of design used in the experiment. Is it experimental or a clinical trial? If a clinical trial what sort of clinical trial was it (prevention, screening, diagnostic, treatment)? In the design section you also need to specify the variables as well as the levels of these variables (i.e. what different aspects occurred within each variable). You also need to explain whether your experiment compares groups of people, i.e. through a control group, (between groups), or whether it studies the same group of people over time (within group). You should also note whether there are any particular controls in place, such as placebo-controlled, randomisation of participants or blind administrations. Don't think of this last list as a checklist; rather try to explain your experimental design within these terms. If you didn't compare groups of people then there is no need to mention it.

Materials

In this section you should describe the materials, measures and equipment used in your study. This may include testing instruments, drugs use, equipment used to record information and technical instruments. However, don't simply list each piece of equipment: you need to make the research clear to the reader. In this section you need to explain how each piece of equipment was used to measure each variable.

Procedure

In this section the researcher should detail how the data were collected. Therefore you should carefully document all the important aspects of the experiment as it was carried out. You need to explain what you had participants do, how you collected data, how you used the materials and the order in which the different stages of the experiment occurred.

Quantitative survey studies

In a quantitative survey you may need to use a slightly different format. For a survey you will again detail the sample as with an experimental study but you may rename the materials section as measures or a questionnaire administered section. In this section you will detail each of the scales administered, who designed them, what they are intended to measure, an example of the items and the scoring method. All this detail is provided so the reader gets a good understanding of what each of the measures used looks like.

A sample section and a measures/questionnaire administered section may be all you see in some research papers. You may also see a design section, highlighting that it was a survey method, but are less likely to see a procedure section, as details such as handing out questionnaires and collecting them back in again is thought of as too much detail, though you might want to include some detail if you think there is something the reader needs to know about the research.

EXERCISE 11.3

We have provided a sample method section. Decide for yourself whether we have provided enough information for you to replicate the study. What extra information would you require?

Method:

Participants
A random sample of 50 nurses was approached out of the population of 75 full-time and part-time nurses employed by the hospital. Agency nursing staff were not approached, as the permanent staff would govern all induction and training in patient assessment and we viewed them as being vital to driving the methods and ethos of patient assessment. Out of the nurses that we sampled, 33 replied to the invitation letter with a completed questionnaire (66 per cent response rate), although only 31 of the forms were useable with complete data.

Materials
We used the Stanislav Falls Assessment Procedures Index (Stanislav, 2005). This comprised a 35-item form that requires respondents to identify the factors they consider when assessing an older person's risk of falling. This questionnaire has been mainly validated with hospital-based older person care (Stanislav and Spector, 2004) and has been found to have subscales tapping into three main concepts – physical health, psychological well-being and the mobilisation process. These three subscales have internal consistencies of 0.89, 0.65 and 0.85 respectively.

Procedure
Posters advertising the study were placed on staff noticeboards near the three wards and the agreement of the staff unions and the hospital management was obtained before commencing the study. Local Research Ethical Committee approval was also granted in November 2005. The research team sent the questionnaire to the sample of nurses via the internal post during the week commencing 12 December 2005. The forms had a self-addressed, stamped envelope for participants to send their completed returns to the team by a two-week deadline.

Analysis
As we were primarily interested in the relationship between type of Care of the Older Person ward and nurses' reported assessment of nutritional problems when examining patient risk of falling, we conducted a chi-square analysis on these two variables.

Qualitative studies

However, with a qualitative research report you will need to use a different set of criteria. Again, the overriding rule is to take the reader through the decisions and method of your research. Again practice does vary but you will tend to see the following areas outlined.

Methods chosen for collecting the data

In qualitative research there is always a rationale lying behind a particular approach, and therefore there should be some statement of why the particular method was chosen. For example, the material being discussed might be of a sensitive nature to discuss in a group, so a one-to-one interview may be preferred. By contrast, some issues might be more amenable to group discussion and it could be justified that a focus group method may help elicit a more in-depth and frank discussion from participants.

Sampling

As with quantitative reports, some detail must be provided on how the sample was recruited and the constitution of samples, i.e. how many people were there, what were their ages, sex and ethnicity. Include any details that are relevant to replicate how the study was conducted and the methods of getting a sufficiently representative and/or sizeable sample.

The research setting

It is also a good idea to give the reader an idea of the research setting, so they have a context to understand the discourse. For example is the interview being carried out by a district nurse in the person's home, or is it being carried out in a hospital or clinic? Providing a context to research may help us understand the discussion. For example, if we are told that the interviews were carried out in the person's home we know that some attempt has been made to carry out the interview in surroundings familiar to the interviewee and one which the interviewee feels most comfortable in.

How the data were collected

In this section the researcher should detail how the data were collected, where conversations were recorded and the method of transcription (e.g. Jefferson method of indicating conversational pauses and when speech between two people blend together). Are there transcripts of a focus group discussion, or notes made from an observation, or from diary records? Most of all these should be detailed very fully so anyone could repeat the data collection method. For example, if you used an interview schedule, was it semi-structured, unstructured or structured? Also, can you give a sample of the kinds of questions asked? This information should be provided so that researchers could use the same approach to data collection, if they so wished.

THINGS TO CONSIDER

Analysis sections in the method/methodology

Sometimes in research papers there may be a subheading in the method section called 'analysis', which outlines any particular analysis procedures that were used in the study. Usually the type of analysis used is detailed in the results section (we discuss this next). However, sometimes, so as to provide a full picture, the method used to analyse the results is provided in this section. This might sometimes be needed, particularly if an unusual or sophisticated technique has been used. Some people/ researchers/journals/lecturers like to see detail of this in the method, while others leave this to the results section. We just thought we would highlight it so if you're reading a research paper and it contains an analysis section it doesn't confuse you.

Results/findings sections

When writing a results section, regardless of whether it is a quantitative or qualitative study, the main aim is to present your findings in as simple a way as possible. It may be that you have waded through a massive amount of output or data, and printed off many graphs or analysed many taped interviews. Therefore the temptation is to place it all in the results. However, you must remember that you are trying to help your reader identify the most important findings. If you make your results long and complicated, it will be hard for the reader (marker) to understand what you have done.

You need to concentrate your writing around your main aims (hypotheses) of your study. Don't get distracted by information that you think would be nice to be in there. There are times when you find something interesting but remember that unless it's directly relevant to your study you should not introduce analysis that falls outside your question. Most of all write your results as a narrative, explaining each of the steps in the analysis, and always assume the reader (even if it is your lecturer) is new to the research.

There are some special considerations to make depending on whether you are writing results obtained from quantitative or qualitative research.

Quantitative data

Sometimes with quantitative data it is a good idea to provide an overall picture of the data by reporting the summaries, such as means and standard deviations of any measures used. If you're going to do this, do it early in your analysis, perhaps making it clear that this is an informative section.

However, the main part of your analysis should be designed to answer your research aims. At all times fully explain your statistics, and most often your choice of statistics. Never assume prior knowledge, or assume that the reader knows what you are talking about. For example when reporting a statistical test do not say something like 'A significant main effect was found for type of health care team and team objective setting.'

If this is all you tell the reader, then you haven't provided enough information to make sense of the data. All you are saying is that type of health care team has some influence on how they set their objectives. This isn't really that helpful – we don't know what teams are involved and the extent to which some teams are better at setting their team objectives than other teams. The following sentence shows a clearer illustration of what the main trends are and how the authors made sense of the results:

> *A further independent groups t-test revealed that multidisciplinary clinic teams (M = 22.87) scored statistically significantly more highly than primary health care teams (M = 9.74) in terms of team objective setting.*

(Williams and Laungani, 1999; p. 24).

Note that there is something missing in the reporting of the mean scores in the results – the standard deviations for each mean. If you look back at what we have covered in Chapter 7, you can see that this is an essential part of knowing how dispersed the scores are, as well as knowing what the scores are on average.

EXERCISE 11.4

We have provided a sample results section. What extra information would you require in this section?

Results:
Table 1 outlines the distribution of nurses who said that they either did or did not consider nutritional problems among their patients when assessing risk of falling on the wards. It is noteworthy that only 16 out of the 31 (51.6 per cent) nurse respondents reported looking out for nutritional problems when assessing falls' risk.

Table 1 Nutritional problems as a risk factor for falls among older patients

'Which ward do you work in?'	'Consideration of nutrition problems?'	
	No	Yes
Spongebury	5	6
Wickham	7	7
Hesham	3	3

A chi-square analysis showed that there was no significant relationship between the type of ward that the nurses worked on and their focus on nutritional problems among patients when conducting falls' risk assessment, $\chi^2(2) = 0.059, p > 0.05$.

What you're looking for is clarity in expressing the identified differences or relationships for a specified variable or between variables. So you need to be clear in showing the direction of differences or strength of the relationships as well.

Finally, graphs, charts, tables and diagrams help your reader identify key results and also allow you to break up long parts of text, or explain it more simply. However, be sure to explain all graphs, charts, tables and diagrams in text highlighting the key findings in the text.

THINGS TO CONSIDER

Do you interpret the results in the results section?

There is sometimes an area of ambiguity regarding how to comment on the results obtained. Basically, it should be remembered that the authors should simply report the main trends and give no speculations as to the reasons for the results in the results section. Any attempts at interpreting the results and making sense of why these results were obtained should solely be confined to the discussion section of the quantitative study report.

Qualitative data

In a qualitative report the reporting of the qualitative data is usually the longest section. There are often a lot of data to wade through so your main skill is to try to reduce all this information into a manageable size, which is largely dictated by your course leaders (e.g. maximum length for a dissertation) or by journal editors. However, it also needs to be detailed enough to convey the themes/categories that you found from your data in a convincing way to the readers. You have to remember that you not only have to produce a narrative of the findings but also clear examples as to why you have arrived at labelling some parts of your data as constituting a certain theme (e.g. Why is a theme about patient–nurse communication that you have found called 'striking up rapport'? Could it be called something else as well?). Try to adopt the following practices to make your qualitative analyses transparent, verifiable and credible to your readers:

- Arrange the findings according to the dominant themes and sub-themes that might have arisen from a thematic analysis. Present one dominant theme first, then any sub-themes that might be connected to this dominant theme before moving on to the next dominant theme.

- If you are reporting on an interview study, bear in mind that it will not be possible to report everything that was said in the interviews. You need to be selective and pick the best examples carefully; try to show that a theme is dominant by providing evidence that this theme arose with a variety of participants and is not evidenced by the data collected from just one person.

- When using quotes, select substantial (not necessarily lengthy) quotes that provide solid evidence of the theme or category that you are aiming to illustrate.

Discussion

This section outlines the interpretation of your results and what they mean in terms of your research objectives and aims, and the wider research literature and practice. Also in this section you may look for opportunities to point out the importance of your findings and the issues that arose out of your study. Regardless of whether the research is quantitative or qualitative, discussion sections comprise three main elements: (1) interpreting the findings, (2) contextualising the findings and the study in relation to the literature, (3) evaluating the study and making recommendations.

Interpretation of the findings

In the discussion section, you should be looking to provide a brief summary of the findings – this is not for the authors to repeat the statistics or verbatim quotes in the results section or to come up with new findings not already covered in the results. This is your chance to give your interpretations as to why certain trends were obtained. For example, if unexpected, non-significant findings were obtained in a quantitative study, there should be an outline of your reasoning as to why this was the case. Also, you will not get good marks from your tutor or positive feedback from colleagues by only highlighting significant results that support your viewpoint. Although nursing research papers are essentially arguments for going in a specific direction in terms of research, theory or practice, you should also highlight alternative explanations for your results. This shouldn't be an endless list, but there may be a rival explanation and this needs to be acknowledged. Try to avoid speculating beyond the results that you obtained and go one step too far by generalising your findings to a wider patient group (e.g. assuming that reasons for non-compliance with glucose testing among diabetic patients are similar to those held by patients with other chronic health conditions).

Contextualising the findings and the study in relation to the literature

Another element that a good discussion should have is that it should clearly define whether the data confirm your hypotheses (as in a quantitative study) or whether a new theory has been generated (often in the case of qualitative studies). If a hypothesis was not supported by the data, are there any alternative ideas for further research and further hypotheses? Could any anomalous findings in a quantitative study lead to an exploratory qualitative study to try to explain such anomalies? Many good researchers will recognise the process of doing research is ongoing, whereby data often throw up more questions than answers, leading to possible new directions for conducting further research and trying out novel health care interventions or health promotion strategies. Therefore, it is essential that you provide suggestions for future studies in the area. Excellent recommendations go beyond simple ideas of getting larger samples (although sometimes this helps when the original study is involving analysis of data for a sample of 20-odd participants!) and try to expand on the ideas of the literature rather than just simply the results. The better research reports entail proposals for more effective designs and alternative methods of analysis. The astute authors will cover limitations of their study to pre-empt the kinds of concerns that readers might have over the data collected. Most importantly, you need make explicit attempts to make sense of their data in terms of care policies and clinical practice procedures. This discussion needs to illustrate the nursing theory and research that has gone before the study took place and that you shouldn't generally cover new research not covered earlier on in the introduction; if you are, think about why you haven't included this in your introduction.

Evaluating the study and making recommendations

Finally, it will be helpful at the end of the paper to make an overall assessment of how good the paper is. Summarise the general strengths and limitations of the study so you can make clearer to the reader the main points you are trying to convey. Another aspect to include is some recommendations. These recommendations might apply to developments in policy, changes to nursing practices or future recommendations for researchers to further study in this area. This section might be better placed before your final conclusion and integrated with other sections, so you will have to make a judgement where it is best placed, either in a separate section or with your final summary. Finally there should be one or two sentences that summarise your overall findings and main conclusion.

EXERCISE 11.5

We have provided a sample discussion section for our paper on falls. Identify which parts of the discussion are addressing the three main components of: (1) interpreting and making sense of the findings, (2) contextualising the results in light of prior research, (3) evaluating the study, with suggestions for future research. If you had to make a recommendation to hospital practices on preventing and managing falls among older people, based on the results of the study, what would it be?

Discussion:

It can be seen from the results that only half of the nurses who responded to our survey of falls' risk assessment practices said that they considered nutritional problems among their patients. This trend is in line with prior research (e.g. William and Hill, 2003) showing that nutrition is a neglected part of inpatient care for the older person and that nutritional well-being tends to be left to the dietician to monitor (Tidy and Meal, 2000). Unexpectedly, there was no link between type of ward and evaluation of nutritional problems as a risk factor, thus indicating that nursing practice seems fairly consistent within a community hospital setting. There are some potential limitations that need to be considered. Although our sample of 31 respondents was a sizeable percentage of the population of nursing staff within the three wards, it needs to be recognised that there may have been fewer senior nurses obtained with random sampling as they constitute a relatively small percentage of the total number of nurses employed in the study sites. Given that it is likely the senior

▶

nurses would be more involved with patient assessment (and falls' risk assessment) than junior nurses, this could explain why only half of our sample had considered nutrition as a factor. Further research could aim at replicating the administration of our questionnaire to staff at other similar wards, but through the use of a stratified sampling method. Nevertheless, the current trends seem to suggest the need for nursing practice to routinely incorporate the nutritional status of an older patient and for nurses to be educated to the impact that poor nutrition among older patients can have on making the patient disorientated and weak when mobilising. As we did not find a link between type of Care of the Older Person ward and reported assessment practices, we would recommend that this education should cover the training of all grades of nursing and in all types of wards

Other things to include: references and appendices

Finally your report will have a reference section and might have a section with one appendix or many appendices. You will have come across references sections before in your research work. Like your other work, it is important that you provide details of all the research and theories covered by other researchers that you have cited in your research report. The format of references differs according to institutions and you will have received direction on how to format references at your institution. Therefore check the convention for referencing on your course. Do also be aware that references sections are very different from a bibliography section, which is not often encouraged as common practice when writing a research report. A bibliography is a list of all the resources that you used when compiling the report, whereas a references section only lists the references that you actually cited from in your report. Although it might be tempting to show the wide range of reading that you've done and the hard work that you've devoted to your report, if a resource wasn't considered important enough to cite in the report, then it's best to list only those you really did use in a references section.

The other section you are likely to have in a research report is an appendix. The aim of the appendix is to contain related information which is not essential to your report but may be important for the reader to get a full understanding of all relevant aspects of your study. This really shouldn't be a licence to fill your report with additional material such as printouts from statistical packages like SPSS or whole transcripts of conversational data. Your lecturer may direct you to include certain additional information in your report. However, you might typically include full details of an interview schedule, a questionnaire/behaviour checklist especially designed for the study, or additional analyses conducted, in this section.

11.2 Presenting your research as an oral presentation

At many stages during your nursing career and during your studies into research and evidence-based practice, you might have to give an oral presentation. It is likely that at some stage during your career and your studies, this will involve presenting some research findings to other health professionals. Unfortunately, there is no way to avoid this and in many ways, they are useful media for presenting your case for a different method of clinical practice or a better way of understanding what your patients and clients are experiencing of your services. Oral presentations of research are really central to developing yourself as a nurse and also in convincing fellow health professionals in your health care team about how to implement evidence-based practice. Not many people like giving an oral presentation and it is a common occurrence to get nervous with worry before presenting at a conference or a journal club or other research symposium. However, there are ways in which you can make sure you make a success of your presentation. The phrase 'if you fail to plan, then you plan to fail' is extremely appropriate to presentations, and you really do need to do the following to make sure you can make the most of your research presentation.

Knowing the objective of the exercise

There are clear objectives when you are giving the presentation. It is unlikely to just to be about your research, but also your ability to present ideas and findings. Therefore you need to understand what is required from the talk. Once you have realised what the objectives are you can make sure that you plan your talk around these objectives. So if it is about presenting research information, then you make sure you present some research information. If it is about talking in front of people, then you make sure that you organise yourself so that you do it properly. Therefore getting a set of answers to the question 'what are the objectives?' will help you shape and plan your presentation. Also find out other information. Be clear about the time allotted for your presentation and who you are presenting too. This will be your biggest challenge as no doubt your first research presentation will be on your course and therefore you will be presenting alongside other students and the time allocated to these sessions will be brief. It will help to write down the objective(s) and other information (time, audience) and plan around that. If you fulfil all the objectives then there is no way you can fail the presentation.

Knowing your audience

It is advisable to know your audience thoroughly. Are they other nurses, non-experts and/or experts in applying the research method you have used, such as using conversation analysis to understand how health professionals and patients interact? Knowing the level of your audience will help you pitch the talk at the right level. Likely at this stage it is going to be other students on your course and at least one lecturer. So think about their expectations. What do they want to hear? And in answer to that, given that you are a colleague, what would you like to hear? Therefore plan around that, don't make it too complicated, keep it interesting and make it as enjoyable as you can for your audience.

Plan, plan, plan and plan again

The next stage is to plan your talk. Do a rough outline of the main points of your presentation, but keep it focused. Even if you are basing your talk on your research report, you will have extensive and detailed material. Remember one of the key academic skills is to be able to identify key points. You're presenting a talk based on your research; you are not presenting your research report. So strip it down to the main points and key elements of the research. What the main ideas, what are the messages, what is the main finding? What is the main conclusion? Just take 10 minutes to sit down and plan the talk, highlighting 7-10 main points you have to get across. You certainly won't have time to have any more.

Structure your talk

When developing your talk it helps if you split it up into distinct parts. If you break up the material in this way then it will help you retain a focus to your presentation, addressing each main component. As such your presentation should contain the following:

- A **title** page (see a sample of one in Figure 11.2a): Introducing yourself and the title of the research.
- A **summary** of the research, briefly stating what you have done.
- An **introduction**. This should provide an overview of the literature. However, if you have a short time to present, such as between 10 and 20 minutes, this has to be incredibly brief. You need to state the problem, the main theory and research informing your research, and a statement of the research aims.
- An outline of the **method**. Again this needs to be brief. Concentrate on a brief description of the sample and the main variables measured and techniques used. There is no need (or space) to go into detail.
- A **results** section that outlines one or two main findings and shows examples of the results. Again don't go into too much detail. You are just trying to get your message across. If you over-complicate this section you may lose time and lose impetus in your talk.
- A **discussion/conclusion** section, listing the main findings of your investigation and perhaps one or two thoughts about how the research could be progressed.

Have a look at some further slides from a sample presentation (Figure 11.2) which used PowerPoint and reported on findings from a qualitative study.

It may not be a good idea to develop the talk in the order of title page, introduction, etc. Instead, perhaps start with the results and discussion and strip this down to the main basic findings, or at the most a couple of findings and main discussion points. Then work back to the method and introduction and use the main points that are addressed in the results and discussion as a guide of what to cover. By starting on

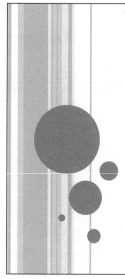

THE RELEVANCE OF 'FLOW' IN EXPLAINING PAEDIATRIC NURSES' SATISFACTION AND ENJOYMENT AT WORK

Kathryn Worrall
Guy's and St Thomas'
NHS Trust

Glenn Williams
University of Nottingham,
School of Nursing, Derby Centre

British Psychological Society's Annual Conference,
Imperial College,
London
15–17 April, 2004

(a) Example of a title slide from an oral presentation of nursing research.

AIMS

- Introduce flow theory and its possible relevance to paediatric nurses' job satisfaction

- Identify whether the theory of flow can explain all aspects of optimal experience among paediatric nurses

- Discuss whether the findings of this study could help increase retention of paediatric nurses

(b) Example of a research aims slide from an oral presentation of nursing research.

THE PROBLEM/LITERATURE REVIEW

- Poor nurse retention (Sheild and Ward, 2001)
- Low retention likely to have negative effect upon staff morale, service delivery and patient health
- Job satisfaction and enjoyment at work have been strongly associated with nurse retention (Shader *et al,* 2001)
- There are very few studies into job satisfaction among paediatric nurses (except for e.g. Holaday and Bullard, 1991)
- Increased understanding could help enhance nurse retention

(c) Example of setting out the problem investigated or a literature review slide from an oral presentation of nursing research.

Figure 11.2 Example of the main points of a PowerPoint presentation.

METHOD

- Qualitative, phenomenological approach
- 8 Paediatric nurses from a large teaching hospital in the East Midlands
- Semi-structured interviews
- Interviews were taped and transcribed
- Voluntary and purposive sampling
- Analysis to match data with categories from flow theory (i.e. challenge, feedback, control, unity, concentration, time)
- Analysis grounded in data only

(d) Example of a methods page from an oral presentation of nursing research.

CATEGORIES THAT EMERGED

- **Intrinsic Work Objectives**

  'I like working with kids, it makes you very humble when they are sick. It's lovely to see them get better and go home.'

- **Keeping Busy**

  '. . . and you think OK, we have been really busy, it has whizzed by but I have actually achieved something.'

(e) Example of a results/main findings slide from an oral presentation of nursing research.

IMPLICATIONS FOR PRACTICE

- Flow theory can contribute to explaining participants' satisfaction at work.
- The findings identified a number of aspects to the participants' work that may have been preventing them from experiencing flow.
- Increasing the likelihood of paediatric nurses experiencing flow by modifying training and work situations may increase satisfaction and therefore retention.

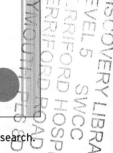

(f) Example of a discussion/implications slide from an oral presentation of nursing research.

Figure 11.2 Continued

the results and discussion, this might give you a better idea of pictures that you might want to include in your presentation or a clearer idea of the main points that you could cover in the introduction of your talk to 'set the scene'.

Keep people's attention: make it interesting

Nothing makes a talk go slower for you, or the audience, than a boring talk. Therefore standing there and just talking, or even reading from a script is potentially not likely to maintain your audience's interest. There are three tricks you can use to make your talk interesting: visuals, simplicity and momentum.

Use visuals

There are many ways to communicate a message and surprisingly speech isn't always the best one. In fact it takes a lot of effort for an audience to follow someone talking and also gives you a lot of pressure as all eyes will be on you. So why don't you at the very least distract the audience from just you and present the visuals.

If you are able to use visuals there are things you can present; pictures, illustrations, diagrams, graphs and statistical tables. Remember the phrase, 'a picture paints a thousand words'. Imagine if there was a difficult concept or idea you need to get across. If it would be simpler to represent that idea or concept in a diagram then that will not only help you explain difficult concepts but also save you time. So at this stage you should be planning to present all of your material accompanied by something such as PowerPoint. It is likely that nurse tutors at university, or fellow health professionals that are listening to your presentation, are expecting you to present using PowerPoint.

However, don't try to overuse PowerPoint. You have lots of detail, but keep it simple. Only use your most essential ideas on PowerPoint. So for example if there is a complicated diagram, simplify it, particularly as it would take a great amount of time to explain the whole diagram. Avoid visual information that contains a lot of data, and the adage 'Less is more' certainly applied here.

In terms of number of PowerPoint slides, as your talk will be short, at least 10 minutes and at most 20 minutes, one PowerPoint slide per 2 minutes of the talk is the most you can probably have. Again, keep it simple, as you have your summary, introduction, method, results and discussion/conclusion to fit into the main aspect of the talk. We recommend no more that two slides for each section. If you need more then this might be an indication that you need to do more editing of your talk.

Keep it simple

It's always tempting to try to show your audience that you know many things and haven't left anything out, but a presentation isn't just about knowledge; it's the ability to present, and the skill of cutting down information into a clear and manageable form when presenting. Try to present your main ideas via PowerPoint. Keep these displays simple, listing the main ideas, but don't go into much detail on the slide. Presenters tend to elaborate on what is on the slide. So if you put all the information on there, it is likely that you will expand even further from what is on the slides and therefore expand the duration of your presentation. As a result, it might be helpful to time how long your talk will take by having a 'dry run' of the presentation before the big day. One other thing to bear in mind is that it will be good to elaborate when talking about each of your slides; this will make it more interesting to the audience as there is nothing more frustrating than sitting in the audience and having to hear someone speak word for word from the PowerPoint slides (sometimes known as PowerPoint karaoke!).

Maintaining the momentum of your talk

Think of your favourite song. It is likely to have many different aspects to it, some sort of verse or chorus, quieter then louder bits. More mellow parts followed by more intense sections. That's the key to a good song, taking your audience with you. So imagine talking for 10-20 minutes; how do you keep someone interested for that long? Well you have to be aware of your speed and the momentum of the talk. Imagine a talk that's very fast or very slow, i.e. the same speed all the way through, the audience knows what to expect and therefore may lose concentration and get bored, so try to think of ways of controlling your talk.

One way of planning for momentum is by starting with a strong opener. This will grab your audience's attention and get them interested in the talk. Also planning an opening will help you get over those nerves because carefully scripting those first lines of your talk will get you (and your audience) into the talk.

It doesn't have to be 'all singing and dancing' because you want to get the main serious points across, but be aware in your talk of where things might be getting a bit the same or you may be losing momentum, and see if you can use a visual example or light moment to change the speed of the talk. Also, one key idea to help the momentum of the talk is transition. Transitions in talks are tools for moving from one slide to another or from one idea to another. Being aware of the transitions in your talk and capitalising on them will help you and the audience focus and ensure that your talk flows. So try to ensure that each section flows from one to another, that ideas being discussed earlier in the talk are addressed and followed through in the talk. If you don't do that perhaps you should ask yourself if they need to be there.

Rehearse and prepare

You rehearsing could make the difference between a good and an average presentation. It's tempting not to rehearse, because it seems to be a waste of time. However, how it sounds in your head and the time you think it'll take you to present it are very different to how it will be on the day. To help, do the following:

● Rehearse your presentation out loud several times. This will not only help you develop the talk, but you will come across problems in the presentation that you weren't aware of. This will allow you to address those problems and rectify them before the presentation, rather than discovering while you are presenting.

- Develop a set of prompt cards to help you in your talk. This should just be the main areas to be covered. It's best not to write a script to be read out as in practice this often leads to stale and monotonous talks. Develop your talk, but have a set of cards, or copies of your PowerPoint slides, to act as a memory aid throughout your talk.

- Time yourself. You can never be sure how long something takes, so while you are rehearsing time yourself. Make sure that you fall within the time that has been provided for your talk. This will also allow you to add parts if you fall way under the time limit or cut things out if you go over.

- As you are rehearsing note where you potentially get stuck. If you find yourself forgetting part, which in all likelihood you are going to, write key starting phrases on your prompt cards/notes, so if you forget in the talk what to say next you have a nice little sentence to get you back into the talk.

- You might also want to give out handouts in your presentation detailing your work. This might be a copy of your slides or a quick summary of your work. This isn't essential in a student presentation, but might be a nice touch to your presentation.

On the day–the presentation

Finally, on to the day of your talk! No doubt you will be filled with excitement and looking forward to your presentation. You have worked hard on it, planned it and rehearsed it. However, there are some things you can do on the day to make your talk go even better than you have anticipated.

- Make sure you have a couple of copies of your talk. Therefore rather than having one USB data stick with your talk on, have two data sticks, just in case one gets damaged. Also email the talk to yourself. Sometimes USB data sticks are not compatible with some computers or you might lose the data stick, whereas if you have emailed it to yourself you still have this as a fallback position if the worst happens. In most places where conferences/symposiums are held, there should be email access on some of the computers that are being used for the presentations, so do take this precaution of emailing it as a back-up plan.

- Don't panic. You will get nerves, but use them to your advantage. Everyone gets nervous before a talk. However, don't let your nerves rule you. Nothing bad will happen in the presentation and you have nothing to fear. The audience and lecturers are on your side and will want you to do well. In fact many people will be glad it's not them up there, or if a few of you are presenting that day, be feeling exactly the same as you.

- When you start the presentation take something with the time on it (a watch, a mobile phone [but switch it to silent]) and put it by you so you can keep to time. It is very important that you keep to time.

- Speak clearly and look at the audience. Try to keep eye contact with people and just talk to them about your work. Looking at the audience can give you clues to how things are going and whether people understand you. However, don't get too distracted by the audience as someone looking uninterested might just be a look of panic as they're up next. Also don't worry if you make a mistake or forget something. Though in your head a mistake might seem crucial or pausing because you've forgotten something might seem a long time in your head, in fact most people won't notice it at all.

- If you have brought handouts, pass them around after you have finished your presentation.

Finally when you've finished your presentation expect some questions. This can be the most fearful part of the presentation, because you are unable to plan for it. However, questions after a presentation are a very good way for you to clear up any potential misunderstanding in your presentation or for you to continue to emphasise the importance of your findings. Here are some key suggestions to handle this part of the presentation well:

- Unless you want to have an open discussion during your presentation, let your audience know that there will be an opportunity for questions at the end.
- When you finish your presentation ask, 'Who has the first question?', and then have the confidence to wait. Someone will probably ask a question, even if it seems a long time, because there will be an embarrassed silence.
- When someone asks a question, the first thing you need to do is repeat it in your own words. This is done for two reasons. The first reason is to check with yourself and the questioner that you understand the question. The second reason is to make sure all the audience has heard. Sometimes the person asking the question won't be heard by the rest of the audience, for example they may be at the front. Therefore repeating the question back makes sure everyone is included in the question/ answer session. The audience will get bored if they have to listen to an answer when they do not know what the question is.
- If you did not understand the question or hear the question, ask the questioner to repeat the question.
- When answering the question, keep it brief. Don't go into another talk, as the audience will get bored. If you can keep it to a one- or two-sentence answer then do.
- If you don't know the answer, don't worry. Just say you don't know, but you can offer to find the answer later, ask if anyone else in the audience knows, or suggest some reading where the answer is most likely to be found.
- If no-one asks a question, don't worry. However, sometimes you can get the session going by saying 'here is a question I'm sometimes asked', or 'here is a question that often arises in this area' and then give your answer. You could prepare such an answer beforehand. This usually gets the question and answer session going and will prompt people to ask other questions. If people don't ask you any questions, don't worry, thank them for their time and end the talk.

And when it's finished, given all the planning, it will hopefully have gone well. You will also find that, having finished the presentation, you may feel relieved, pleased with yourself and still buzzing with excitement!

EXERCISE 11.6

The key to a good talk is planning and organisation. In the section above we have out-lined the things you should do. However, sometimes the best way to learn something is to learn what not to do. Therefore imagine if you wanted your presentation to go badly, what five things could you do to make them go really badly? Write them in the space below.

1. _____

2. _____

3. _____

4. _____

5. _____

OK. Now, DO NOT do these things!

11.3 Presenting your research in a poster

It is likely during your career as a nurse (with the pressure to show that you are imple-menting evidence-based practice) for you to be required to present your work in the form of a poster, which might often be at a conference or research symposium. A poster is simply a large piece of paper or board that you use visually to communicate your research. The difference between a poster presentation and oral presentation is that the poster should convey most of the presentation - not you.

If you ever go to a nursing conference you are likely to see a number of poster presentations, in which people can go around (as in an art gallery) and view the re-search. Usually what happens is researchers stand by the poster and give delegates a chance to inspect the poster and ask the researchers any questions that arise. This process allows for a greater number of topics to be viewed at any one time. Overall they are sometimes preferred by the audience and presenters over oral presenta-tions because they allow people to learn and talk about research without having to sit in a series of presentations whilst waiting for the presentation that they really want to listen to.

Your research poster

Research posters require a lot of time to prepare and in the next sections we are going to provide you with the techniques for creating a good poster, based on: (1) gen-eral content, (2) design and presentation and (3) creating the content.

General content of the poster

The content of the poster is largely the same as a presentation, with a title, a summary, introduction, method, results, and conclusion sections (see Figure 11.3a). It is likely the organisers of the poster session might also supply a list of sections that your poster should include, which are unique to just that session.

However, like the oral presentation, you must make hard and fast decisions on what information to present. You must decide which parts of the research would best be shown visually and have most impact. Unlike the oral presentation, you can provide sections of writing, even with detail but these should be short because people don't have the time or patience to read large sections of text. Therefore, the main aim should be clarity in the type of ideas and number of messages that you want to present. Think of yourself like an advertiser who needs to sell their research, and ideas that have sprung out of the research, to other people. Be keenly aware that, by using the poster as your medium, you need to capture the attention of passers-by as quickly as possible; once they have walked by your poster and gone on to the next one, it is too late. As a result, visual impact is key, as well as having a clear and simple message from your research. Before constructing your poster, a crucial part of its success is being clear about the main messages that you want to convey in it. You will need to have a go at making that message one that can be communicated with an economy of words and perhaps with one or two main graphics. Have a look at the following examples of research posters (Figures 11.3b and 11.3c)

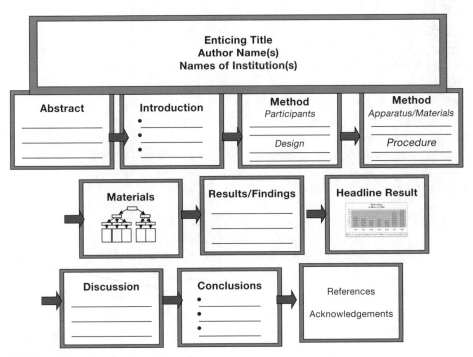

(a) Sample layouts of a research poster.

Figure 11.3 Examples of research posters.

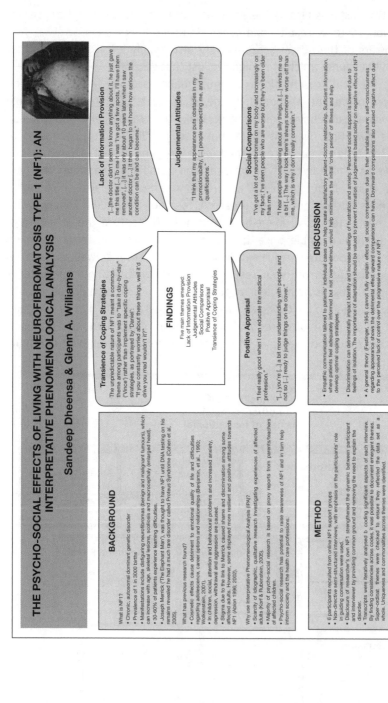

(b) Example of a qualitative study poster: coping with neurofibromatosis.

Figure 11.3 Continued

NEUROTICISM BIASES LINKS BETWEEN WORK STRESSORS AND STRAINS

Glenn A. Williams & Ian P. Albery

Context of Study

There has been much debate about the role of the 'third' variable in work stress research (e.g. Zapf et al., 1996). These variables could include personality traits like Neuroticism that might interfere with accurate assessment of how stressors could be linked to strain. Neuroticism has been found to have an important influence as a possible third variable (Brief et al., 1988; Payne and Morrison, 2002; Spector et al., 2000).

Method

Participants: 76 National Health Service employees were surveyed. They were based in one general hospital within South East England.

Instruments: We used the Job Stress Survey (Spielberger and Vagg, 1999), the Short Form of the EPQ-R (Eysenck and Eysenck, 1991) and the Job Satisfaction scale of the Occupational Stress Indicator (Cooper, Sloan and Williams, 1988).

Analysis: A four-step strategy was used.

Step 1: Was Neuroticism correlated with the predictor and the dependent variable (DV)?

Step 2: Did Neuroticism contribute a significant proportion of variance in DV scores?

Step 3: Did other predictor predict the DV to a greater extent than Neuroticism did?

Step 4: Is there a reduced correlation between the predictor and the DV after partialling out Neuroticism?

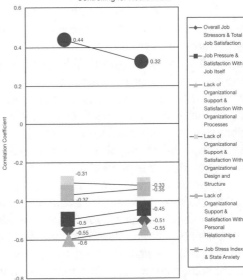

Fig. 1. Work Stressor-Strain Links Are Generally Weakened After Controlling for Neuroticism

Results

Neuroticism **was related** to the links between:
(1) Overall Job Stressor Index scores and Total Job Satisfaction levels;
(2) Job Pressure Index scores and levels of Satisfaction with Job Itself; and
(3) Lack of Organizational Support Index scores and Satisfaction with Organizational Processes.
With all three sets of stressor-strain links, Steps 1, 3 and 4 were fulfilled.
Neuroticism was not related to Lack of Organizational Support Index scores and Satisfaction with:
(A) Organizational Design and Structure and (B) Personal Relationships.

Conclusions

1. Neuroticism should be regularly measured and statistically controlled. Without doing this, the true strength of the relationship between a work stressor and a work strain may be masked.
2. Stress prevention and management should target staff groups with the highest levels of Neuroticism.
3. If the relationship between work stressors and strains remains strong, even after controlling for Neuroticism, psychosocial hazards may be a problem within these types of organizations.

(c) Example of a quantitative study poster: stress in the health service.

Figure 11.3 Continued

and judge whether the messages are clear. Is there too much jargon? Is the title short and sweet (i.e. no more than 15 words long) and is there a clear message about the major findings?

Design and presentation of the poster

So, what design are you looking for? Posters have to be done well, and it's simply not a case of writing some things on several pieces of A4 paper and pinning them up. It's about taking a large piece of paper or board (about the size of a large poster that you may have had in your bedroom) and placing the story of your research on that board. Generally, depending on the size of your poster, you'll have space for between 500 and 1500 words. It would be a good idea before starting to find out what size limits you must adhere to.

If you are looking to make an excellent presentation you are looking for an impressive overall appearance. An excellent presentation should have a coherent structure with transition between different parts, that has excellent images, graphics with the text well integrated supporting the pictures with a narrative. Most of the entire poster should provide a clear explanation of the research. If you need some indication of what a poster shouldn't be, a poor poster would be something that has a poor presentation that looks as if it has been hurried and not thought through. A poor presentation might have little coherence and lack a clear logical flow to it; the sections might seem disjointed for instance. In poor posters, each section might contain too little information to give enough of an idea about what the main messages of the research are, whereas an equally poor poster might be so jam-packed with information that it's difficult to sort out what the researchers' main messages are.

The overall design of your poster should be a series of components or small components. Imagine the front page of a good newspaper. There are different sections that go to make up that front page. The editor of that newspaper will have spent some time making sure that the front page works well and you should try to do the same. Develop a page that is made up of different boxes (rectangles). Make sure areas are balanced on the page and this will allow you to group the areas around the page in an appropriate fashion. Plan a theme for your design: what is the overall style, the font, the colours you are going to use? For example you need to use colours sparingly and only to differentiate and add interest. Try to avoid garish colours, like bright green or pink. Try to have a light background (as used in newspapers) and avoid dark backgrounds. However, the main point is that you should have some idea of how your poster is going to be laid out, before you start filling in the boxes.

Ensure you have a consistent style (i.e. font, font size, headings, formatting). An inconsistent style will interrupt the flow of your presentation. Make sure your font is not only consistent but of a similar size. Also ensure that the font size is readable from a short distance. You should aim to have a font size at least 20pt, if not slightly larger. Make sure all the headings are the same style and appear in a similar way. If you use bold text or italicise aspects of the text make sure it is consistent throughout.

When presenting figures, diagrams or a table make sure the captions for each of these are consistent and positioned consistently in terms of the figure.

Finally, if you can, develop your presentation on a computer with an appropriate software package, like Microsoft PowerPoint or a desktop publishing package like Microsoft Publisher®. This will allow you to develop the presentation sensibly, allowing you to make changes quite easily to text and poster design, whilst getting an overall impression of what the poster will look like before you get it printed.

Creating your poster

And now, on to the actual content . . . When writing your content, you need to decide on the central message, which is most certainly the conclusion that you have obtained from having done the study. All aspects of your presentation should focus on that conclusion. Therefore all other aspects of the presentation should be planned around this point. You should view the poster as a short story, telling the audience about your work leading up to the ending, your conclusion. Make sure your poster includes a clear statement of your research aims, a brief description of your method, and a summary of your main results leading to your conclusion and suggestions for future research.

You haven't got space for long explanations of each of these things. Keep all aspects short and direct, but ensure each box is interesting to read in itself. Therefore you must make the clarity of each section a top priority. You must decide on what information would be most interesting and informative for each section (e.g. introduction, method) and present that. Set yourself the target of one or two points you want to get across in each box. Most of all keep the material simple, when using text use short and direct sentences. When showing your results or diagrams, only illustrate the main findings or the points or aspects of the model or the theory.

Also, it takes a long time to develop a poster; it is not something you can create in an evening. Give yourself plenty of time to create your poster. If you are working with other people, meet a long time before the presentation date and plan and allocate your time around developing the design of the poster, the content of the poster and when you are actually going to create it.

Self-assessment exercise

Below is the paper we have discussed a number of times in this chapter, 'Assessment of nutritional problems and risk of falling in hospital-based older person care: brief research report'. For this exercise we would like you to read the paper again, and pretend you have to present an oral presentation in which you can use seven PowerPoint slides. In the spaces indicate what information from the paper you would put on each of the slides that would provide the basis of your talk.

Assessment of nutritional problems and risk of falling in hospital-based older person care: brief research report.

Abstract

Falls among older people are problematic in the hospital environment and a cause for concern among administrators, patients, relatives and health professionals alike. In the current study, the views of 31 nurses on falls' risk assessment were obtained from a randomly selected sample of 50 nursing staff working in three Care of the Older Person wards. We focused on nurses' consideration of poor nutrition among patients as being a major factor for making falls more likely and hypothesised that there would be a relationship between the type of ward that a nurse was based on and acknowledging nutritional problems as being implicated with falls. No significant link was found between ward type and nurses looking at nutrition. We outline the implications for staff training with needing to ensure that more nurses see nutrition as a falls' risk factor. It is also recommended that this education does not need to be targeted to those working in only one type of Care of the Older Person ward.

Introduction

Falls among older people contribute greatly to mortality and morbidity throughout this country and the government (Department of Health and Health Care, 2003) has been implementing action plans to target this growing problem. The Dietetic Society (2007) has claimed that one of the major risk factors for falls among older people is that many of them are undernourished, thus leading to dizziness when older people are mobilising. In the hospital environment, there should be less chance of older patients not having sufficient nourishment, as there should be more control over what food is administered to them. However, there is evidence that the older patient has problems with diet and feeling hungry due to polypharmacy (i.e. needing to take a cocktail of prescribed drugs throughout the day) (Jefferies and Dealer, 2006). In the current study, we were aiming to see whether nurses involved with care of the older patient were taking poor diet/malnourishment into account when considering a patient's risk of falling. This study focused on the reported falls' risk assessment practices of a sample of registered general nurses working at three Care of the Older Person wards in a community hospital based in a city within the New Pleasant state. We also sought to explore whether there was a relationship between the type of ward that the nurses worked on and the reported assessment practices. It was hypothesised that there would be a link between ward and assessment of diet when examining risk of falling. This hypothesis was grounded in observations by the research team that one of the wards (Spongebury) appeared to have patients with higher dependencies than in the other two wards, which dealt mainly with rehabilitation, and that staff would thus have less time to consider nutrition as an issue.

Method

Participants

A random sample of 50 nurses was approached out of the population of 75 full-time and part-time nurses employed by the hospital. Agency nursing staff were not approached, as the permanent staff would govern all induction and training in patient assessment and we viewed them as being vital to driving the methods and ethos of patient assessment. Out of the nurses that we sampled, 33 replied to the invitation letter with a completed questionnaire (66 per cent response rate), although only 31 of the forms were useable with complete data.

Materials
We used the Stanislav Falls Assessment Procedures Index (Stanislav, 2005). This comprised a 35-item form that requires respondents to identify the factors they consider when assessing an older person's risk of falling. This questionnaire has been mainly validated with hospital-based older person care (Stanislav and Spector, 2004) and has been found to have subscales tapping into three main concepts – physical health, psychological well-being and the mobilisation process. These three subscales have internal consistencies of 0.89, 0.65 and 0.85 respectively.

Procedure
Posters advertising the study were placed on staff noticeboards near the three wards and the agreement of the staff unions and the hospital management was obtained before commencing the study. Local Research Ethical Committee approval was also granted in November 2005. The research team sent the questionnaire to the sample of nurses via the internal post during the week commencing 12 December 2005. The forms had a self-addressed, stamped envelope for participants to send their completed returns to the team by a two-week deadline.

Analysis
As we were primarily interested in the relationship between type of Care of the Older Person ward and nurses' reported assessment of nutritional problems when examining patient risk of falling, we conducted a chi-square analysis on these two variables.

Results

Table 1 outlines the distribution of nurses who said that they either did or did not consider nutritional problems among their patients when assessing risk of falling on the wards. It is noteworthy that only 16 out of the 31 (51.6 per cent) nurse respondents reported looking out for nutritional problems when assessing falls' risk.

Table 1 Nutritional problems as a risk factor for falls among older patients

	'Consideration of nutrition problems?'	
'Which ward do you work in?'	*No*	*Yes*
Spongebury	5	6
Wickham	7	7
Hesham	3	3

A chi-square analysis showed that there was no significant relationship between the type of ward that the nurses worked on and their focus on nutritional problems among patients when conducting falls' risk assessment, $\chi^2 (2) = 0.059, p > 0.05$.

Discussion

It can be seen from the results that only half of the nurses who responded to our survey of falls' risk assessment practices said that they considered nutritional problems among their patients. This trend is in line with prior research (e.g. William and Hill, 2003) showing that nutrition is a neglected part of inpatient care for the older person and that

▶

nutritional well-being tends to be left to the dietician to monitor (Tidy and Meal, 2000). Unexpectedly, there was no link between type of ward and evaluation of nutritional problems as a risk factor, thus indicating that nursing practice seems fairly consistent within a community hospital setting. There are some potential limitations that need to be considered. Although our sample of 31 respondents was a sizeable percentage of the population of nursing staff within the three wards, it needs to be recognised that there may have been fewer senior nurses obtained with random sampling as they constitute a relatively small percentage of the total number of nurses employed in the study sites. Given that it is likely the senior nurses would be more involved with patient assessment (and falls' risk assessment) than junior nurses, this could explain why only half of our sample had considered nutrition as a factor. Further research could aim at replicating the administration of our questionnaire to staff at other similar wards, but through the use of a stratified sampling method. Nevertheless, the current trends seem to suggest the need for nursing practice to routinely incorporate the nutritional status of an older patient and for nurses to be educated to the impact that poor nutrition among older patients can have on making the patient disorientated and weak when mobilising. As we did not find a link between type of Care of the Older Person ward and reported assessment practices, we would recommend that this education should cover the training of all grades of nursing and in all types of wards.

PowerPoint presentation

In the spaces below indicate what information from the paper you would put on each of the slides that would provide the basis of your talk.

SLIDE 1

SLIDE 2

SLIDE 3

SLIDE 4

SLIDE 5

SLIDE 6

SLIDE 7

Summary

We hope this chapter has provided you with some useful pointers on how to share findings from your research in a written format through a report, as an oral presentation, or in the form of a poster. In the following chapter, we will take you through some of the advanced thinking that you will need to engage in to become more proficient in conducting nursing and health care-related research.

Chapter 12

Advanced thinking in research methods and practice: From novice to expert nurse researcher

KEY THEMES

Mixed methods research • Working with others when doing research • Reflexivity • Applying theory and research to nursing practice

LEARNING OUTCOMES

At the end of this chapter you will be able to:

- See the strengths and limitations of conducting mixed methods research to combine quantitative and qualitative methods of data collection and analysis

- Understand how researcher–researcher and researcher–participant interactions can be successfully negotiated when dealing with groups of people

- Reflect on the influence of your role as a researcher and the progress of the research process

- Explore ways of applying findings from nursing research to practical situations.

Introduction

IMAGINE THAT . . .

You are an infection control nurse who has just completed a small-scale survey of methods that staff members are using to control infections in a hospital ward. However, you think that this survey has not got 'under the skin' of the subject matter. You worry that you haven't got the entire picture of adherence to infection control procedures throughout the entire hospital and are wondering about how representative the ward in your dissertation was. In addition, despite the staff saying that they did all the right things when adhering to infection control procedures, it still worries you that infection rates within the ward are still relatively high. Are staff members saying that they're doing one thing and then doing something different? What about if you wanted to look at staff practices in the rest of the hospital? How could you move beyond doing a small-scale piece of research to doing something that could have a massive, beneficial impact on practice? Who would you need to involve in taking that next step and what kinds of approaches could you take? Would it be better to combine a range of data collection techniques to get a better understanding of the whole phenomenon of infection control in this hospital?

With this chapter, and the following chapter, we will be equipping you with skills to gain confidence in coming into contact with more advanced research techniques and skills to become a more proficient research-informed nurse. With the imaginary scenario that we have just presented, this may become a reality for some of you. There will be pressing clinical issues that you will want to resolve, such as in tackling hospital-acquired infections, and we are going to encourage you to move beyond any approach that seems like it has a tried and tested formula. Instead, we are going to be encouraging you to move beyond the student researcher role and enable you to see the imperfections that often may arise when carrying out nursing research. This chapter will present less of a black and white 'cookbook' method for being a more experienced nursing researcher. Instead we will offer to you a 'smorgasbord' menu to choose from a variety of research methodologies and methods that you can adapt and shape depending on the research problems that you might encounter. We will show you that you can use a variety of methods to look at the same phenomenon. For example, study of the well-being of nurses in your hospital could involve focus groups, one-to-one interviews, participant observation or the use of a stress survey. We will look at the so-called divide between quantitative and qualitative research and will show you that this divide is less important to have once you are proficient in using both of these approaches. After a while, it may be more important to get a holistic picture of the phenomenon concerned, such as infection control practices, by asking a range of questions and matching each question to the most appropriate research method. We will show you some of the issues that you need to resolve to become a more proficient nurse researcher, such as deciding whether to look at qualitative or quantitative data (or both), how to reflect on your role in the research, and how the research has been progressing, among many more other advanced techniques.

12.1 Bridging the qualitative/quantitative divide

As nurse researchers there are a number of central questions that you need to consider in terms of the actual application of research within the health care setting before we start. A crucial point relates to the rationale or motivations that drive the research in the first instance and what you hope to achieve. As nurses, you are working during an era of needing to promote and implement evidence-based nursing practice where actions at a practice level, and practice development in a wider sense, are driven by evidence. You might then need to fully understand as to what forms the evidence might take and how this evidence can be acquired or known. It also raises questions regarding the utility of the research, for example, as part of a practice-based profession, you need to consider how the proposed research that you intend to do will enhance or add to present understanding on what is acceptable nursing practice. Most importantly, you need to know how to disseminate your findings to let others know about any improvements that can be made to practice in order to enhance patient care and patients' health.

Historically, the preoccupation with comparing quantitative and qualitative research has led to the notion that these two methodologies occupy opposite ends of a methodological spectrum. The implications of such a distinction have meant that traditionally qualitative research has been perceived by some disciplines (e.g. by some people working in the biomedical sciences) as less rigorous and less credible than its quantitative counterpart.

In Figure 12.1 you can see the kind of hierarchy of evidence that traditionally was used to put randomised controlled trials (RCTs) on a pedestal as one of the most credible and rigorous method of research in the health field, with qualitative research not even being placed on the hierarchy by some people! From the biomedical researchers' perspective, the RCT design is seen as important for studying the clinical effectiveness of an intervention through minimisation of bias and being able to generalise the findings to other settings. However, we will also show you later that the way in which researchers have used the RCT design is not without its limitations, particularly in neglecting the all-vital human element to studying patients' or service users' experiences of health and illness. You may also notice that systematic reviews or meta-analyses are put at the top of the hierarchy; this is because this type of research is meant to produce even more generalisable findings by pooling the results of many RCT studies into one large data set and analysing this pooled information. However, even this approach is not without its limitations, as it depends on what research questions are most relevant to you. Petticrew and Roberts (2003) have argued that a hierarchy is less useful than a matrix of typical questions that are matched with research designs. By using the earlier case example of hospital infection control practices and policies, we have adapted Petticrew and Roberts' (2003) matrix approach in Table 12.1.

Nowadays, nurse researchers are more enlightened in knowing that qualitative research can coexist comfortably with quantitative research in shedding new light on

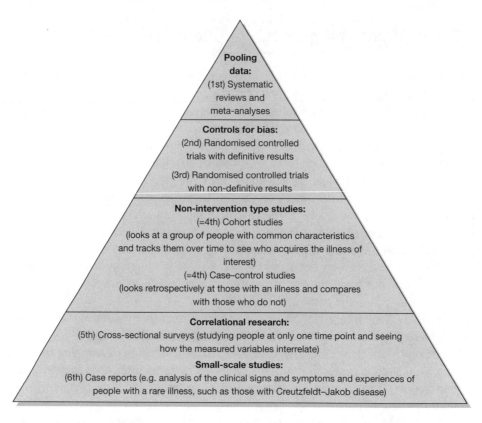

Figure 12.1 A traditional hierarchy of evidence in descending order of credibility and rigour (adapted from Petticrew and Roberts, 2003).

phenomena that are of interest to nurses. There are some who would argue that qualitative research is important as a stand-alone approach to researching the experiences of service users or how health professionals deliver health care; still others view qualitative research as being a supplement to quantitative research and a few people seem to believe that qualitative research is not a vital component for nursing research and that one should rely solely on quantitative studies when researching health care and service users' recovery from illness.

In Table 12.2, you should be able to see how quantitative research and qualitative research both have their limitations but they also have their strong points, which we need to use to get a better insight on the whole phenomenon being investigated.

We need to use different ways of 'seeing' the issue that we're interested in. We want to use an illustration of these different ways of seeing, which one of the authors was first introduced to by Professor Paul Thomas, a Professor of Research, Training and Education for Primary Care at Thames Valley University. In Figure 12.2, we have adapted the way in which he demonstrated that there are different 'truths' and ways of knowing and that we cannot rely on just one source of knowledge to knowing truly about the domain that we want to study.

Table 12.1 Questions to ask about reducing hospital acquired infections – a matrix approach

Research question	Qualitative research	Cross-sectional survey	Case-control studies	Cohort studies	RCTs	Systematic reviews or meta-analyses
Effectiveness Does alcohol rub work better than soap and water? Are some alcohol rubs better than others in reducing infection transmission?				*	**	***
Acceptability How comfortable is alcohol rub compared to other methods of hand-washing? Are there unexpected side effects of using certain types of rubs?	**	*			*	***
Cost-effectiveness Are certain types of alcohol-based rubs more cost-effective than others?					**	***
Satisfaction What are Muslim patient and health worker concerns with using alcohol-based rubs? How inconvenienced are some staff or patients in using soap and water versus alcohol rub?	**	**	*	*		*

Key: *** = highly appropriate; ** = somewhat appropriate; * = could be used.

Source: adapted from Petticrew and Roberts, 2003

Table 12.2 The strengths and limitations of quantitative and qualitative research

Issues	Type of research	
	Qualitative	Quantitative
Methods	Observations, interviews	Experiments, surveys
Major questions	What is X?	How many Xs exist?
Reasoning	Inductive (i.e. works from observing the **specifics** of a situation and helps in developing a more **general** theory, often through the development of themed-type influences)	Deductive (i.e. works from a **general** model of how treatment should work effectively and then tests out **specific** hypotheses to see if the treatment works as expected)
Strengths	• Validity • Can help explain why participants in quantitative studies have done unexpected things (e.g. dropping out of a clinical trial, not complying with their medication regime) • Can give insights into sequences of events and possible causal factors to behaviour among service users	• Reliability • Breadth of coverage • Ability to see whether trends in one sample are similar to those found in other settings
Weaknesses	• Might be too specific to certain situations and not generalisable to various settings • Could be open to alternative interpretations so needs to have transparency in how the data are coded	• Too reductionistic and sometimes artificial by being separated from everyday events in 'the field' • Humans may not think, act and feel in uniform ways at all times • Ignores the role of situational and contextual influences

Source: adapted from Mays and Pope, 1996

In the next section, we will encourage you to be open to using quantitative and qualitative approaches to getting more insights into the area that you're interested in, rather than solely using one type of methodology.

12.2 Mixed methods in nursing research

As the discussions surrounding the qualitative-quantitative divide highlight, there are often quite stark differences between the opposing ends of the methodology spectrum. However, it is equally important to consider the value of combining approaches or undertaking a 'mixed methods' approach to the research enquiry process.

For example, imagine that you would like to design a research project to explore the experiences of older carers in the community setting (McGarry and Arthur, 2001). The specific focus of the enquiry may be towards asking the following questions:

● What is it like to be an older, informal carer?

● And (from a nursing or health perspective) is there an impact later in life on the carer's health and well-being as a result of providing informal care?

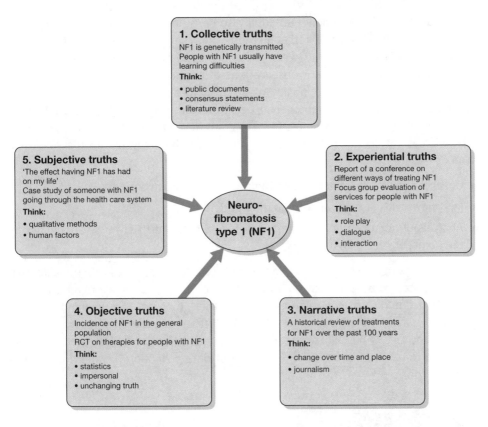

1. Collective truths
NF1 is genetically transmitted
People with NF1 usually have
learning difficulties
Think:
• public documents
• consensus statements
• literature review

5. Subjective truths
'The effect having NF1 has had
on my life'
Case study of someone with NF1
going through the health care system
Think:
• qualitative methods
• human factors

Neuro-fibromatosis type 1 (NF1)

2. Experiential truths
Report of a conference on
different ways of treating NF1
Focus group evaluation of
services for people with NF1
Think:
• role play
• dialogue
• interaction

4. Objective truths
Incidence of NF1 in the general
population
RCT on therapies for people with NF1
Think:
• statistics
• impersonal
• unchanging truth

3. Narrative truths
A historical review of treatments
for NF1 over the past 100 years
Think:
• change over time and place
• journalism

Figure 12.2 Different ways of 'seeing': five truths about neurofibromatosis type 1
(ideas adapted from Thomas, 2006).

These are arguably both important questions which, as a whole, provide a more complete picture of caregiving, but they also involve quite different research approaches. For example, to explore the experiences of older people may require a more open approach with in-depth interviews, whereas assessing the impact of caregiving on health and well-being could entail quantitative analysis of the differences in health and well-being between carers and non-carers.

12.3 Triangulation and complementary approaches to understanding the area being researched

Triangulation is a concept that first originated in the field of mathematics and cartography (i.e. creating maps). To use triangulation in that conventional sense would mean calculating the distance to any given geographical point by using triangles and two reference points around the point of interest. Triangulation in nursing research does not mean measuring things in 'threes'; instead, all that is emphasised is incorporating more than one data collection method. It also does not mean solely employing one quantitative method and qualitative method; it may involve, for example, the use of several qualitative or quantitative methods, such as by collecting data through focus groups and making participant observations of clinical practices. One of the main advantages of using triangulation lies in getting a more comprehensive and trustworthy understanding of the phenomenon being studied. For example, in a qualitative study exploring the ways in which district nurses develop and experience successful relationships within the patient's home, the researcher may obtain the following sources of data:

● Observation of district nurses and their interactions with patients,

● Interviews with district nurses and their patients, and

● Analysis of documentary data (e.g. policies on how a district nurse should act in the home, or care plans).

In this way, the researcher attempting to capture these experiences within the district nursing process is able to draw on a wide range of data to provide a rich account of such district nurse–patient relationships. Another thing to bear in mind when it comes to triangulation is that there are many different kinds in health care research (see the box below) but, when researchers talk about this concept, it is usually with reference to having more than one method of data collection (i.e. methodological triangulation).

THINGS TO CONSIDER

Four types of triangulation

Although the common assumption about triangulation is that it is all to do with having more than one data collection method, there are those (Denzin, 1978) who have argued that triangulation can also come in other guises, all of which can help to boost the credibility of the research that is being conducted. These kinds of triangulation are as follows:

1. Investigator triangulation: having data collected and/or analysed by more than one researcher.

2. Theory triangulation: using more than one theory to make sense of the data collected about a specific phenomenon.

3. Data triangulation: collecting data in different contexts (e.g. various times, clinical settings, different health care users).

4. Methodological triangulation: using more than one method to get information about the research problem of interest.

Overall, when using any of the different kinds of triangulation you will be better equipped to obtain a full understanding of the phenomenon that you're studying, but do be conscious of the fact that this might often require more time and resources to do well. Do bear in mind that it takes a great deal of time, expertise and skill to carry out one research method in a competent manner (e.g. when designing a questionnaire, this usually means pre-testing the items, trialling the items with a small group of participants, going through various phases of validation, etc.). If considering triangulation for any research that you're involved with, try to make sure that you have sufficient expertise and experience in executing the methods of data collection and analysis; or, if needs be, co-opt a more experienced co-researcher to work with you. Let us move on to the next issue when it comes to being a more advanced researcher, namely how to collaborate with others in an effective way.

12.4 Collaborating with others

When collaborating with others in research there are five aspects to consider:

- Managing interpersonal relationships in nursing research
- Managing possible role conflicts in being a nurse and a researcher
- Managing relationships among co-researchers
- Working in, and with, stakeholder groups
- Iterative group-related research – the Delphi technique

We will now consider each of these in turn.

Managing interpersonal relationships in nursing research

However, even within a particular research tradition, e.g. qualitative, the nature of the research will to a greater extent influence how relationships are established. In ethnography for example, the relationship that exists between the nurse both as ethnographer, i.e. the person carrying out the research, *and* as part of a shared profession (nursing) as the focus of the research arguably has particular significance due to the proximity or mutuality of the field of observation.

This of course may have both positive and negative consequences for the researcher. For example, prior knowledge of the professional language used and the nuances of working practice may enable you to 'fit' in to the environment and to have 'insider' knowledge. However, it may also have disadvantages as you will be viewing the environment with a 'professional eye' and therefore a certain 'bias' when perhaps a more neutral perspective is needed. At times when conducting qualitative studies, it is important for nurse researchers to expose their assumptions so that others who read about the study can verify the authenticity of the account. Also, as a nurse researching within your own professional group, you will need to be mindful of the potential conflicts that may occur in terms of alliance. By contrast, it may help to be viewed as an 'outsider' and be less familiar with the jargon and ways of working within a health care setting. The following quote from Howard Becker's (1993) observational study of medical students' language used about patients is an excellent illustration of how this outsider role can help provide a fresh perspective to how health professional language is used and its impacts on patient care:

> One morning as we made rounds [of the hospital wards], we saw a very talkative patient, who had multiple complaints to tell the doctor about – all sorts of aches and pains, and unusual events. I could see that no one was taking her very seriously, and on the way out, one of the students said, 'Boy, she's really a crock!' I understood this, in part as shorthand for 'crock of shit'. It was obviously invidious. But what was he talking about? What was wrong with her having all those complaints? Wasn't that interesting?. . . So when Chet [the medical student] called the patient a crock, I made this theoretical analysis in a flash and then came up with a profoundly theoretical question: 'What's a crock?' He looked at me as if to say that any damn fool would know that. So I said, 'Seriously, when you called her a crock, what did you mean?' He looked a little confused. He had known what he meant when he said it but wasn't sure he could explain it . . . I got all the students interested in the question, and, between us, with me asking a lot of questions and applying the results to succeeding cases [of patients who could possibly be seen as 'crocks'], we ended up defining a crock as a patient with multiple complaints but no discernible physical pathology. (pp. 31-32)

In the above quote, the thing to bear in mind is that having an outsider's perspective could be extremely helpful as it can assist in getting an alternative view on why health care workers do the things they do. Overall, we would argue that you need to be aware of your role as nurse researcher, your professional role as a nurse and also be open to the twists and turns that a research project might take. Imagine that you are interviewing a nurse as part of a study and during the interview the nurse becomes visibly distressed and starts to tell you about how much she dislikes one of the managers in the hospital. Is this permissible as data or does it fall outside of legitimate data that can be used within the study? Should you proceed or stop the interview? Should you include the interview transcript in the findings of the study?

With this in mind, discussion in the nursing literature surrounding the role of the nurse as researcher has developed at a number of levels, ranging from the technical or practical aspects of engaging in fieldwork or gaining competence to more in-depth consideration of the mechanisms and relationships through which such roles are accomplished in practice. These are the issues and dilemmas that need to be carefully considered and addressed in the process of becoming an informed, authentic and ethical nurse researcher. We will revisit the practical and ethical issues of doing nursing research in the next chapter too, as there are many complex things to consider when doing research in a practice-based environment. But let us now turn to the problems that might be encountered in wearing two hats – the one of a nurse and the one of a researcher.

Managing possible role conflicts in being a nurse and a researcher

As nurses conducting research in our own profession we are also governed by a professional code of conduct (NMC, 2008). We then need to be clear about our responsibility both as a researcher and as a nurse. This duality has the potential to raise tensions, for example, we have a clear responsibility to report instances of bad practice if this is observed. As a nurse researcher, most of the time you are meant to be an observer rather than someone who intervenes in what you are witnessing. It may be wise to meet this role without having to feel the need to intervene in situations that you are witness to, unless it were a medical emergency and you were the only person available to intervene. However, we realise that the ethics of being an ethical and effective nurse researcher is rarely black-and-white so you may wish to consider what you would do in the case scenarios in 'Things to Consider'.

THINGS TO CONSIDER

Ethical dilemmas for nurse researchers

As nurses conducting research, often as observers of your own profession, you are governed by a professional code of conduct (NMC, 2008). You then need to be clear of your responsibility both as a researcher and as a nurse. This duality has the potential to raise tensions. For example, you may have a responsibility to report instances of bad practice, if this is observed.

1. Imagine that you are a nurse who is conducting an observational study of district nurses. As an experienced nurse you note during one visit that the nurse has applied a dressing in a way that is in conflict with recommended guidelines. How would you proceed?

2. Imagine that you are a nurse who is conducting an observational study of nurses working in an acute ward. One evening, as you are walking out to the car park and chatting with a group of nurses from the ward, one of the nurses makes a racist comment about a patient on the ward. How would you proceed?

3. Imagine that you are conducting a study observing nurse–patient relationships on a busy surgical ward. While you are observing you see a nurse ignoring a patient's requests to be assisted to the toilet. What would you do? Who would you inform? Would you approach this nurse, and how? What might be the impact on research relationships?

Managing relationships among co-researchers

It was once written that 'No man is an island, entire of itself' (Donne, undated). Although these sentiments were perhaps not originally intended for the trials and tribulations of doing nursing research, it is apt to remind us that while research can sometimes be a singular endeavour, collaboration can be much more enriching professionally and personally. However, it is also worth remembering that while collaboration brings with it inherent benefits, there are some important factors to consider before embarking on this particular enterprise.

Working in, and with, stakeholder groups

There are certainly some things to remember when working with groups (within the nursing profession and among other different health care professions) and between groups (as part of a collaboration) and much will depend upon the size and scope of the project to be undertaken in terms of how this will work overall and like any relationship what is crucial is that you will be able to 'get on' with each other over an extended period of time. This is not to say that there isn't scope for constructive challenges but rather that the foundations of the relationship are strong enough to weather the storm.

Doing large-scale projects

If the project is large scale you may need to think about the formation of a steering group. The function of a steering group is largely to help to keep the project on time and on target in terms of resources. It is also there to help to manage the general direction. The people who are usually part of a steering group have credibility and authority within the particular subject area and are representative of all key stakeholders within a particular field. It is also worth thinking about the time commitment needed for a steering group and the importance that your colleagues may or may not attach to it.

Doing smaller-scale projects

While you may not enlist or form a steering group for smaller-scale projects you will still need to be aware of and acknowledge other people who are both able to offer valuable support and knowledge with the development of the project and who may also have influence in terms of access 'gatekeepers'. A gatekeeper, within the context of health service research, is the term used to describe a person/or people who control access to potential study participants, such as patients or health professionals. For example, imagine that you would like to undertake a project in another NHS Trust, who might you need to approach in order to gain permission to approach the staff and/or patients? It might in the first instance be the manager of a particular service. However, it is also worth remembering that gatekeepers can also limit access, by for example pre-selection of participants or areas of study.

Iterative group-related research – the Delphi technique

While most group-based research requires face-to-face meetings this is not always the case, and the Delphi technique is a case in point. This method describes the particular process whereby individuals could form a 'virtual' panel of experts (participants) and are surveyed on a particular topic or issue. Particular survey instruments are used and distributed to the individuals involved in several rounds and the role of the researcher is to analyse and collate responses and then provide feedback and elicit further information through further rounds of questions. The advantages of this approach are that it is possible to form a group of expertise from across a wide geographical area without the problems of physically meeting, and the anonymous nature and distance may facilitate a greater openness among members. The disadvantages are that this approach is time-consuming for the researcher and there may be issues in terms of commitment and attrition on the part of survey group members.

12.5 What is reflexivity?

In some texts on research methods, you may come across the concept of reflexivity. Being a reflective researcher relates to the ability to take a step away from carrying out the nuts and bolts of doing a study. Reflexivity is to do with being able to 'hold a mirror up' to what is going on in the study and to reflect on the researcher's role in the research process, why the researcher has chosen the specific topic and the level of influence that the researcher might have over the research participants. Reflection also involves the researcher considering whether their choice of topic or method of interpretation is justified. In this section, we will take you through the use of a systematic framework of reflection to illustrate what takes place when you reflect on your research practices. We will use a qualitative study as an example but we hope you will see the potential for using reflection in quantitative research as well by also briefly taking you through an instance of using reflection in this type of research.

Reflection should be an integral part of the process of becoming a proficient practitioner in any profession and you will undoubtedly have been introduced to the process and function of reflection during your nursing career. Although one could argue that reflection is something that we automatically do on a regular basis, it is something that we rarely do regularly and in a systematic way unless an extreme situation might make the need for reflection appear necessary. Kolb (1984) distinguished between four main stages in the cyclical process of learning new skills. These were: (1) going through the experience itself, (2) reflecting on what happened in the experience, (3) generalising from this experience to similar types of experiences and (4) testing out this generalisation. As can be seen, the construct of reflection appears to be of pivotal importance to learning and there are a variety of ways that it can be undertaken. Although there are a broad range of tools that the reflective practitioner can use to reflect, we will use the term 'reflection' to mean a staged, systematic process that may have a retrospective (i.e. looking backward) and/or prospective (i.e. looking forward) focus. This represents the simultaneous analysis of looking backward to 'immediately past experiences, and forward to experiences which are imminent' (Cowan, 1998, p. 36).

Reflecting on your role as researcher and on the research process

There are two main areas of focus when engaging in reflection: (1) analysing your role in the research process and (2) examining the research process itself. By having a focus on the research process and the extent to which the study is meeting your original aims and objectives, this enables you to carry out more rigorous research, the findings of which may have massive implications for clinical practice. Sometimes you may need to revisit the aims and objectives and the methods being used in the study to see whether everything is going to plan. For instance, what if patients in a study that you're conducting are regularly omitting to answer certain questions in a questionnaire? Is it because they are getting too tired towards the end of filling out the questionnaire? Or are they finding that the subject matter of some of the questions is too sensitive for them? If you're finding that non-completion of the questionnaire is a recurring problem, it may be wise to be flexible and make decisions about whether to continue with the study design as it stands and what to do with the data collected so far. On a more extreme level, it is a question that may arise when administering a new drug to study participants during an RCT and finding that some of the participants in the experimental group are experiencing unpleasant side effects. When, and how often, do you reflect on the way the study is going and whether to terminate it?

Identifying good times to engage in reflection

Here are a few things to consider when needing to use reflection in your nursing research. Some novice researchers tend not to worry about being reflexive as they may be more concerned about mastering a new data collection or analysis technique. The research **protocol**/process that the novice researcher has agreed with their supervisor will be one that they feel honour-bound to stick to. In the researcher's mind, there is little need to be reflexive or look to the possibility of adapting to how participants are responding. In the novice researcher's mind, the supervisor knows best and any participants that behave in an anomalous way are just being 'awkward'.

More expert researchers revisit the research at various points during the study. When an expert researcher does a pilot study as a prelude to the real thing, the researcher goes through a systematic process of focusing on what occurred and whether participants reacted in unexpected ways. All too often, as academics, we have been regularly surprised by the neglect of reflexivity by students doing their dissertation studies and leaving any reflection until they are writing up the discussion section. To avoid leaving reflection to the last minute, we would recommend keeping a diary of the research as it is progressing, or at least a log of critical incidents that have occurred. See if you can regularly use a reflective framework like Gibbs' (1988) when doing research, just as you would do when reflecting on incidents from practice as part of updating your professional nursing portfolio. You need to realise that the research environment is rarely going to follow a perfectly designed scenario. When working with these imperfections, you need to challenge yourself by engaging with the critical questions of: is the study going as anticipated? What could affect the progress of the study? Do you need to get more skills (e.g. in interviewing patients or with recruiting potential participants by learning graphic design skills to develop posters to advertise your study in GP surgeries)? If some skills are beyond your reach at the present time, who might you need to approach to see if they could collaborate with you?

Using reflection to be clear about your role

Ensuring that you are reflecting on your role as researcher and on the research process is crucial and very different from you reflecting on your role as a nurse and the nursing process. At times, you may find yourself caught between the positions of being a nurse and being a researcher, and these roles might start to blur. For example, you might find that you are witness to a patient that you're interviewing who becomes extremely upset during the interview and wants to talk about his personal problems, rather than the subject matter of the research. As a nurse, you may feel compelled to counsel the patient regarding the personal issues that have arisen rather than stay on track with the research-related enquiries. Although ethical researchers are meant to look after the well-being of their participants, it is also vital to ensure that the point of doing the research is not disregarded. Although research participants should always have the option to withdraw from a study at any point, the researcher should also ensure that the whole point of doing the research is not significantly deviated from too.

Using reflective frameworks to reflect

You will remember from an earlier chapter that we introduced you to the use of Gibbs' (1988) reflective framework when doing critical appraisal. We would also urge you to use it for reflection when doing any type of research and will take you through two instances of its use. First, we will use it with a qualitative study and then secondly we will use it with quantitative research. As a reminder, there are six major stages to undergo with the reflection – description, feelings, evaluation, analysis, conclusion and an action plan. With description, it only needs to be a brief account of an incident or situation. An incident can be a one-off event that has made the nurse researcher stop and think, whereas a situation could be ongoing. The feelings component of the reflection could be an assortment of emotions that are experienced at the time or being felt as a result of reflection on what is ongoing. Evaluation entails looking at the possible good or bad points of the event/situation. Analysis involves focusing on theory or previous research or other related experiential evidence that could help to explain the situation or event. The conclusion is an opportunity for the nurse researcher to consider what the most prominent points of the reflection have been; this is important, especially for a complex process of reflection in which sometimes the person doing the reflection may not be able to 'see the wood for the trees'. As a result of the whole process of reflection, the research nurse would then construct a plan of action to face this event/situation. This is a cyclical process with the possibility of another phase of reflections in which the research nurse is able to reflect on how successful the action plan from a previous cycle of reflections has been when encountering the consequences of this action plan on another occasion (Example 12.1).

Example 12.1

Reflecting on a qualitative study

1. DESCRIPTION:

I am research nurse employed by a hospital trust to analyse the impact of a shift to a more patient-focused way of working with the development of multidisciplinary teams centred around the patient's experience rather than only working in a team of just one professional group. I am interviewing a nursing sister who is implementing the organisational changes in her newly formed multidisciplinary team. The nurse complains of feeling burnt out and overwhelmed by the stress that has been brought on by this organisational change. The sister also relates to me that many of her colleagues in the team are feeling uncertain about their jobs and are unclear about the roles and responsibilities that they are meant to fulfil.

2. FEELINGS:

I feel **curious** about why this nurse has told me this. Does she expect me to tell her senior managers about her troubles and the concerns of her colleagues? What is her agenda? Is she just keen to let off steam? How does she see me? Is she keen to tell a fellow nurse about these issues in the hope that I will understand? Does she see me as being located away from the changes that have been introduced but still able to make an impact on these changes? I feel **worried** about the well-being of the staff and **concerned** about the knock-on effects on patient care. Are the patients getting a poor deal out of these changes? I am a little **confused** about my own role and what I should be reporting. The focus should have been on the effects of these changes on patient care and patient well-being and I have conflicting feelings about where the direction of the research might be going. I am **interested** to know how these organisational changes were planned and what the perceptions of the health care workers have been about these changes.

3. EVALUATION:

Good points:
It is helpful to find that the staff are so open with me about their thoughts and feelings. I can start to identify where the changes have impacted on staff health and working practices.

Bad points:
I am employed by the Trust and may face a conflict of interests if I gather too much information that is critical of the Trust and what it has done. I could get too distracted away from the original focus on assessing how patient care is being delivered and how the patients may be benefiting from these changes. The patients should, after all, be my main focus. It also looks like some of the staff don't have an outlet for venting their feelings about the change and they may not have sufficient social support to help them cope. Some of the sources of stress, with worries about job security or lack of clarity over roles and responsibilities, could have been pre-empted by the managers who implemented this change.

Example 12.1 continued

4. ANALYSIS:

In terms of the conflict of interest issue, I need to get more information on this. I need to look at similar examples in which hospital Trusts have employed a researcher who has found things that could have been critical of the Trust's practices – what did they do? I can talk to some of the other research nurses in my department and also to some of those working at a nearby hospital. Regarding the processes of changing health care organisations so that they adopt more patient-focused practices, I should look at how staff have been introduced to these changes and the reactions that might occur among them. I've seen a study by Schoolfield and Orduña (1994) that has talked of reactions by health care staff to organisational change as being akin to bereavement. There are also some useful articles in the professional and academic press about how to implement a more patient-focused way of caring with less upset for patients and staff concerned. I've also seen in the literature how patient care can be adversely affected if the organisational change is not planned in a way that encourages front-line staff and also patients to inform the planning of the change at various stages of its implementation.

5. CONCLUSION:

I have found that the Patient-Focused Care programme that has been introduced in the hospital has had some influence on staff and there is a potential for these effects as having an adverse set of consequences for how patient care is delivered. I can justify broadening the focus of the research to incoroporate analysing the impact of changes to implement patient-focused care in relation to staff as well as patients.

6. ACTION PLAN:

I need to contact the manager of my research department and talk to my research nurse colleagues about expanding the focus of the project. I also need to get approval from my manager regarding what I can and can't report when writing up the study results. I need to make it clear to prospective participants about what my role is and what I can and can't do in terms of reporting on the findings. If some staff members are experiencing stress over the changes that have been implemented, I need to make sure they can approach someone for help by enlisting the support of the hospital's occupational health department. I need to ensure that I also have enough emotional support during this study, especially if participants are venting unpleasant emotions to me. I need to have regular talks with my manager and my partner. Finally, I will revisit the action plan and see how well it has worked in subsequent reflections on this project.

We hope you will have seen from the reflective process in Example 12.1 that it should not be too time-consuming (it took 30 minutes to think about the situation and write it up) and it should be a good excuse to stop and think, rather than carry on regardless when unexpected things happen during the duration of your study. In Example 12.2 you can also see another example of reflection, but this time the reflection deals with issues of having a poor response rate with a questionnaire study of health care staff.

Example 12.2

Reflecting on a quantitative study

1. DESCRIPTION:

I am a nurse who is doing a dissertation study to look at the impact that moving to a patient-focused way of working has had on nurses working within a hospital. I have sent out a stress survey to all nurses who are likely to be affected by these changes. The survey has 40 items that need to be rated from '0' (no stress) to '10' (very high stress). The items outline 40 possible sources of stress that may have occurred since these changes were put in place in the hospital. After distributing questionnaires to a random sample of 500 nurses from my list of 1,000 that work in the hospital, I've only had 60 back in the past month. Why?

2. FEELINGS:

I'm irritated. Don't the staff see that I want to get information that could help to fight their cause? I can help identify areas for intervention to make their working lives less stressful. I'm concerned. Did I have the right list of nursing staff from the Human Resources department? I've had 50 unopened questionnaire packs returned to me with notes on the outside saying that the staff member has left the Trust or is off on a long-term absence.

3. EVALUATION:

Good points:

I'm not pressed for time. I have another month to still collect data until I need to start doing the data analysis and write-up for submitting my dissertation. I have sufficient financial support and resources to send reminders to the entire sample, along with a copy of the questionnaire in case some people have misplaced it.

Bad points:

It is possible that I didn't get sufficient support from the staff unions to see if they can encourage staff to take part in the survey. Perhaps they are suspicious of my intentions in doing the study or they doubt that anything will result for the better from their participation in the survey. It is also possible that I've been sent an out-of-date staff list from the HR department. Perhaps the response rate is not as low as I originally thought. Staff may also be deterred from filling out the survey if they think it's going to take too long or perhaps they think their views won't be listened to by their managers.

4. ANALYSIS:

I need to look at similar studies in which the researchers have done stress surveys of health care staff who have been affected by large-scale organisational changes. It is possible that stress survey research typically has low response rates, with highly stressed and overworked staff having too little time to take part and staff with hardly any stress believing that the survey isn't for them since they're not stressed out!

I have found out about some of the things that might be deterring the sample from taking part by having had informal chats with some of the staff who weren't sampled. I can also get more information from them about whether support from the staff unions or from the hospital's occupational health department would have prompted them to take part in a survey of this nature. Perhaps these people would have been able to inform me as to whether a prize draw would have been a useful incentive as well.

Example 12.2 continued

5. CONCLUSION:

There seems to be a low response rate to this survey of staff stress but I need to find out more about whether this is truly the case and I also need to explore different ways of providing incentives or reminders to the sample to enable them to take part.

6. ACTION PLAN:

- Check the accuracy of the staff lists from the HR department.
- If the staff list is generally accurate, generate a random sample of 50 further possible participants from the list to make up for the 50 people who couldn't take part due to leaving the organisation or being absent in the long term.
- Re-visit the entire sample with a mailed copy of a reminder to take part, along with another copy of the survey and a clear two-week deadline to return it completed on the front page of the request to take part. I will also ask those who have already taken part to ignore this request but will include a telephone number on the information sheet in case any potential participants have queries about the content of some of the items or whether they are experiencing difficulties in meeting the two-week deadline for returning the survey.

A fundamental difference between qualitative and quantitative approaches lies in the proximity of the researcher to the study participants. For example, in RCTs the researcher specifically seeks to minimise or negate their influence or potential bias on the research. Likewise, if you consider historical accounts of qualitative research you may notice that the presence of the researcher to a large extent is also absent or minimised. By contrast, in contemporary accounts of qualitative research the researcher and their role in the research is usually clearly illuminated and this is because nowadays the role of the researcher in qualitative research is largely accepted and acknowledged as an integral part of the research process as a whole.

In qualitative research the researcher's connection and subsequent effect on the research is at its broadest level known as 'reflexivity'. However, as a whole reflexivity encompasses a number of complex strands, for example, the role of the researcher in the actual 'production' of the data and the way in which information is shaped by the particular perspective of the researcher, so for example, the reasons why the researcher has chosen to pursue a particular topic may have personal as well as professional resonance and may influence the way the research is shaped or viewed through a particular lens. This does not make the research less credible *per se* but rather requires that the researcher makes these links explicit and transparent.

Reflecting on the need for establishing rapport with participants

Moreover, broadly speaking, in qualitative research the researcher has a closer proximity to the research by virtue of the methods used. In ethnographic research for example, it is probable that the researcher will have formed relationships with the participants in order to gain access and also in terms of carrying out data collection which is largely conducted through observing and/or participating in a particular culture or setting. These relationships are known as building up a rapport with the participants and showing that the presence of the researcher is not a threat to them. The whole issue of having a rapport with participants in nursing is a complex one. McGarry (2007b) has written about the dynamics of having this rapport relationship in terms of the nurse researcher being perceived by the participants as trustworthy and someone worthy of respect, and possibly of friendship. However, it may sometimes be best to avoid trying to have a rapport with the research participants, particularly if the nurse researcher is likely to find out things that could be critical of fellow nurses' ways of working or dealing with patients. McGarry (2007b) has quoted examples in which researchers in one study (Russell *et al*, 2002) even did not seem to develop rapport with the participants at all; if anything, there was a degree of distrust and sometimes hostility towards the researchers. Despite this state of affairs, the participants in the study seemed to see the researchers as still having a job to do and were relatively frank in what they were willing to disclose. McGarry (2007b) has also reflected on her own role in her research field notes after an interview with a nurse. She has observed that, although she was deemed to be trustworthy and have had some form of rapport with her informants, she was still perceived as not being an explicit part of the nursing team.

> *I had not expected this response to my question and it was obviously very difficult for [name of participant] to tell me about this; the emotion she was feeling was clearly evident . . . I reflected on this interview and whether this candid account would have been uncovered to me had I not been viewed as a colleague, as someone who would understand. However, as I listened [to the interview] and read my earlier field notes, it was perhaps because I was explicitly perceived as not being a colleague that this very private account was shared with me.*
>
> (McGarry, 2007b, p. 13)

In this reflection, it is apparent that McGarry saw her role as being one in which the nurse who disclosed an unpleasant experience might have seen the researcher as someone who could act as a temporary confidante with limited repercussions likely to occur from making these disclosures. In general, it is possible that some participants may see you in a different way to which you would like to be seen as a nurse researcher and it may help to be aware of these differences, especially when you want to disseminate your findings to others.

12.6 Applying your research findings to nursing practice

Consider the following quotation on how important it is to ensure that nurse researchers translate their theories and findings into demonstrating some clear links to clinical practice:

Nursing is essentially a practice-based discipline, and the knowledge generated by nursing research must somehow be translated into nursing practice if it is to help us decide, if not how to live, then at least how to nurse.

(Rolfe, 1998, p. 673)

Notice the 'if not how to live' part to the quote as this is quite crucial to being an effective nurse researcher. At times, you may do research that shows the kinds of health-related behaviours that could be damaging or physically and emotionally enhancing in their nature. As a nurse, many of you would undoubtedly be keen to know how to promote a healthier lifestyle amongst the general population to prevent them from becoming ill; this is tied up in knowing how to live, with patients' lifestyles often making it more complicated for a nurse in terms of doing things that could be problematic for one's health, such as not regularly checking blood glucose levels if a patient is a diabetic or not adhering to advice on appropriate diet or exercise after recovering from a heart attack. In this section, we will look at the ways in which you can become a more expert nurse researcher by knowing how to translate a theoretical model or some research findings into a practical situation. We will also discuss the barriers that might impede you from translating theory/research into practice and will explore ways of overcoming these barriers.

Answering the 'so what?' question

All too often you may read an article in a journal like *Nursing Times* or *Journal of Advanced Nursing* and wonder what the implications of a research project are for your everyday nursing practice. Some journals may have a section in the article for the authors to identify why the area that has been researched is relevant to the reader. We will show you how to make it transparently obvious when writing about a theory or results from a study that you've undertaken. The first example will use a general theory of how people cope with stressful situations and will attempt to apply it to the clinical field. Alongside this, we will also introduce you to findings from a series of studies and encourage you to consider how these findings are relevant to the nursing that you do every day.

Have a look at Figure 12.3. It outlines a general theory of stress and coping, which was proposed by Richard Lazarus and Susan Folkman (1984) and is called the cognitive appraisal theory. It has been applied to a range of areas, such as in looking at how students cope with the stress of sitting an examination (Folkman and Lazarus, 1978) and in various areas of health care too. The theory introduces three main evaluations (or appraisals) that people might undertake when faced with a potentially stressful situation. In the first evaluation, known as primary appraisal, a person may weigh up a situation and attempt to decide whether it is a threat to their well-being, a challenge, or something quite trivial. Then there is the secondary appraisal, which is when the person decides to try to cope with a situation once it is seen as being a threat and potentially stressful. Finally, after deciding how to cope with a stressful situation, tertiary appraisal (or reappraisal) happens when the person evaluates whether the attempt to cope has worked. It then becomes an ongoing process until the situation is no longer seen as a threat.

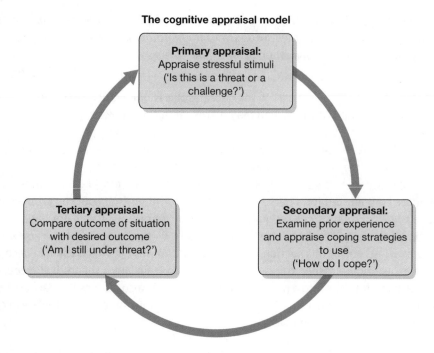

Figure 12.3 A general model of stress and coping

(adapted from *Stress, Appraisal and Coping*, Springer, New York (Lazarus, R.S. and Folkman, S., 1984) © Springer, New York).

Now, let us see how we can translate this theory into practice. Imagine that you are a nurse working in a ward that involves preparing patients for elective surgery and you may need to enable the patients to cope better with what they may perceive as the real threats of surgery to their health. They might go through a cost-benefit analysis to decide whether the surgery is worthwhile and, having done so, they may be very fearful of what the surgery entails; they may also worry about whether they will feel much pain and may be concerned about the long-term risks to their health and quality of life after having undergone the surgery. Think about the following questions that could be asked when using each stage of Lazarus and Folkman's (1984) cognitive appraisal theory:

- *In the primary appraisal stage:* how do patients appraise threats to themselves?
- *In the secondary appraisal stage:* how do they attempt to cope with the threat?
- *In the tertiary appraisal (or reappraisal) stage:* do the patients regularly check the success of their coping strategies?

Here is what you could do in this situation by using the cognitive appraisal theory to help the patients who are getting more concerned about their operation:

In the primary appraisal stage:

- Help patients to 'reframe' the situation so that they can see the risks of the operation in a less extreme, and less catastrophic, way
- Give more information so that the patients are aware of all of the risks involved

In the secondary appraisal stage:

● Help the patients to adopt the coping strategy that best works for them and allows them to feel less stressed; some patients may prefer to see the operation as more of an intellectual exercise, whereas others might prefer to do things to quell excessively anxious feelings.

In the tertiary appraisal stage:

● Enable patients to try out different ways of coping with the stress of the perceived threat to their well-being and allow them to build up confidence in knowing that some of the coping strategies that they try out will be more effective than others.

With this approach, we have been able to show you how to dissect what is going on when trying to apply a *general* theory of stress and coping to a more *specific* area of helping patients to cope with the stress that may occur when preparing for surgery. There is a wide range of possibilities for this theory to be used in health care contexts, such as if you were a paediatric nurse who needed to prepare children for admission to hospital. However, although it has been said that 'there is nothing more practical than a good theory', we do need to make sure that we test out the theory to see what parts of it work well in nursing practice. To this extent, you may need to collect data to see if the theory translates into the practice setting where you work. In other instances, you may not have the time (or the energy) to do your own research so you may need to consider previous studies that have been done in a similar area.

Self-assessment exercise

Applying research to practice

Look at the summary of published research below and consider how research can be applied to practice in this specific situation of reducing teenage pregnancies.

Reducing teenage pregnancies (Arai, 2003)

In the UK, youthful pregnancy and parenthood is considered an important social and health problem and is the focus of current government intervention. Contemporary policy approaches depict early unplanned pregnancy as a consequence of relative deprivation and a lack of opportunity, leading to 'low expectations' among youth, and as the result of sexual 'mixed messages' or poor knowledge about contraception. This small-scale, qualitative study explores how well these explanations accord with accounts of pregnancy and motherhood provided by young mothers and Teenage Pregnancy Local Co-ordinators in diverse English localities. The results suggest that structural factors may be more important in explaining early pregnancy than those relating to sexual attitudes and knowledge. The tension between the idea of early motherhood as problematic, or even pathological, and early motherhood as rational is also considered.

Imagine that you're working in a primary care trust as a nurse who is targeting the high number of teenage pregnancies in your catchment area. What might this study tell you about the role of social class in influencing the high level of teenage pregnancies in the area? Is it possible that young girls in your locality also hold attitudes that view early motherhood as a rational and viable choice? How might you persuade them otherwise?

Once you have had a go with this exercise, try a few more exercises using the following three research examples. For each example, look at the summaries and consider what nurses could do to change their practice to help patients with specific health problems.

Example 1: Falls among older people (Rosendahl *et al.*, 2003)

Reference: Rosendahl *et al*. (2003) Prediction of falls among older people in residential care facilities by the Downton index. *Aging Clinical and Experimental Research, 15(2)*, 142-147.

BACKGROUND AND AIMS: Falls are frequent among older people living in residential care facilities. The aim of this study was to investigate the prediction accuracy of the Downton fall risk index among older people living in residential care facilities at 3, 6 and 12 months, and with two different definitions of falls. METHODS: Seventy-eight residents in one residential care facility, 56 women and 22 men, mean $+/-$ SD age 81 $+/-$ 6 years, participated in this study. Forty-seven percent of participants had dementia, 45 per cent depression, and 32 per cent previous stroke. Forty-one percent of participants used a walking device indoors, and the median score of the Barthel ADL Index was 16. At baseline, the Downton fall risk index was scored for each individual. A score of 3 or more was taken to indicate high risk of falls. Participants were followed up prospectively for 12 months, with regard to falls indoors. RESULTS: At 3, 6 and 12 months, and using a fall definition including all indoor falls, sensitivity ranged from 81 to 95 per cent with the highest value at 3 months, and specificity ranged from 35 to 40 per cent . The prognostic separation values ranged from 0.26 to 0.37. Within 3 months, the risk of falling was 36 per cent in the high-risk group (index score $>$ or $=$ 3) and 5 per cent in the low-risk group. The accuracy of predictions did not improve when applying a fall definition in which falls precipitated by acute illness, acute disease, or drug side effects were excluded. CONCLUSIONS: Already after 3 months, the Downton fall risk index appears to be a useful tool for predicting falls, irrespective of their cause, among older people in residential care facilities.

Question What do you think are the main things that you could do in your everyday nursing practice if you were involved with older people living in residential care facilities?

Example 2: Use of bandaging for wound care (Castonguay, 2008)

Reference: Castonguay, G. (2008) Short-stretch or four-layer compression bandages: an overview of the literature. *Ostomy/Wound Management, 54 (3)*, 50-55.

Venous ulcers are a common, costly occurrence. Treatment typically includes the use of short-stretch and four-layer bandages — both with demonstrated ability to increase venous return and healing rates. Which is superior is unclear. To determine whether short-stretch bandages or four-layer compression systems provide shorter healing times and fewer adverse events when used in adults with venous ulcers, a search of English-language literature was conducted using the search terms short-stretch bandages and wound care, compression bandages and wound care, compression and venous ulcers, four-layer compression and venous ulcers, and multilayer compression and venous ulcers. Data from 25 studies published between 1997 and 2006 were examined. Short-stretch and four-layer compression bandages were found to be equally as effective in managing the oedema that compromises venous ulcer healing. Time to healing was found to be shorter using four-layer or one- to two-layer compression when compared to paste compression in 24 studies. Ankle brachial index is an important factor to consider in determining compression appropriateness. Generally, use of any compression system is better than no compression at all.

Question What do you think are the main things that you could do in your everyday nursing practice if you were involved in wound care?

Example 3 Infection control in hospitals (Pittet *et al.*, 2007)

Reference: Pittet, D. *et al.* (2007) Double-blind, randomized, crossover trial of three hand rub formulations : fast-track evaluation of tolerability and acceptability. *Infection Control and Hospital Epidemiology, 28 (12)*, 1344-1351.

OBJECTIVE: To compare health care workers' skin tolerance for and acceptance of three alcohol-based hand rub formulations. DESIGN: Double-blind, randomised, crossover clinical trial. SETTING: Intensive care unit in a university hospital. PARTICIPANTS: Thirty-eight health care workers (HCWs). INTERVENTION: A total of three alcohol-based hand rub formulations (hereafter, formulations A, B and C) were used in random order for 3-5 consecutive working days during regular nursing shifts. Formulations A and B contained the same emollient, and formulations B and C contained the same alcohol at the same concentration. Use of each test formulation was separated by a 'washout' period of at least two days. A visual assessment of skin integrity by a blinded observer using a standard six-item scale was conducted before and after the use of each formulation. Univariate and multivariate analyses were used for the assessment of risk factors for skin alteration, and product acceptability was assessed by use of a customized questionnaire after the use of each formulation. RESULTS: Thirty-eight HCWs used each of three formulations for a median of three days (range, 3-5 days). The mean amount of product used daily (+/–SD) was 54.9+/–23.5 mL (median, 50.9 mL). Both subjective and objective evaluation of skin conditions after use showed lower HCW tolerance for product C. Male sex (odds ratio [OR], 3.17 [95 per cent confidence interval {CI}, 1.1-8.8]), fair or very fair skin (OR, 3.01 [95 per cent CI, 1.1-7.9]), skin alteration before hand rub use (OR, 3.73 [95 per cent CI, 1.7-8.1]), and use of formulation C (OR, 8.79 [95 per cent CI, 2.7-28.4]) were independently associated with skin alteration. CONCLUSIONS: This protocol permits a fast-track comparison of HCWs' skin tolerance for different alcohol-based hand rub formulations that are used in health care settings. The emollient in formulation C may account for its inferior performance.

Questions

- What are the implications of these findings for using alcohol-based hand rubs in hospital?
- Which hand rub might you use if you were working in a hospital?

Summary

In this chapter, we have given you some of the advanced research techniques and issues for consideration in order to become a more expert nurse researcher. Many of these techniques and approaches have been helpful to us in our research endeavours. We hope you will be the wiser about the advantages and disadvantages of using quantitative and qualitative research methods and can see potential in adopting mixed methods approaches and various kinds of triangulation when doing your research. We have encouraged you to be reflective researchers, irrespective of which type of research methodology and method you are employing. We have also shown you how research findings, and theories emerging from research, can have a massive impact on your nursing practice and on the practice of others in your health care team. Next, we will take you to the final chapter of this book, which will take you, step-by-step, through all of the processes that you will need to undertake when progressing from research idea to research reality. We will take you from the initial stages of thinking about research ideas from your everyday encounters in nursing practice all the way to the step of submitting an application to an ethics committee to do a research study.

Chapter 13

Going forward:
A step-by-step guide from research idea to ethics application

KEY THEMES

Generating research questions • Doing more refined literature searches • Preparing a research proposal • Ethical principles • Making an application to a Research Ethics Committee

LEARNING OUTCOMES

At the end of this chapter you will be able to:

● Use the criteria of SMART to develop and evaluate appropriate research questions

● Understand the best ways to do a literature search to become more focused in your literature reviewing

● Consider the people who might have a stake in your research idea (i.e. stakeholders) and who could be potential collaborators when doing the research

● Know the main issues to address when developing a research proposal

● Identify the four major ethical principles to gauge the acceptability of a proposed nursing research project

● Understand some of the processes required to make an application to a local Research Ethics Committee.

Introduction

IMAGINE THAT . . .

You are a nurse working in the community as part of a district nursing team based in a GP surgery and wanting to do research into inappropriate referrals from hospital staff to yourself and your district nursing team. As such, you begin by considering why the referrals are generated in this way and with this in mind you start to think about role perception in terms of how hospital staff and other agencies might view the role of the district nursing service (McGarry, 2003) and your own team's portrayal of their roles and responsibilities to others in the GP surgery and to other agencies.

In this chapter we are going to look at the kinds of things that you will need to do when undertaking your first research project; this might be a dissertation as part of a course of study or a project that you wish to carry out to be a research-informed nurse. As a reminder of some of the topics that we've covered in previous chapters, we will be showing you how effective development of research questions and comprehensive, focused literature searches can enable you to prepare a successful research proposal to receive support from your NHS Trust or from a funding body. We will also show you some of the key issues to consider when submitting an ethics committee application, which will be an essential part of the process in some studies that you might wish to carry out. We have used real-life instances of nursing research that we have been involved with to illustrate the different stages of taking a research idea and making it a research reality. We have changed the names of the researchers and the NHS Trusts concerned to avoid embarrassment as all too often good researchers look back on their work and realise how they could have done a much better job!

The following imaginary scenario provides a starting point as you progress from stages of initially identifying an issue worth investigating to the preparation of a research proposal or ethics application. We will return to this scenario at various times within the chapter in order to illustrate the key points highlighted within the discussion as a whole.

13.1 Defining your research question or area of enquiry

If we use the example of wishing to address how hospital staff view district nurses' roles and responsibilities we need to see whether this is a researchable and meaningful question. To decide on this, we would recommend that you use the following acronym of SMART, which stands for:

- Specific
- Measurable

- Answerable
- Relevant
- Taxing or time-focused.

When being *specific,* you need to consider whether the question that you wish to pose about district nursing roles is one that is too broad and whether it is a question at all. For example, if you had decided to say that the research question is 'how do hospital staff members view district nurses' roles?' at least this is phrased as a question; some nurse researchers simply start with a general topic like hospital staff members' views on district nursing roles. There might need to be an elaboration of which types of hospital staff members perceive the district nurses and what the district nurses do; also, there would need to be a consideration as to why this question might crop up. The district nurse who has decided to study this area is feeling disgruntled that some of the hospital staff are referring patients who have been discharged from the hospital with little understanding as to what the district nurses can do to support these patients. This is the problem and should guide the formulation of a more refined question, namely, 'When hospital workers refer patients to district nurses, what are the hospital workers' perceptions of what district nurses can do for these patients?'

Note that this is a much more advanced question - it relates to what is going on in the referral process - and it is a lot more specific. However, we still haven't resolved another issue. Who are the hospital staff members in the question? What level of seniority or expertise do the nurses who are making these referrals have? When are they doing this referring of patients to the district nurses? There are further questions that still need resolving to make it more specific.

In terms of being *measurable*, you need to have a clear idea as to how you're going to collect information and the potential group of people you're going to collect the data from. In terms of measurement, this is where you need to decide whether it is a question that needs a quantifiable answer by the use of quantitative methods or whether more in-depth, richer answers are needed via qualitative methods. Alternatively, you might need to use a mixed methods approach by using qualitative and quantitative methods to get more comprehensive ways of measuring your answers. Perhaps you might want to use data already collected by a hospital or primary care trust so you will need to do secondary data analysis of data collected by other people. The main thing to decide at this early stage is, 'Can I measure it and if so, how?'

By having *answerable* questions, you need to bear in mind that your research question should ideally be phrased as a question, rather than a general topic. For example, it would be more appropriate and more focused to ask an answerable question such as 'Which method is best for healing of venous leg ulcers - short-stretch bandages or high-compression bandages?' This approach is much more effective than having a general topic of interest such as leg ulcer care because you need to show others how or why the research questions that you're developing are *relevant* for clinical practice. Rather than looking at something that is just an intellectual curiosity, you need to show why the research question is of vital importance for your health care organisation to support you to do the study. By being relevant, the research question will be sufficiently interesting to other members of your health care team that it will energise them to work with you to give you access to participants or to help in collecting or analysing the data that you collect.

Finally, excellent research questions need to be *taxing*. By taxing, we mean that your research question needs to require some active involvement in systematically collecting, analysing and interpreting data and finally reporting on your findings. Research projects are rarely ones that take a matter of weeks (this may be possible at a stretch, although you may need to watch out for how rigorous the study can be). If the question is too simplistic and does not require much depth or breadth in collecting and analysing data, then this may not be sufficient to base any major shifts in how you organise and provide health promotion or health care. With the SMART abbreviation, 'T' has also been used to represent *time-focused* and this is also a good discipline to adopt when developing a research question. By what date do you need to have finished the project in terms of reporting it to those who have supported you (i.e. an NHS Trust or funding body) or is there a course requirement to have the research question answered by a specific date when submitting your dissertation? If there is no time limit, it might be still wise to place a limit on when you need to have come up with an answer as this can keep you focused on getting the work done on time. Make sure your time limit is agreed with your research collaborators too. The focus on time could be crucial for a piece of research that is mainly documentary or involves a systematic review of data in the form of published studies. Such a time-centred question could mean addressing areas like how the role of the district nurse has changed over the past ten years. Or you could be enquiring whether the same period of time has seen specific initiatives within NHS Trusts to radically change district nursing roles to take on new activities or to eliminate certain duties from the role.

13.2 Conducting a search of the literature and reviewing the evidence

The things to remember about doing a literature review are that you need to start broadly and then become more specific. For example, you might be generally interested in the area of depression among patients and how to combat this problem amongst them. This is still quite a general area because depression could impact on your patients in a wide range of situations and health care settings. To become more specific, think about the issues that arise in your clinical role as a nurse. Perhaps you are a health visitor and you have seen postnatal depression as a problem amongst South Asian women in the locality that you work in. These women may be relating experiences that appear to you to be symptoms of depression, but you may be unclear about how a South Asian woman's experience of depression would manifest itself. Your literature review then needs to start to become more specific and narrow down into a more closely circumscribed area. You would look for literature into whether depression is higher in women than in men and also how the symptoms of depression may vary according to a person's sex. You could also look to find out whether South Asian women experience different kinds of depression when compared to women from other ethnic groups. There is also peripheral literature that might be related to your area of interest in terms of how women from various Asian ethnic groups exhibit emotional problems, such as one study that showed South and South East Asian women as experiencing more psychosomatic problems (i.e. tension headaches, other aches and pains as signs of stress) when compared with Caucasian women (Williams, 2002). Your literature review could then move beyond looking at differences between men and women or between ethnic groups to focus specifically on variations in experiences of postnatal depression (PND) and whether PND is uniquely different from the experience of depression in general. Finally, the literature review could become even more specific to see whether the Asian and Caucasian women's experiences of PND differed and, if so, what might be the reasons for this. If there are not many studies that have explored this specific field, then perhaps this might help to justify the rationale for doing a study in this area. Perhaps there is quantitative research to show that South Asian and Caucasian women have different rates of PND with South Asian women having lower levels, on average. How could this be explained and how might South Asian women recognise, and cope with, PND differently from those of other ethnic groups? As a result, there may be scope for doing a qualitative investigation into the possible reasons for such differences between South Asian and Caucasian women in terms of the ways in which PND shows itself and how women from different ethnic groups cope with PND on a collective or individual level.

Literature searching – a case example

Let us go back to the case example at the beginning of this chapter in terms of awareness of roles and responsibilities of district nurses by hospital staff. There may not be many previous studies that have tapped into this issue. However, you can still see whether there is relevant literature by starting from the general, and more peripheral, literature and becoming more focused on any related studies once you have cast this wider net. Before doing a literature search of the electronic databases, it would be best to pose sufficiently broad but comprehensive questions to address this area. Here are a few possible queries to pose:

- Who are district nurses? Who defines their role? Is it defined by an NHS trust or by a professional body such as the Royal College of Nursing's (2003) guidance for referrals to district nursing services? Do the roles and responsibilities of district nurses vary according to each NHS trust?

- With which professional nursing roles do district nurses have things in common? Are they similar to practice nurses or health visitors with the activities that they undertake or might they have similar client groups? (see Beech, 2002). How are they different from other nursing groups?

- What kinds of contact do district nurses have with people working in the hospital sector? Do they rarely meet with each other or are there schemes that have been organised that transcend the boundaries between the hospital and the district settings such as with the services provided by a bridging team, which 'bridges' the gap between the hospital and home environment and enables patients to have a smooth transition to their homes when being discharged from hospital? An orthopaedic bridging team in Dartford and Gravesham NHS Trust (undated) is just such an example, in which nurses and a physiotherapist co-ordinate discharge from hospital to home and the provision of continued care to them. Other similar schemes involve district nursing-type health care, such as the 'Hospital at Home' service that is provided for older adults by Johns Hopkins Medicine in Baltimore, Maryland, in the USA (Johns Hopkins Medicine, undated). These kinds of schemes help to enable hospital nurses and district nurses to exchange knowledge about patients and have clear lines of responsibility for health professionals in either the hospital or the home.

- Which decision-making processes are undertaken when making a hospital patient referral to the care of a district nurse? There is an article (Davies, 2003) on how referral criteria are developed and this could give a few clues as to how appropriateness of referrals are decided and whether certain decision-trees are being developed to reduce the possibility of misplaced referrals.

- How do some trusts work to reduce the number of inappropriate referrals? Have a look at Brent Teaching Primary Care Trust (TPCT)'s (2004) efforts at doing so by having a list of what the district nursing can and cannot do.

All of these questions should help in guiding you to decide whether there is enough known about this issue to be able to make adjustments to the district nursing service without needing to conduct research. Perhaps a preliminary piece of work is still needed even after considering that there is seemingly sufficient information available to all services on what the district nursing team does. Maybe you want to see what the perceptions of your own district nursing team are in relation to what they can and can't do and you want to compare their views with those of the hospital staff who regularly refer to your team. Where might there be areas of agreement and disagreement? If we look at the list of activities that are covered in the Brent TPCT district nursing guidelines that we referred to above, there are several things that might be ambiguous. For starters, the concept of 'guidelines' seems to suggest that what you're about to read is not necessarily black and white. For example, there is a section in the guidelines that mention activities like health promotion and education. What might this involve? Health promotion and education might mean different things to different people. Perhaps this might be a good starting point to ask questions of your district nursing colleagues and the hospital staff who make their referrals about this. Are both groups clear in terms of what they see as being the sorts of health promotion and education that district nurses might do and what they are currently seen to be doing? How well do district nurses think that they communicate different parts of their roles and responsibilities to others and how well is this communication received? As you can see, there is plenty of scope for exploring these issues after having done a literature review by using some of the principles that we have covered in earlier chapters within this book and within this chapter.

13.3 Identifying potential stakeholders and collaborators and others who will need to be involved in the development of your research

I keep six honest serving-men (They taught me all I knew);
Their names are What and Why and When
And How and Where and Who.

(Kipling, 2001)

The above quote by Kipling from the *Just So Stories* is all about curiosity of one kind or another and is apt for this chapter as a whole, as it is here that you start to consider the specific issues in terms of developing your skills as an independent researcher. However, crucially while we talk about becoming an *independent* researcher, you should also be mindful that this does not mean that you always need to be working away from others and that often you need to be an *interdependent* researcher; you do this by consulting with and collaborating with colleagues, stakeholders and other researchers to develop research questions that everybody can identify with, to plan out and execute the research and finally to disseminate your findings. In fact, as you will remember from the previous chapter, interactions of this kind are crucial to the quality of the research you carry out, particularly in getting findings from a study integrated into everyday nursing practice.

Once you have decided upon the focus for your research, you will need to consider not only the particular research question(s) (*what, why, how, where and when*) but also *who* in terms of who you will need to approach to discuss your research ideas prior to developing your proposal, both to help you to develop your thinking and planning and also practically, for example in terms of accessing a particular group of individuals. These groups of people and individuals are probably best encapsulated through the terms 'stakeholders' and 'collaborators' and we will define and discuss these groups in greater detail here.

Identifying stakeholders

Stakeholders in a general sense are an integral part of any research endeavour and it is essential that you identify and involve stakeholders in the development of your research from the outset. In the broadest sense stakeholders are the people who, collectively or individually, will benefit in one way or another from the outcomes of your research. There are different kinds of stakeholders and we have listed examples of the two main groups below – although after reading this section you may want to add to this list based on your own research proposal.

Organisational stakeholders

Stakeholders in this context are the organisations or individuals who have commissioned or funded your research, for example your local trust may have identified a particular issue that warrants exploration and are seeking to commission someone to undertake a piece of research in this area, or it may be an organisation or charity which funds research into a particular area or field of health care. Organisational stakeholders therefore will benefit from your research in terms of organisational outcomes, for example carrying out a piece of research to address a particular deficit in care delivery or service. Imagine for example that you are a hospital manager and through the audit process you have identified that there are significant delays in discharging patients home following routine surgical procedures. You therefore want to commission a piece of research to find out why this is happening and more importantly how the delays can be minimised in terms of improved patient service delivery and organisational efficiency.

Service users and others who might be affected by your research

Stakeholders in this context are the individuals or groups of people who will ultimately benefit from the findings of your research, the most obvious example is service users and/or carers. This particular kind of stakeholder is crucial to the research endeavour: not only are they the recipients of the research but also they are highly likely to be the most informed and hold the expertise in a particular area, for example expert patient groups – they also know what they would like or expect from a particular intervention or service! Consider for example the development of the National Service Framework for Older People (Department of Health, 2001). This has been described as a *stakeholder* policy, which means that during the development of the NSF for Older People (2001) a range of individuals and organisations with a particular interest, for example service users, carers and key organisations and expertise in this area, formed an integral part of the development from design through to inception.

Identifying potential collaborators

As well as stakeholders, collaborators will also form part of the groups of people who will be involved in the development of your research and have a different role to that of the stakeholders. Collaborators therefore may be defined as the individuals or groups who work together towards a common goal – in this case developing and conducting a successful research project. Working collaboratively means working together in terms of sharing knowledge and expertise and can be on a small or larger scale. For example, you may consider collaborating with colleagues from another department in the health care organisation within which you work or maybe with someone from a local university, such as someone who has taught you. If you are undertaking formal study this may present an opportunity to develop collaborative links with individuals within a particular organisation, for example a local university department with the requisite experience and expertise in data coding or analysis. In larger-scale projects, you may consider collaborating with different organisations or similar organisations across regions.

Aside from stakeholders and collaborators there are also a number of other individuals or groups that you will need to approach prior to and during your research, for example your local trust's research and development (R&D) department. In the following section, we will consider the process of developing your research proposal and this will also give you the opportunity to consider *who* you will need to consider and work with during your research.

13.4 Developing your research proposal

Preparing a good-quality proposal is crucial from the onset of any well-organised project. The reasons for doing this are threefold.

First, the production of a clear proposal of the research will help you to clarify in your own mind the aims and objectives of the research, rather like a research diary. This will be of help to you when you come to write your final project report. For example, writing a proposal, even if this is amended several times in the process of development, will provide a record of your original thinking, and the motivations and ideas that you had in the first place. The production of a proposal will often include a list of the costs incurred when carrying out the research (e.g. stationery and postage, phone calls, tapes and transcription production of reports, needing to register to attend seminars and conferences and disseminate the findings). In Example 13.1 on the next page you can see an example of a research proposal, with comments on it from a person who has provided feedback on this draft.

Second, depending on the scope of your project you may want to enlist a 'critical friend', for example a colleague with previous experience of research or this area of expertise who will be able to read through the proposal and advise on clarity, feasibility, potential difficulties and gaps in information - all of the things that a potential funder and the ethics committee will be looking for. Taking the time to prepare a good-quality research proposal has the potential to pay dividends in terms of saving time later and more importantly a successful outcome. In Example 13.1, we have also included examples of comments typed in the margin by such a critical friend.

Example 13.1 A sample research proposal with critical friend's comments (in the margin)

RESEARCH PROPOSAL

Please structure the research proposal under these headings (1) Aim of project, (2) Background, (3) Plan of investigation and (4) Application of study results.

1. AIM OF PROJECT

- To analyse factors that contribute to the uptake of complementary and alternative medicines with a view to informing commissioning of complementary and alternative medicines (CAMs) in East Staffordshire.

Objectives:

To achieve this aim, we have developed the following objectives. We plan to:

- Conduct two focus groups with users of CAM – one group will be with CAM users who are health professionals and one group will be members of the general public who are not health professionals;

> **Comment [p1]:** What is your rationale for looking at people who have used CAM and are not health professionals versus those who are health professionals? Why do you think they will have different perceptions?

- Develop a questionnaire, which has a range of closed questions relating to themes obtained from the focus groups and from a comprehensive literature review;

- Distribute the questionnaire to a convenience sample of 200 users of CAM within East Staffordshire;

> **Comment [p2]:** This could be problematic. Why not have a random sample so it will be less biased and perhaps more representative of the CAM users in the region?

- Conduct 30 semi-structured interviews with users of CAM in East Staffordshire to obtain more in-depth data regarding complementary therapy use and the types of CAM that they believe should be commissioned in the National Health Service;

- Stage an open forum with key stakeholders to discuss the main trends and to obtain their perspectives on complementary therapy usage and commissioning.

> **Comment [p3]:** The first three activities are all involving collection of data from people who will presumably be sympathetic to using CAM and having it provided on the NHS. Surely you should collect data from a group of people who have lukewarm opinions or who are very against the use of CAM?

2. BACKGROUND

CAM has become a popular choice for the British public over the past 10 years. This trend has developed to such an extent that a Select Committee is currently reviewing the regulation of such therapies and the accreditation of complementary practitioners. This difficult task has been compounded by the diversity of definitions of CAM, which could include a wide range of therapies from homeopathy and relaxation techniques to traditional Indian or Chinese medicines. One definition of complementary and alternative medicines has divided therapies into manipulative (e.g. osteopathy, acupuncture) and non-manipulative (e.g. homeopathy, aromatherapy) treatments although this taxonomy may ultimately not be that informative for understanding why some people are drawn to some therapies rather than others. In addition, as East Staffordshire has an ethnically rich population, there may be some health care consumers who view their traditional ethnic therapies as part of their mainstream health care. It is therefore highly likely that East Staffordshire may become an area that is under particular pressure from consumers to provide less 'conventional' medicines and therapies

> **Comment [p4]:** This area is very broad. It might be better to look at people's experiences on a limited number of complementary and alternative medicines, rather than looking at such a broad range of therapies. People's motives for using one therapy for pain, such as using acupuncture, might be very different to using other therapies, such as homeopathy.

Example 13.1 continued

as part of standard NHS service provision. An analysis of current patterns of, and reasons for, complementary therapy use within East Staffordshire may be especially helpful in planning and commissioning NHS care for the future. Furthermore, although decision-making for commissioning health services has become more overt in recent times, public consultations regarding the provision of certain types of therapies or medicines have not been that well-developed in the UK. The Oregon Experiment in the United States has been a useful means for dialogue and debate on the rationing of health care, although decisions into the commissioning and provision of CAM in the NHS have not been widely discussed. A study into why people turn to CAM and a healthy debate on how traditional medicines offered in primary care *and* CAM can coexist within the NHS is clearly needed, especially as the demand for self-care and complementary medicines is increasing rapidly.

> **Comment [p5]:** Should we be responding to consumer demands or should we be looking at whether the therapies actually have a beneficial effect? Perhaps the issues that could be explored in this proposed study could focus on looking at whether the patients have felt that the treatments have actually worked.

Although there has been a growing body of critical appraisal into the efficacy of CAM (e.g. Cawthorn, 1995; Royal London Homeopathic Hospital, 1999), there has been relatively little research into why people access CAM. In those studies that have reviewed complementary therapy provision by health professionals, the main methodology adopted has been quantitative and has involved the use of postal questionnaires (e.g. Rankin-Box, 1997; Wearn and Greenfield, 1998). Other quantitative surveys have involved analysing prevalence of usage of CAM (e.g. Ernst, 1998). These studies have been informative about complementary therapy provision and use; however these approaches have been less helpful for explaining in-depth issues such as possible barriers to accessing CAM and satisfaction with 'conventional' health care. Qualitative studies into the use of CAM for some types of illnesses have been useful in illustrating underlying processes, barriers and levels of satisfaction among users (Adewuyi-Dalton and Walker, 1999; Adler, 1999) although these studies are usually the exception. Overall, a triangulated approach to people's use of complementary therapy and their preferences regarding the types of therapies to be offered in the NHS could offer a more rigorous appraisal into the commissioning and provision of CAM.

> **Comment [p6]:** This is useful justification on why the study is needed. The possible problem that might arise is whether studying users of CAM in East Staffordshire is too geographically focused for something that might be influenced by popular national trends to use CAM for all sorts of health complaints. Would it be possible to compare your samples with those in other parts of the country?

3. PLAN OF INVESTIGATION

Our study will have three data collection phases and one phase in which key stakeholders will be able to comment on the findings obtained.

Phase 1: focus groups

We will be conducting two parallel focus group sessions. One focus group will be carried out with approximately 15 users of at least one complementary therapy and who do not have a health professional background. The other focus group will involve health professionals who have used at least one complementary therapy for their own health. The focus groups will be semi-structured and participants will be asked to relate their narratives regarding their usage of CAM. These narratives will enable us to understand a range of factors including the context of complementary therapy use, the process of referral and barriers to accessing CAM. We will obtain the consent of participants to audiotape their conversations. Tapes will be transcribed verbatim and their content analysed. This process will take about 3 months.

> **Comment [p7]:** Again, the rationale for looking at these two separate groups (health professionals and non-health professionals) isn't that clear.

> **Comment [p8]:** Will it be enough to just do content analysis? What about doing a thematic analysis or an interpretative phenomenological analysis?

Example 13.1 continued

Phase 2: postal questionnaires

By extracting the main factors of complementary therapy use from the focus group data and with a comprehensive literature review, we will develop, pilot and distribute a questionnaire. This phase will enable us to explore how prevalent such factors have been among a sample of 200 complementary therapy users within East Staffordshire. Our convenience sample will be drawn from a wide range of users (health professionals and lay persons) with whom the research team comes into contact in the course of our work. Questionnaires will be handed out and administered face-to-face. Users will be offered the opportunity to be entered into a prize draw if they return a completed questionnaire. Completed questionnaires will be entered onto a statistical computer package (SPSS) and a range of descriptive analyses will be carried out. Phase 2 should take about 4 months.

> **Comment [p9]:** Possible ethical concerns arise – do participants get a chance to take away the questionnaire and consider whether they want to take part or is there a possibility that they might be pressurised into taking part? Would it be appropriate to get the team handing it out to their patients when conflicts in role as health professional and researcher may arise? Might it be best to get an independent person to collect the data, especially if some of the participants may be saying less than complimentary things about the services that they receive from GP surgeries?

Phase 3: interviews

This phase will involve approaching a sample of 30 participants from the questionnaire respondents who expressed an interest in being interviewed: 15 of the participants will be health professionals and the other 15 will be lay members without a health professional background. These participants will be invited to an interview by one of the research team. The interviews will be semi-structured and will enable us to adopt a deeper analysis of themes that may not be amenable to discussion in a group setting. We will audiotape the interviews and carry out verbatim transcription of the conversations. We will then thematically analyse the interview data and see how these trends complement findings from Phases 1 and 2.

> **Comment [p10]:** Again, this rationale of splitting them up into two groups hasn't been made clear.

Phase 4: presentation/open forum

We will be staging a presentation of some of the key trends to about 50 invited key stakeholders within East Staffordshire who are involved in the commissioning, provision and receipt of CAM in primary care. This phase will provide us with the opportunity to disseminate results but also to obtain a wide range of perspectives regarding our findings. Comments from the open forum will be incorporated into the final report to be submitted to East Staffordshire PCT and in presentations to other PCTs within the West Midlands region.

References

Adewuyi-Dalton, R. and Walker, G. (1999, March) *A qualitative investigation of users' experiences of group relaxation classes and aromatherapy massage in a cancer support and information centre.* Mount Vernon Hospital: Internal Report.

Adler, S.R. (1999) Complementary and alternative medicine use among women with breast cancer. *Medical Anthropology Quarterly, 13 (2)*, 214–222.

Cawthorn, A. (1995) A review of the literature surrounding the research into aromatherapy. *Complementary Therapy, Nursing and Midwifery, 1 (4)*, 118–120.

Ernst, E. (1998) Complementary therapies for asthma: what patients use. *Journal of Asthma, 35 (8)*, 667–671.

Example 13.1 **continued**

Rankin-Box, D. (1997) Therapies in practice: a survey of assessing nurses' use of complementary therapies. *Complementary Therapy, Nursing and Midwifery, 3 (4)*, 92–99.

Royal London Homeopathic Hospital (1999) *The Evidence-base of Complementary Medicine*, 2nd edn. London: The Royal London Homeopathic Hospital.

Wearn, A.M. and Greenfield, S.M. (1998) Access to complementary medicine in general practice: survey in one UK health authority. *Journal of the Royal Society of Medicine, 91 (9)*, 465–470.

4. APPLICATION OF STUDY RESULTS

Please detail generalisability and relevance of proposed study along with plan for dissemination of the results and implications for health care.

Transferability

Although the study has a large qualitative component, the methods of our study and our analysis strategies could be transferable to other studies and other settings. We will adhere to a rigorous process of conducting and analysing the interviews and focus groups (i.e. using several people for classifying data into themes and checking with interviewees to ensure that the themes agree with their interpretation of the data). The issues raised and the processes of discovering underlying beliefs and practices may be transferable to a mixture of ethnic groups as our sample will attempt to reflect the diversity of ethnicities within the area. Prevalence data from the questionnaire survey should also allow us to analyse the extent to which our sample is comparable with samples obtained in other studies into complementary therapy use.

> **Comment [p11]:** As mentioned earlier in the comments on this proposal, it might be better to have a survey of some users of CAM outside of the local region too in order to find out how generalisable these findings are

Relevance

The project outcomes could affect the attitudes and practices of a wide range of stakeholders involved in primary care and the provision or receipt of CAM. GPs, users, commissioners, providers of 'conventional' health services and providers of CAM may all be affected in a number of different ways.

With the recent changes in the way that primary care services will be commissioned by PCTs and the increased awareness about CAM among users and practitioners, it will be important to ensure that the findings of our research are at the forefront of primary care commissioning.

We are anticipating that our study could be influential in:

- Commissioning and marketing complementary therapy in primary care settings;
- Highlighting the health beliefs and practices of lay and health professional users of CAM;
- Identifying barriers to accessing appropriate health care (complementary or otherwise).

Dissemination

We will be looking to disseminate the findings at a wide range of forums and conferences. We will be staging a presentation/open forum of key findings to key stakeholders for discussion and action, and this will also act as part of the dissemination process. We will also be submitting our work to a number of peer-reviewed academic and applied journals.

Third, in producing a clear proposal you will also need to consider your timescales (the project begins at the thinking stage so ensure that you build in the time for all of the administration, for example ethical approval). One method that may help you to think about the project and plan time is a Gantt chart. Gantt charts provide useful tools for planning and timetabling projects. The role of a Gantt chart is to keep the research project on target in terms of timescales and help to schedule the various component parts of a project in a sequential manner, for example, you will need to receive ethical approval before you can recruit study participants. Importantly, Gantt charts also enable you to identify the 'critical path' of the project, that is the sequence in which tasks will need to be completed at a particular point in time in order for the project to be successfully completed by the project end date.

There are a number of ways of producing a Gantt chart and we have included two examples below. Gantt charts can be produced in Microsoft Excel for example and there are also a number of computer-assisted software packages available – depending on the size and complexity of the project. Figures 13.1 and 13.2 illustrate two examples of Gantt charts that have been used with a professional project management computer program. In Figure 13.1 you can see that the duration of each task is indicated with a shaded box. Some tasks have what are known as 'milestones', these are specific dates by which certain activities need to be done. By 23 October, activity Number 13 needs to be achieved and there are several other activities that have deadlines, like activity Number 32 (the production of the final report), which needs to be done by 4 July. The last couple of activities (Numbers 35 and 36) involve telling others about the research findings.

In Figure 13.2, this is an example of a study that has the use of two major types of methods – analysis of data that have already been collected (see activities numbered 14-33) and the running of two sets of focus group interviews (see activities numbered 10-13 and 35-39) with the first set of focus groups informing the analysis of currently existing quantitative data and the second set of focus groups acting as a resource to get stakeholders to comment on the quantitative data analysis, in a way similar to the conducting of Delphi studies that we mentioned in the previous chapter. In this way, the informants or stakeholders in the first round of focus groups are helping to set the agenda and posing certain research questions whilst the second round of focus groups acts as a forum for the stakeholders to critique the validity and usefulness of the quantitative data that have been analysed.

13.5 Ethical considerations

As a general rule, quite a few proposed studies with patients/service users often require ethical approval from a local Research Ethics Committee (REC) before the research can be carried out. Some studies, like systematic reviews of data in a publicly

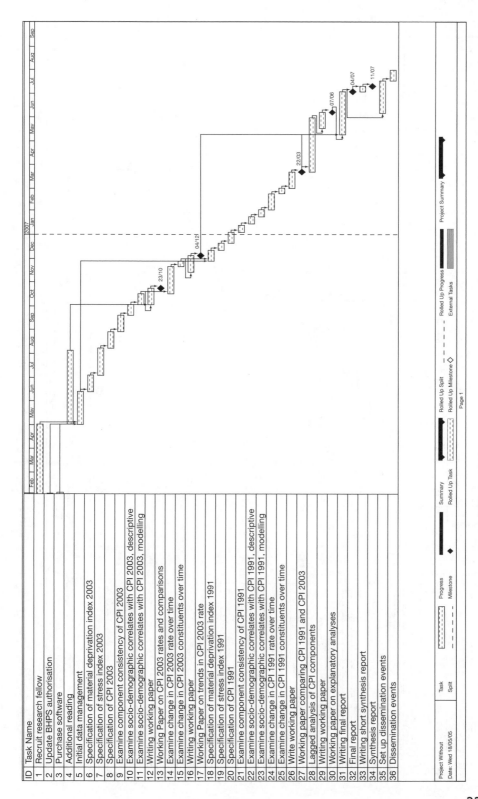

ID	Task Name
1	Recruit research fellow
2	Update BHPS authorisation
3	Purchase software
4	Additional reading
5	Initial data management
6	Specification of material deprivation index 2003
7	Specification of stress index 2003
8	Specification of CPI 2003
9	Examine component consistency of CPI 2003
10	Examine socio-demographic correlates with CPI 2003, descriptive
11	Examine socio-demographic correlates with CPI 2003, modelling
12	Writing working paper
13	Working Paper on CPI 2003 rates and comparisons
14	Examine change in CPI 2003 rate over time
15	Examine change in CPI 2003 constituents over time
16	Writing working paper
17	Working Paper on trends in CPI 2003 rate
18	Specification of material deprivation index 1991
19	Specification of stress index 1991
20	Specification of CPI 1991
21	Examine component consistency of CPI 1991
22	Examine socio-demographic correlates with CPI 1991, descriptive
23	Examine socio-demographic correlates with CPI 1991, modelling
24	Examine change in CPI 1991 rate over time
25	Examine change in CPI 1991 constituents over time
26	Write working paper
27	Working paper comparing CPI 1991 and CPI 2003
28	Lagged analysis of CPI components
29	Writing working paper
30	Working paper on explanatory analyses
31	Writing final report
32	Final report
33	Writing short synthesis report
34	Synthesis report
35	Set up dissemination events
36	Dissemination events

Project Without
Date: Wed 18/05/05

Task
Split
Progress
Milestone
Summary
Rolled Up Task
Rolled Up Split
Rolled Up Milestone ◇
Rolled Up Progress
External Tasks
Project Summary

Page 1

Figure 13.1 A Gantt chart for a study mainly involving data analysis.

337

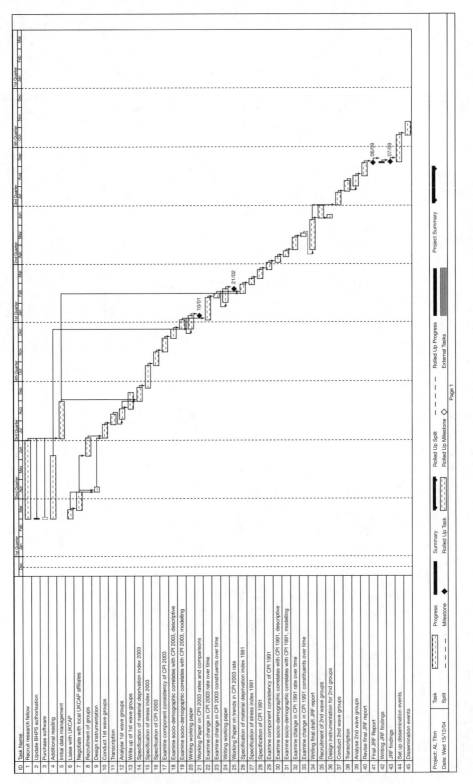

Figure 13.2 A Gantt chart for a mixed methods study.

accessible archive, will usually not require ethical approval and other pieces of work could be reasonably defined as clinical audit or service evaluation. If your proposed work is either clinical audit or evaluation, then ethical approval should not be sought either. The National Research Ethics Service (NRES) is part of the National Patient Safety Agency (NPSA) and provides helpful guidance on its website: **http:// www.nres.npsa.nhs.uk/**. This guidance can help you decide if your project can be suitably defined as research, or audit, or service evaluation.

THINGS TO CONSIDER

Is it research, audit or evaluation?

The NRES (2008) has published a document outlining the decisions to be made before approaching a local REC. If clinicians are carrying out activities of quality assurance such as clinical audit or assessing whether a service meets a specific standard, then ethical approval is not needed. However, as the NRES (2008) highlights, research may involve greater risks to patient well-being and satisfactory practice. To help decide whether your work is research, audit or evaluation, consider the following four issues: (1) intent, (2) treatment, (3) allocation of treatments, and (4) randomisation.

With **intent**, by its very nature, research might be testing or developing new knowledge and this could mean putting patients in a novel, and possibly uncomfortable, position beyond the usual care that they might receive. By the definition of research that the NRES is adopting, research is often aimed at finding out what *should* be done, whereas audit and evaluation should be intended to track what *is* being done.

With assessment of **treatment**/care techniques, audit and service evaluation will only involve analysing treatment that has a satisfactory evidence-base to support it; by contrast, research may involve developing this evidence-base and trialling new treatments.

In terms of **allocation** of patients into intervention groups to receive a specific treatment, this is mainly likely to happen with research and to follow a protocol of allocating participants into control groups or intervention/treatment groups. Conversely, audit and evaluation will only be analysing care that has been agreed upon between health professional and patient.

Finally, **randomisation** is another means of differentiating research from audit/ evaluation. In research, patients might sometimes be randomly assigned to groups that are studied, whereas audit and evaluation should not have any persons being randomly allocated to various treatment or control groups.

The NRES can also point you in the direction of your local REC by identifying the different RECs available by Strategic Health Authority and by country (England, Wales, Scotland and Northern Ireland). Another thing to bear in mind is that the criteria that local RECs will use to assess the acceptability of an ethics application might vary by the type of study that is being proposed. For instance, there are only certain RECs that can review applications made to do a Clinical Trial of an Investigational Medical Product (or CTIMP, for short). There are other criteria to be borne in mind if your research includes prisoners, children, adults who might not have the mental capacity to give consent to take part in research, medical devices, or ionising radiation.

From 1 April 2009, it has been a requirement for all new applications to National Health Service (NHS) RECs to be made through the online Integrated Research Application System (IRAS). This is available from the website: **https://www. myresearchproject.org.uk/** Likewise, all applications for an NHS Trust's R&D department to support a research study also need to be submitted via IRAS. The IRAS is a very handy system as it standardises the forms that you need to fill out, irrespective of which local REC you apply to. There are different forms that are available from IRAS for applying to do clinical trials, clinical investigations of medical devices and studies involving ionising radiation. The types of forms that will probably be more of interest to many of you are the ones dealing with questionnaires/interviews for quantitative analysis or mixed quantitative/qualitative methodology. There is also a specific form for those who wish only to use qualitative methods and there is another form for those who are doing a student project (not for a doctorate but for other levels of qualification). For non-doctoral students to do a project involving NHS patients/service users, this will require the chief investigator (usually the student's supervisor) to fill out most sections of the form in conjunction with the student. At present, a student who is doing research for a doctorate is expected to be the chief investigator and largely responsible for maintaining appropriate ethical standards throughout the study.

IRAS provides some example application forms to give applicants an idea of the questions that are being asked, depending on the type of study that is being proposed. You will need to give yourself sufficient time to draft your application and get feedback from colleagues or your supervisor before you complete your application online. You will also need to consider the underpinning ethical principles that guide the decision-making of ethical committees and which help to inform your decisions, as a researcher, while the study is underway. To get an idea of the kinds of questions that need to be answered, we have provided you with excerpts of the online ethics form in Example 13.2. Please note that we have drafted these excerpts to illustrate the issues that are being considered by the local REC and there are some sections that have not been completed in this example. Usually, all sections need to be filled out. It is also worth noting that the ethics form is a relatively lengthy document, but do not let this deter you; this is because there needs to be a range of safeguards to protect the people who are taking part in your research and the welfare of participants (and researchers!) should always be borne in mind. We will revisit the ethics form in Example 13.2 when discussing the four main ethical principles for conducting acceptable research.

Example 13.2 Research Ethics Committee applications using the Integrated Research Application System (IRAS) form

[Note to reader: Below is a draft of an ethics application for a study using the application form template entitled, 'Questionnaires/interviews for quantitative analysis or mixed quantitative/qualitative methodology – including children'.

Only some of these sections are completed, for illustrative purposes. Please note that the sections in the forms do not follow a wholly sequential order, as some of the sections are only included in forms for certain types of studies].

Please enter a short title for this project (maximum 70 characters)

Acceptability of Pupil-Held Record to Students, Parents and Health Professionals

1. **Is your project an audit or service evaluation?**

   ○ Yes   • No

2a. **Select one category from the list below:**
   - ○ Clinical trial of an investigational medicinal product
   - ○ Clinical investigation or other study of a medical device
   - ○ Combined trial of an investigational medicinal product and an investigational medical device
   - ○ Other clinical trial or clinical investigation
   - • Study administering questionnaires/interviews for quantitative analysis, or using mixed quantitative/qualitative methodology
   - ○ Study involving qualitative methods only
   - ○ Study limited to working with human tissue samples, other human biological samples and/or data (specific project only)
   - ○ Research tissue bank
   - ○ Research database

   If your work does not fit any of these categories, select the option below:
   - ○ Other study

2b. **Please answer the following question(s):**

   (a) Does the study involve the use of any ionising radiation?

   ○ Yes   • No

   (b) Will you be taking new human tissue samples (or other human biological samples)?

   ○ Yes   • No

   (c) Will you be using existing human tissue samples (or other human biological samples)?

   ○ Yes   • No

3. **In which countries of the UK will the research sites be located? (Tick all that apply)**
   - • England
   - ○ Scotland

Example 13.2 continued

○ Wales

○ Northern Ireland

4. In completing this form, which bodies are you making an application to?

- NHS/HSC Research and Development offices
- Research Ethics Committee
- ○ Patient Information Advisory Group (PIAG)
- ○ Ministry of Justice (MoJ)

5. Will any research sites in this study be NHS organisations?

- Yes   ○ No

6. Do you plan to include any participants who are children?

- Yes   ○ No

7. Do you plan to include any participants who are adults unable to consent for themselves through physical or mental incapacity? *The guidance notes explain how an adult is defined for this purpose.*

○ Yes   • No

8. Do you plan to include any participants who are prisoners or young offenders in the custody of HM Prison Service in England or Wales?

○ Yes   • No

9. Is the study, or any part of the study, being undertaken as an educational project?

○ Yes   • No

10. Will identifiable patient data be accessed outside the clinical care team without prior consent at any stage of the project (including identification of potential participants)?

○ Yes   • No

PART A: Core study information

1. ADMINISTRATIVE DETAILS

A1. Full title of the research:

How Acceptable Is a Pupil-Held Record ('Health Fax') to Students, Parents and Health Professionals?

A2. Chief Investigator: Mr Graham A. Parker
                                     Title Forename/Initials Surname

Post: Professional Lead for School Nursing

Qualifications: RGN, RSN

Example 13.2 **continued**

Employer:	East Staffordshire Primary Care Trust
Work Address:	East Staffordshire Primary Care Trust, Riddlestone, Greyhawkings,
Post Code:	ST96 7GH
Work E-mail:	graham.parker@espct.nhs.uk
* Personal E-mail:	
Work Telephone:	(017565) 862 4558
* Personal Telephone/Mobile:	
Fax:	(017565) 962 4548

* This information is optional. It will not be placed in the public domain or disclosed to any other third party without prior consent.

A copy of a current CV (maximum 2 pages of A4) for the Chief Investigator must be submitted with the application.

[Note to reader: Sections A5-1 and A5-2 cover research reference numbers and whether the current application is connected to previous applications].

2. OVERVIEW OF THE RESEARCH

To provide all the information required by review bodies and research information systems, we ask a number of specific questions. This section invites you to give an overview using language comprehensible to lay reviewers and members of the public. Please read the guidance notes for advice on this section.

[Note to reader: Sections on Lay Summary and Summary of the Main Issues precede Section A10 onwards.]

A10. What is the principal research question/objective? *Please put this in language comprehensible to a lay person.*

The principal objective of this project will be to:

- Examine the acceptability of a pupil-held record (the 'Health Fax') for 11-year-old children in mainstream schools and for 'looked after' children aged 7 years.

A11. What are the secondary research questions/objectives if applicable? *Please put this in language comprehensible to a lay person.*

The secondary objectives of this project will be to:

- Assess how the Health Fax is being used by a sample of East Staffordshire schoolchildren.
- Analyse the perceived usefulness of the Health Fax and make amendments to the format and content of the Health Fax in light of comments made by pupils, parents and health professionals (General Practitioners and School Nurses).

▶

343

Example 13.2 continued

A12. What is the scientific justification for the research? *Please put this in language comprehensible to a lay person.*

The Health Fax is an innovative health record booklet for schoolchildren, which was originally developed by School Nurses in Optimum Health NHS Trust (McAleer and Jackson, 1994). It was piloted in 1993 by Optimum Health with 17 schools in Lewisham and Southwark (North). The rationale of the Health Fax was to provide the School Nurse and the pupil with a framework for discussion about the pupil's health needs during the one-to-one health interview, which was usually conducted at Year 7 for children (at age 11) in mainstream schools. The Health Fax was primarily aimed to empower schoolchildren and to encourage them to take a shared responsibility for their health. The Health Fax was also seen by School Nurses at Optimum as providing the potential for enhancing communication between different agencies that may come into contact with the child and may have similar beneficial effects as the Personal Child Health Record in Health Visiting (McAleer and Jackson, 1994). The ethos of the Health Fax has been supportive of policies such as the Department for Education and Skills and Department of Health (1996)'s circular on 'Supporting Children' and the Children's Charter, as set out by the United Nations' (1992) Convention on the Rights of the Child. The Health Fax was seen as incorporating the recommendations of the Polnay Report (British Paediatric Association, 1995) in which the following topics, among others, were recommended as part of a core programme for 11–12-year-olds, many of which are included in the Health Fax: (1) adjustment to school, (2) road safety, (3) water safety, (4) diet, (5) smoking, (6) exercise, (7) personal hygiene, (8) dental health, (9) sun protection, (10) sexual health and education, (11) drugs, (12) alcohol, (13) stress, and (14) referring oneself to a School Nurse or GP. The Health Fax was also seen as following the basic principles of health policies such as the Hall Report (e.g. Hall and Elliman, 2006), which recommended moving away from blanket screening to a more targeted approach by setting clear objectives and measurable outcomes. East Staffordshire PCT's Child Health Promotion Group has considered adopting the Health Fax as standard practice, with the permission of the Health Fax developers, but the PCT is as yet unclear about the benefits or difficulties that might be encountered in using it. The Health Fax will be given out to a pilot sample of 11-year-olds in mainstream schools and to children looked after. In this study, we are seeking to find out how the pupils in the pilot areas have experienced using the Health Fax and what parents and health professionals also think about it.

References:

British Paediatric Association (1995) *Report of a Joint Working Party on Health Needs of School Age Children*. Chaired by Leon Polnay. London: British Paediatric Association.

Department for Education and Skills and Department of Health (1996) *Supporting Pupils with Medical Needs: A good practice guide*. London: DfES.

Hall, D.M. and Elliman, D. (2006) *Health for all Children*. Revised 4th edn. Oxford: Oxford University Press.

McAleer, M. and Jackson, P. (1994) The school health fax. *Nursing Times, 90 (31)*, 29–31.

United Nations (1992) *Convention on the Rights of the Child*. Available via: http://www.everychildmatters.gov.uk/_files/589DD6D3A29C929ACB148DB3F13B01E7.pdf, accessed 5 August 2009.

Example 13.2 continued

[Note to reader: After Section A12, Section A13 then requests a full summary of the methodology and design of the study.]

A14–1. In which aspects of the research process have you actively involved, or will you involve, patients, service users, or members of the public?

- ○ Design of the research
- ○ Management of the research
- ○ Undertaking the research
- • Analysis of results
- • Dissemination of findings
- ○ None of the above

Give details of involvement, or if none please justify the absence of involvement.

4. RISKS AND ETHICAL ISSUES

RESEARCH PARTICIPANTS

A17. Please list the principal inclusion and exclusion criteria.

Inclusion criteria:
Pupils will need to have had some experience in using the Health Fax so that they can talk about how it may have helped, or hindered, their ability to have health- and well-being-related dialogue with health professionals, parents or guardians. The experience of using the Health Fax should be for at least the duration of the trial period of 3 months.

Parents/guardians and other health professionals (e.g. General Practitioners) will need to have come into contact with at least one pupil who has used the Health Fax during the trial period.

Exclusion criteria:
As being able to assess the utility of the Health Fax is the primary concern of this study and the questions in the survey only relate to the Health Fax, we will only be looking to get feedback from people who have come into contact with using the Health Fax, either as a pupil or responsible adult.

RESEARCH PROCEDURES, RISKS AND BENEFITS
Sections A18–A26 cover the following questions:

A18. Give details of all non-clinical intervention(s) or procedure(s) that will be received by participants as part of the research protocol. These include seeking consent, interviews, non-clinical observations and use of questionnaires.

1 survey.

A21. How long do you expect each participant to be in the study in total?

The survey should take about 20 minutes to complete.

▶

Example 13.2 **continued**

A22. What are the potential risks and burdens for research participants and how will you minimise them?

For all studies, describe any potential adverse effects, pain, discomfort, distress, intrusion, inconvenience or changes to lifestyle. Only describe risks or burdens that could occur as a result of participation in the research. Say what steps would be taken to minimise risks and burdens as far as possible.

No major risk and burdens are anticipated for the participants. We do not expect there to be a significant amount of intrusion, inconvenience or change to lifestyle as a result of taking part.

A23. Will interviews/questionnaires or group discussions include topics that might be sensitive, embarrassing or upsetting, or is it possible that criminal or other disclosures requiring action could occur during the study?

○ Yes   • No

If Yes, please give details of procedures in place to deal with these issues:

A24. What is the potential for benefit to research participants?

Through this research, we will be able to gauge the utility of certain sections of the Health Fax among this pilot sample of schoolchildren. We will also be able to assess how the Health Fax might help, or hinder, effective health- and well-being-related communication between the pupils and health professionals/parents/guardians.

A26. What are the potential risks for the researchers themselves? (if any)

No major potential risks are anticipated.

RECRUITMENT AND INFORMED CONSENT

In this section we ask you to describe the recruitment procedures for the study. Please give separate details for different study groups where appropriate.

A27–1. How, and by whom, will potential participants, records or samples be identified?

See response to A29.

A28. Will any participants be recruited by publicity through posters, leaflets, adverts or websites?

• Yes   ○ No

If Yes, please give details of how and where publicity will be conducted, and enclose copy of all advertising material (with version numbers and dates).

A29. How, and by whom, will potential participants first be approached?

Students will be approached in class by the school nurse who will hand questionnaires to everyone in class. At the same time, a questionnaire for parents/guardians will also be given to the students to hand to their parents/guardians. For approaching children

Example 13.2 **continued**

looked after who will have used the Health Fax, this will be done through liaising with the appropriate health and social care professionals who will circulate the survey to those children who have used the Health Fax. A sample of General Practitioners (GPs) in the locality will be randomly selected from a list of GPs in the area and they will be mailed a copy of the survey.

A30–1. Will you obtain informed consent from or on behalf of research participants?

- Yes   ○ No

If you will be obtaining consent from adult participants, please give details of who will take consent and how it will be done, with details of any steps to provide information (a written information sheet, videos, or interactive material).

Arrangements for adults unable to consent for themselves should be described separately in Part B Section 6, and for children in Part B Section 7.

If you plan to seek informed consent from vulnerable groups, say how you will ensure that consent is voluntary and fully informed.

If you are not obtaining consent, please explain why not.

Please enclose a copy of the information sheet(s) and consent form(s).

A30–2. Will you record informed consent (or advice from consultees) in writing?

- Yes   ○ No

If No, how will it be recorded?

A31. How long will you allow potential participants to decide whether or not to take part?

The participants can decide to take part during any time within the two-month study period, after having received a copy of the questionnaire in the class or by mail.

A33–1. What arrangements have been made for persons who might not adequately understand verbal explanations or written information given in English, or who have special communication needs?(e.g. translation, use of interpreters)

If appropriate in some schools, questionnaires will be translated into the pupil's native language and back-translated into English, to check whether there is sufficient conceptual and functional equivalence. We will be using the local interpreting services for this purpose.

[Note to reader: After Section A33-1 in the IRAS form there are several further sections. These sections include questions on: confidentiality of data, storage of data, incentives and payments, publication and dissemination of findings, scientific and statistical review of the proposal, management of the research, insurance/indemnity to carry out the research and considerations relating to the inclusion of children in research.]

Four ethical issues to consider

Four main moral principles (based on Beauchamp and Childress, 2001) underpin bio-medical research as reflected in the *Declaration of Helsinki* (WMA, 2000) and you will need to consider these guiding principles when you are constructing your research study and putting together your research proposal. We have listed these principles below, providing examples of how they are applied within practice so that you can consider them within the context of your own developing research.

Autonomy

All researchers are required to respect individual autonomy of study participants. This is evidenced, for example, through the process of informed and ongoing consent – ongoing consent is informing individuals of the right to withdraw from a research study at any time – and through recognising and respecting an individual's right to anonymity, confidentiality and privacy. In the sample ethics proposal in Example 13.2, you can see that informed consent is emphasised and the researchers will usually show how they obtain consent with a copy of the form that prospective participants would need to see before they decided to take part.

In order to gain fully informed consent, you will need to look at how well your prospective participants can understand the information about the study. You need this information to be accessible to people who may not have English as a first language and you may need to consider ensuring that the questionnaire items are phrased in a simple and comprehensible way. In Example 13.2, you can see the researchers considered the possibility of translating the questionnaires into a range of languages. The researchers haven't mentioned whether the information sheet would be translated into some of the most commonly spoken languages as well, so this might need to be made clearer before ethical approval can be given to this proposed study.

Beneficence

This principle is based on the requirement to benefit the individual or patient. In the context of a research study therefore there is a requirement to safeguard the welfare of all study participants, for example clients, patients, colleagues and fellow researchers. It is also considered unethical to undertake research that will be of no potential benefit to either participants or wider society. The ethics proposal in Example 13.2 makes a strong case for the Health Fax as having a variety of potential benefits, particularly in enabling the children concerned to be more aware of issues relating to their health. The ethics proposal highlights the importance of having the Health Fax as a vehicle for schoolchildren to discuss their health concerns with their school nurse, although it would appear from the proposal that it is not clear what parts of the process of using the Health Fax provide the most optimal benefits in promoting schoolchildren's health.

Non-malfeasance

This consideration is also closely associated with beneficence and assumes that no harm will come to the individual as a result of taking part in the research study. However, all research carries with it some risk of harm, however minimal. Depending on the nature and scope of the study the potential harm may be physical, such as being involved in a drug trial, or risks to emotional well-being (e.g. exploring a patient's experiences of a particular illness or care experience and the impact for the individual in revisiting past experiences). It is therefore necessary to consider the possible risks and to identify, minimise and address these when considering the scope of your research study. In the example that we gave in Example 13.2, you can see that many of the questions in the ethics form are concerned with looking at possible risks to the well-being of the participants. The REC application form asks about whether participants are likely to be at risk of physical and psychological harm, and the researchers attempt to show how the schoolchildren will be protected when taking part. It is not likely that participants in a study involving questionnaire surveys or interviews will be at risk of a great deal of psychological harm, but this all depends on the questions being asked as some enquiries may be intrusive and upsetting. As a result, it is usually common practice to have a copy of the survey or interview schedule enclosed in the ethics application, so that the REC can gauge the acceptability of the questions to be asked.

Justice

This principle is concerned with 'fairness' and translated within the context of research will always require the needs of participants to come before the objectives of the research, for example that participants are not coerced or feel obliged to take part in a research study by virtue of the pre-existing relationship (e.g., a nurse–patient relationship) and as such the relationship between the researcher and the person being researched must always be considered. In the sample proposal in Example 13.2, this is something worth considering as the application outlines the school nurses as being the persons responsible for handing out the questionnaire to the schoolchildren. This is potentially problematic as some of the children may feel pressurised to take part due to their pre-existing relationship with the school nurse. Some RECs may argue that it would be best to have an independent researcher who would take responsibility for administering and organising the collection of the questionnaires so that the nurse–patient power dynamic does not lead to an unfair context within which the research will take place.

Based on these principles, the rationale for seeking ethical approval stems from a clear obligation to carry out research that recognises and protects the safety, well-being and dignity of study participants while at the same time enabling high-quality research to be undertaken. As such, obtaining ethical approval prior to undertaking your research study is paramount to ensuring the efficacy of your study and an ethics committee will closely review the research protocol, and other relevant project documentation to ensure that the dignity, rights, safety and well-being of research participants will be protected throughout the research.

The nature and scope of your research will determine the procedures and level of approval that you will need to obtain prior to undertaking the research. The research and development department in your NHS Trust or your local REC will be able to advise you on procedures to be undertaken prior to starting your research study. The NRES (2007) has published a leaflet, 'Guidance for applicants to the National Research Ethics Service' and this takes you through some of the terminology commonly used in the ethical review process, considerations to bear in mind before you apply for approval, and a decision flow-chart on how and were to make your application. The NRES has identified that RECs should usually aim to come to a decision on an ethics application within the period of 60 calendar days, although this timeline of activities could be affected by the REC needing to get clarification on the content of your application.

We would strongly advise you to ensure that you spend time to complete your application as thoroughly as possible as an ethics committee will make their decision regarding your application on the basis of the information that you have supplied. Before submitting your application you may want to enlist the help of a critical friend who may be able to identify potential ambiguities in your application. The NRES (2007) also requests that it is a desirable thing for proposed studies to have confirmation that any resources necessary to fund a project have already been agreed, and that the proposed study will also have been subjected to peer review (i.e. critiqued by others with sufficient expertise to comment on the scientific quality of the study). Some studies might only pose a minimal risk to patients or involve examining routine treatment; if this is the case, the researchers could apply to be exempt from requiring site-specific assessors to inform the REC about the suitability of the research team and the research environment. Most importantly, the research and development department will also need to have approved of the proposed study before it can begin.

As you can see, there are a number of requirements that need to be satisfied before research can be carried out in the UK's National Health Service (NHS). You will need to bear in mind that the requirements, criteria and processes for approving health care research might vary in other countries so you might need to familiarise yourself with these systems before you carry out your research. Overall, although these systems of ethical adherence might seem like a number of hurdles that need to be jumped over before you can even speak to patients/service users about your research, the welfare of these people should remain paramount in your mind before taking those first steps.

Self-assessment exercise

Reviewing a research proposal

Have a look at the following brief research proposal. Imagine that you are part of a panel making decisions on whether different health care studies can be funded.

User and carer involvement in nurse education programmes: developing a meaningful participant framework

Background

The involvement of users and carers in the planning, delivery and evaluation of health service provision is increasingly being recognised as a central component in assuring the maintenance of, and informing the ongoing improvement of, the overall quality of care delivery (Brooker 1997). In a general sense user involvement is not a new concept, with the World Health Organization (WHO) identifying the importance of patient's involvement in their own health care over two decades ago (Flanagan 1999). Recently a number of national policy initiatives (DoH 1989, 1994) and other documentation (English National Board 1996) have provided greater clarity regarding both the scope and direction of user involvement within health care provision, with user participation in education and training programmes for health care professionals being recognised as an essential component within this process. However, although user and carer participation in the development of education programmes and care delivery is now well established, there have also been important questions raised regarding the extent to which user and carer involvement has been translated into meaningful 'active' partnerships rather than 'tokenistic consultation' (Forrest *et al.* 2000). In addition, it has also been recognised that the nature of the user–professional relationship, in terms of perceived balance of power, raises issues regarding the necessity to provide clear reciprocal structures for successful participation in the future (Forrest *et al.* 2000).

Aims of the project

The aims of the proposed project are:

- To provide an in-depth review of the salient literature in this area
- To explore the current situation regarding evaluation of user and carer participation in nurse education
- To identify key areas where user and carer participation may be further developed
- To develop a clear supportive framework for active user and carer participation in nurse education programmes in the future.

Methods

Phase 1

Phase 1 of the project will involve an in-depth review of the literature surrounding user and carer involvement in the development of care delivery in general and more particularly, in the continuing development of educational programmes for nurses (with an onus towards pre-registration education programmes). In addition, there will an evaluation of Student Evaluation of Module (SEM), with regard to user and carer involvement and other relevant school documentation. Phase 1 of the project will provide an evaluation of the present situation and will serve as a foundation for Phase 2 of the overall project.

Phase 2

Using Phase 1 of the project as a foundation, Phase 2 of the study will involve the collection of empirical data through focus groups with nursing students and lecturers from within the School of Nursing. In addition, focus groups will also be undertaken with a number of users and carers. It is envisaged that analysis of focus group data will inform the development of a clear supportive framework for active user and carer participation in nurse education programmes in the future.

▶

References

Brooker D.J. (1997) Issues in user feedback on health services for elderly people. *British Journal of Nursing, 6,* 159–162.

Department of Health (1989) *Working for Patients: Department of Health: Official Publications.* London: HMSO.

Department of Health (1994) *Nurse, Midwife and Health Visitor Education: A Statement of Strategic Intent.* London: Department of Health.

English National Board (1996) *Learning from Each Other.* London: English National Board.

Flanagan J. (1999) Public participation in the design of educational programmes for cancer nurses: a case report. *European Journal of Cancer Care, 8,* 107–112.

Forrest S. Masters H. and Brown N. (2000) Mental health service user involvement in nurse education: exploring the issues. *Journal of Psychiatric and Mental Health Nursing, 7,* 51–57.

Questions

- What do you think are the main strengths of the proposal?
- How could the proposal be strengthened or which areas need further clarification?

Summary

Overall, this chapter has taken you through many of the initial stages that need to be satisfied before you carry out your nursing research. We have aimed to equip you with the skills to develop practice-informed research questions and to then ask searching questions of the literature. You should be able to identify people who are possible stakeholders in your research and potential collaborators. From there on in this chapter, you will have been given some tools for developing a research proposal and you are encouraged to invite colleagues to critique your proposals once you've drafted them. Finally, we have enabled you to be more aware of the nuances of assessing whether a proposed study is ethical by using four key principles of autonomy, beneficence, non-malfeasance and justice. You have been shown the system that currently exists in the NHS for centrally regulating processes of ethical adherence in England, Wales, Scotland and Northern Ireland.

Final comments: taking those first steps to becoming an independent nurse researcher

Before you start on your research project we would like to remind you of some of the fundamental questions to address when you're deciding whether to embark on a research project. These questions are related to many of the issues that we've raised throughout this chapter and we would urge you to revisit them as often as possible at different stages of the research process. This approach should enable you to be a more reflective and effective nurse researcher in the future.

The key questions to consider are:

- Is it an important and relevant area to be researched?
- Can the research have an impact on clinical care, specifically the well-being of patients and the well-being of those who provide care to them?
- Is the research area amenable to measurement? How would you analyse the data collected and how would you interpret the findings?
- Can the research be done in an ethical way?
- Can the research be supported with sufficient human and financial resources?
- How might you put some of the implications from your study findings into changes to practice? What if the study uncovers the need for spending more resources to improve clinical care? Can the health care organisation that you work in help to finance these potential improvements?

We trust this book will have given you all of the essentials that you need to be an effective, ethical and efficient nurse researcher and wish you well in your research endeavours!

Answers to self-assessment exercises

Chapter 1

Extract 1: Difficulties in administering medication to older mental health inpatients (Dickens *et al.*, 2007)
Answer: analysis/presentation, research and quantitative.

Extract 2: NICE guidance on antenatal and postnatal mental health (Hairon, 2007)
Answer: literature, research and quantitative.

Extract 3: A study on effects of working unsocial hours. (Crew, 2006)
Answer: analysis, research and qualitative.

Extract 4: Procedural restraint in children's nursing: using clinical benchmarks (Bland *et al.*, 2002)
Answer: literature, theory.

Chapter 2

Study 1
Answer: cohort study. It is a cohort study because it is measuring people over time (longitudinal design) and looking forwards in the measurements (i.e. having a prospective focus).

Study 2
Answer: RCT. This is because there was random assignment of participants to treatments. Patients were measured before and after treatment was received.

Study 3
Answer: Cross-sectional survey. This is because surveys were done on groups of children in a specific age group but the same children were not studied over different years. Over two years of the study period, the researchers took 'snapshots' of net ownership and the presence of parasites in the blood of children aged under the age of 2.

Study 4
Answer: Cross-sectional survey. This is because participants were only measured at one time point. The researchers are only looking at the relationship between the number of cups of green tea consumed and measurements of health through taking blood samples from participants.

Study 5:
Answer: Case-control study. This is because people with lung cancer (i.e. the 'cases') were selected and compared with a control group who did not have lung cancer (i.e. the 'controls'). The measurements were retrospective (i.e. looking backwards) by examining the medical history of the cases and the controls.

Chapter 7

The main issues that we could find from the dialogue included:

- Involvement of all stakeholders
- Confidentiality of data collection
- Communicating findings to stakeholders
- Arranging sufficient time to execute the project properly
- Getting organisational support to do the project
- How people's bad experiences of the recommendations of action research may deter people from taking part in future studies (i.e. the problems in working with the pharmacists)
- Importance of agreeing roles and responsibilities: making it clear how the project is being led and how participants are facilitated to take part without fear of recrimination
- Making it clear as to what can or can't be changed organisationally as a result of the action research
- Being committed to the agenda as it evolves throughout the duration of the action research
- Being open to the idea that cultural change, as a result of action research recommendations, may need to occur at all levels in an organisation and not just among one group of staff.

Act II. Issues to consider when involving patients and relatives/carers in action research

Question: Having read through this scenario, what are the main issues concerned with involving patients and carers in action research?

Suggested answers:

- **Think about the power dynamics involved and the inequalities between nurses and their patients.** There might be difficulties in getting patients to be open in their views when talking to a researcher if they think that what they say could get back to the health care team and adversely affect the quality of care that they receive. Often patients are resistant to changes to their health care, particularly if they are already satisfied with what they're receiving. As a result, some patients could be defensive in their responses in order to maintain the status quo with their care.

- **Consider the importance of the context of action research and how it's presented to the patients.** Do the patients think that all comments they make will be incorporated and acted upon? Do the patients have a clear idea as to what you want to study and how does this overlap with what they want you to research?

- **Relative/carer participation.** To what extent could you, or should you, involve relatives/carers in setting the agenda of the action research, in collecting data from them and in getting them to comment on the findings for the study? In which circumstances might relative/carer participation be especially important?

- **Think about the ways of collecting data from patients and the things you're asking from them.** Some topics might be highly sensitive (such as the one touched upon in this scenario) and very problematic to discuss in a group. Is a one-to-one interview or a questionnaire more appropriate? Might you want to offer a variety of ways in which participants can voice their opinions and perceptions?

- **What sorts of questions are you aiming to ask?** Questions on their experiences and how they feel? Or questions on their views concerning service improvement and are you then wanting to look at whether the improvements should be systemic or related to the behaviour of staff?

- **Think about fatigue that patients might feel if involved in too many studies all at once.**

- **Look to addressing misperceptions of what can realistically be achieved and what are realistic expectations of a health service.** Is it realistic to expect nurses to escort all older patients to the bathroom? Is it feasible to presume that older patients will have no risk of falling when in hospital?

- **Think about what needs to be done if a patient/carer/relative reports unsafe/ unethical/criminal practice.** What is your role as a researcher and how might this conflict with your role as a registered nurse?

- **Consider the viability of future possible actions arising from data collected from patients/relatives/carers.** Is cultural change needed? Do staff need additional training or do new administrative and monitoring systems require setting up to make bad practices more noticeable? Being able to monitor bad practices may be particularly difficult outside of the hospital setting so do watch out for the problems involved with this.

Act III. Issues to consider when involving staff in action research

Question: Having read through this scenario, what are the main issues concerned with involving staff in action research?

Suggested answers:

- **Setting the agenda as to what to study and how to study it.** How do the staff members view the action research agenda? Do they perceive that they can have some input into it? Do they see the action research agenda as being mutually beneficial to both patients and themselves? Consider the ultimate purpose of the study – do you want staff to be made more aware of the issues around a certain problem in clinical practice? If so, is action research the most appropriate method to do this or are there alternative ways of getting staff to discuss and explore these issues?

- **Collecting information from staff:**
  - Think about the extent to which you wish to get staff taking part in the action research and the amount of time that they would have available to commit to participation. Is it too much to ask to get staff to take part in focus group or one-to-one interviews that may take several hours? Are there other means of obtaining their views in a rigorous and non-intrusive way?
  - Also, consider issues relating to confidentiality and anonymity, particularly if you are asking staff to report instances of poor practice. Would some staff members be more comfortable talking in a more general way? If so, how useful could this still be for your research?

- **Implementing actions after feedback has been received.** Consider the ways in which some staff may prefer to be informed about the action research's findings and recommendations. Would you want to communicate this through a newsletter or through posters or guidance leaflets? Would you want to stage regular sessions with staff or with people who can filter the information to all levels within the health care team? Could you use a train-the-trainer type of approach by getting influential members to help change attitudes or practices within the team?

Chapter 10

Suggested answers:

[CA1]: Issue 2 – Aims: The aims seem relatively clear. It is not clear whether the authors will be able to deliver on all of these aims so we'll need to look at how they do in the findings and discussion sections.

[CA2]: Issue 4 – Design: The use of qualitative research methods looks appropriate, given the exploratory nature of the study and the lack of knowledge into the ways in which first-time fathers perceive their experiences of being depressed after the birth of their children.

[CA3]: Issue 6 – Sample and sampling: How else could the researchers have accessed the potential participants? It may be that the authors could have contacted local antenatal groups, although some fathers may not go to these groups. Also, the fathers who may be depressed before the birth may not be the same ones who are depressed after the birth.

[CA4]: Issue 6 – Sample and sampling: Inclusion and exclusion criteria seem clear.

[CA5]: Issue 5 – Ethics: It looks like the authors have taken great care to address the general ethical issues of getting ethics committee approval and to focus on the specific needs of the participants in terms of protecting their well-being. What are the other ethical issues associated with this topic area? Could stigma surrounding mental health and the cultural aspects associated with men's health make it difficult for the participants to speak out about this?

[CA6]: Issue 7 – Data collection and analysis: What other methods might be used before carrying out the full study? For example, a pilot study could be conducted to test out the acceptability of some of the questions posed and could aid in the development of the semi-structured questionnaire used in the actual study.

[CA7]: Issue 7 – Data collection and analysis: The interviews seem quite brief. Although it is transparently clear about the process of collecting the data, it is not likely that the interviews have been long enough to provide in-depth, 'rich' data.

[CA8]: Issue 7 – Data collection and analysis: It isn't clear whether grounded theory is an appropriate approach to take with the data. From later on, it appears as if the three so-called 'themes' of cognitive, affective and behavioural symptoms of postnatal depression among fathers are purely a function of the questions being asked rather than of what the participants are saying.

[CA9]: Issue 7 – Data collection and analysis: The cognitive, affective and behavioural 'themes' don't appear to be themes at all because these were the sorts of issues that were already put down in the interview schedule for discussion. There needed to be more of a focus on the actual content of what the participants have said and a drawing out of themes from this content. For instance, in the so-called theme of 'cognitive symptoms', there are a couple of quotes on the ways in which the participants see their role and how their world-view has been altered after becoming fathers; these sorts of insights seem to suggest that there is a possible theme regarding the role of the father and the place of this role within society and the family unit.

Glossary

Action research A part of qualitative research which involves a reflective process of problem solving led by individuals working in teams to improve the way they address issues and solve problems.

Alternative hypothesis A hypothesis that refers to a statement that the results found in a study are expected to show a statistically significant relationship.

Bar chart A bar chart is a graphical display of frequencies of scores used commonly with categorical-type data.

Case-control designs Research designs that researchers use to identify or study the possible variables that may contribute to various health factors.

Categorical data Data comprises categories that have no numerical value or order.

Categorical-type data A term used specifically for this book that describes data that has been put in categories and does not have any numerical properties.

Chi-square The chi-square test of association allows the comparison of two categorical-type data to determine if there is any relationship between them.

Clinical trial A study that is conducted to allow safety and efficacy data to be collected for new drugs or treatments.

Cohort study design A study that examines a common characteristic among a sample of individuals.

Cohort Group of people.

Confounding variable An unforeseen, or unaccounted-for, variable that jeopardises the validity of an experiment's outcome.

Construct validity This is a kind of validity that refers to the underlying concepts (or 'constructs') that are being measured. For example, if a researcher studying the mental health of service users with depression has a theory that depression has two main components (or 'constructs'), then this researcher will want to see if these two components surface in how the service users think, feel and act.

Constructivism The principle that knowledge is developed (or 'constructed') according to frameworks and ways of seeing the world. This knowledge is continually shaped and re-shaped, depending on any new information and new situations that are encountered.

Continuous data A set of data is said to be continuous if the values/observations belonging to it may take on any value. Continuous data, unlike discrete data, can have decimal points.

Continuous-type data A term used specifically for this book that describes data that has been ordered numerically or given numerical properties in some way.

Control group The standard by which experimental observations are evaluated by using a set of participants in which they either receive no treatment/intervention or a placebo.

Criterion validity This is a kind of validity that refers to the measuring of a new assessment tool in relation to a benchmark or gold standard. For instance, if a researcher is developing a new tool to measure preoperative anxiety in patients, the researcher will examine how strongly a patient's score on this tool corresponds with another measurement, like the Anxiety subscale of the Hospital Anxiety and Depression (HAD) scale.

Cross-sectional survey A research design that provides the researcher with a picture of what might be occurring in a sample or population of people at a particular time.

Descriptive statistics Statistics that are techniques used to summarise/describe data.

Diagnostic trials A type of clinical trial where research methods are designed for developing tools that can be used for recognising or detecting a particular disease.

Discrete data Continuous-type data. A set of data is said to be discrete if the values are distinct and separate and represent whole numbers. Discrete data, unlike continuous data, cannot have decimal points.

Double-blind A clinical trial or study design in which neither the participating individuals nor the study staff knows which participants are receiving the experimental drug and which are receiving a placebo (or another therapy).

Ecological validity A form of validity. The extent to which the findings can be generalised beyond the current situation.

Effect size The term given to a group of indices that measure the magnitude of a statistical finding.

Empirical Data based on research, not on a theory.

Ethnography A type of qualitative research which treats a group of people as an anthropologist would an unknown tribe, with detailed descriptions of how they live.

Ethnomethodology This relates to the general philosophy of seeing the world and doing research, which involves looking for the formal and informal rules and practices that operate among a group of people.

Evidence-based practice An approach where the best, most appropriate, most suitable methods are used based on theoretical and empirical evidence.

Expected frequencies In a contingency table, Crosstabs in SPSS, the expected frequencies are the frequencies that would be expected to be obtained in each cell of the table from the sample if everything was random. Expected frequencies are spread evenly across the cells. Most commonly used with a chi-square test.

External validity If a study has external validity, its results will generalise to the larger population.

Face validity This is one of the weakest forms of validity and is sometimes called 'acceptability'. Face validity refers to whether a measurement appears to be assessing the concept in question. For example, using a thermometer to establish a person's depression levels might be seen as having relatively low face validity as, on the face of it, the thermometer doesn't seem to be tapping into a person's mental well-being.

Focus group A group discussion, in which a moderator encourages a small group of people to focus on and discuss a topic.

Frequency table A frequency table is a way of summarising data by assigning a number of occurrences to each level of variable.

Genetic tests A type of screening test that looks for inherited genetic markers.

Grounded theory Practice of developing other theories that emerge from observing a group and their observable experiences. Researchers then add their own insight into the existence of those experiences.

Histogram A histogram is a graphical display of frequencies of scores used commonly with continuous-type data.

Hypothesis/hypotheses Suggested explanation or statements of the possible relationship between variables.

Imaging tests A type of screening test that uses X-rays, radioactive particles, sound waves or magnetic fields whose information can be analysed after passing through tissues of the body and that produce pictures of areas inside the body.

Independent samples Independent samples are those selected from the same population or different populations but which are considered independent of each other (for example, men and women).

Inferential statistics Comprises the use of statistical tests to make inferences concerning the nature of the relationship between variables.

Interpretative phenomenological analysis (IPA) An approach in qualitative research which is designed to offer insights into how a person, in a particular context, makes sense of a phenomenon.

Interval data/variables Have levels that are ordered and numerical. Interval data is distinctive from ratio data as interval data have no absolute zero (i.e. absence of what is being measured).

Intervention study A study where the researcher assesses or measures the effects of an intervention.

Longitudinal survey A research design in which the same surveys are observed repeatedly over a period of time.

Mann-Whitney *U* statistical test A non-parametric statistical test for comparing scores of two groups on a continuous-type variable.

Mean An average statistic worked out by adding all the values together, and then dividing this total by the number of values (e.g. the mean of 6 and 4, would be 10 divided by 2, which is 5).

Median The median is the value that appears halfway in a set of data when that data has been ordered by value (e.g. in the set of values 1, 2, 3, 4, 5 – 3 is the median).

Mode The mode is the most frequently occurring value in data (e.g. in the set of values 1, 2, 2, 2, 5 – 2 is the mode).

Negatively skewed distribution A distribution of scores in which the majority of scores fall to the right of the distribution.

Non-parametric statistical tests Non-parametric tests are often used instead of parametric counterparts when certain assumptions about the underlying population are questionable, for example when continuous-type data is not normally distributed.

Normal distribution A distribution of scores shaped like a bell curve in which the same number/percentage of scores fall on either side of the centre of the distribution.

Null hypothesis A hypothesis that refers to a statement that the results found in a study are no different from what might have occurred as a result of chance.

Observational study A study where the researcher observes the effects of a phenomenon.

Observed frequencies In a contingency table, Crosstabs in SPSS, the observed frequencies are the frequencies actually obtained in each cell of the table, from the sample. Most commonly used with a chi-square test.

Ordinal data Data with values/observations belonging to it can be ranked (put in order) or have a rating scale attached.

Paired-samples *t*-test (also known as dependent-groups *t*-test) A paired-samples *t*-test is used to determine whether there is a significant difference between the average values of the same variable made under two different conditions among the same sample.

Pearson correlation coefficient A correlation coefficient (*r*) is a number between −1 and 1 which indicates the degree to which two variables are statistically significantly related.

Percentile Percentiles are values that divide a sample of data into one hundred groups (i.e. 100 per cent), each representing 1 per cent.

Phase I trials A phase in a set of clinical trials that comprises initial studies to gain early evidence of the effectiveness of drugs and their side effects.

Phase II trials A phase in a set of clinical trials that comprises controlled clinical studies conducted to evaluate the effectiveness of the drug and to determine the common short-term side effects and risks.

Phase III trials A phase in a set of clinical trials that comprises controlled and uncontrolled trials after preliminary evidence suggesting effectiveness of the drug has been obtained.

Phase IV trials A phase in a set of clinical trials that comprises post-marketing studies to gain additional information including the drug's risks, benefits, and optimal use.

Phenomenology A qualitative research approach concerned with understanding a population's behaviours from that population's point of view.

Pie chart A pie chart is a pictorial way of summarising a set of categorical-type data.

Placebo A placebo is an inactive pill, liquid or powder that has no treatment value.

Population A population is any entire collection of people.

Positively skewed distribution A distribution of scores in which the majority of scores fall to the left of the distribution.

Prevention trials A type of clinical trial where research methods are designed to look for better techniques to prevent disease.

Probability value (*p*-value) The probability value (*p*-value) in a statistical hypothesis test is the probability of getting a value of the test statistic higher than that observed by chance alone.

Protocol A study plan on which all clinical trials are based.

Qualitative Aspect of the research process that may be estimated by meaning or language. Results are expressed in non-numerical terms.

Quality of life trials A type of clinical trial where research methods are designed to explore ways to improve the quality of life for individuals with an illness.

Quantitative Aspect of the research process that may be estimated by quantity or numbers.

Quartile. Quartiles are values that divide a sample of data into four groups containing equal numbers of observations.

Quasi-experiment Similar to randomised experiments but uses nonrandomized groups.

Random sample Data that have been drawn from a population in such a way that each piece of data that was selected was done so that each piece of data had an equal opportunity to appear in the sample.

Randomisation A method based on chance by which study participants are assigned to a treatment group.

Randomised controlled trial A study in which participants are randomly assigned to one of two or more treatment conditions of a study/clinical trial.

Ratio data/variables Have levels that are ordered and numerical. Ratio data is numerical, but is distinctive from interval data because ratio data can have an absolute zero (i.e. absence of what is being measured).

Sample A sample is a group of units/cases (e.g. people, test results) selected from a larger group (the population) of units/cases. Researchers study samples in the hope of drawing conclusions about the larger group.

Screening trials A type of clinical trial where research methods are designed to develop and assess screening tools to detect certain diseases.

Semi-inter quartile range (SIQR) The semi-inter quartile range is a measure of the ranges of scores between the upper and the lower quartiles divided by two. Also a measure of the extent to which a set of scores vary. Often accompanies the reporting of the median.

Single-blind A study in which one party, either the investigator or participant, is unaware of what drug/treatment the participant is taking.

Spearman correlation coefficient A statistical test that produces a correlation coefficient (*rho*) used with non-parametric data that produces a number between −1 and 1, which indicates the degree to which two variables are related.

Standard deviation A measure of the extent to which a set of scores vary. Often accompanies the reporting of the mean.

Statistical inference. Statistical inference makes use of information from a sample to draw conclusions (inferences) about the population from which the sample was taken.

Statistical significance A result is statistically significant if it is probable not to have occurred by chance.

Stratified sampling A method of sampling from a population based on the characteristics of the population on which the selection is based.

Symbolic interactionism Researchers use this approach to examine how people interpret and react to a variety of labels and symbols that exist within a social world.

Survey A research tool that includes questions (either open-ended or forced choice) and employs an oral or written method for asking and answering the questions.

Treatment trials A type of clinical trial where research methods are designed to test new drugs or new combinations of drugs, new treatments, or new types of surgery.

Type I error When the use of a statistical test incorrectly reports that it has found a statistically significant result where none really exists.

Variable Phenomena that vary.

Wilcoxon sign-ranks statistical test A non-parametric statistical test for comparing scores on the same continuous-type variable on two occasions (or for comparing matched groups).

References

Abdulla, S., Schellenberg, J.A., Mukasa, O., Marchant , T., Smith, T., Tanner, M. and Lengeler, C. (2001) Impact on malaria morbidity of a programme supplying insecticide-treated nets in children aged under 2 years in Tanzania: community cross-sectional study. *British Medical Journal, 322*, 270-273.

Ahmed, Q.A., Memish, Z.A., Allegranzi, B. and Pittet, D. (2006) Muslim health-care workers and alcohol-based handrubs. *The Lancet, 367 (9515)*, 1025-1027.

Alspach, G. (2006) Editorial. Nurses' use and understanding of evidence-based practice – some preliminary evidence. *Critical Care Nursing, 26 (6)*, 11-12.

Arai, L. (2003) Low expectations, sexual attitudes and knowledge: explaining teenage pregnancy and fertility in English communities. Insights from qualitative research. *The Sociological Review, 51 (2)*, 199-217.

Barr, W. (2000) Characteristics of severely mentally ill patients in and out of contact with community mental health services. *Journal of Advanced Nursing, 31(5)*, 1189-1198.

BBC News (2005a) Epidurals increase birth aid need. Available at http://news.bbc.co.uk/1/hi/health/4371552.stm, accessed 31 July 2009.

BBC News (2005b) Fresh drive to wipe out superbug. Available at http://news.bbc.co.uk/1/hi/scotland/4370730.stm, accessed 31 July 2009.

Beauchamp, T. and Childress, J. (2001) *Principles of Biomedical Ethics,* 5th edn. New York: Oxford University Press.

Beck, A.T., Steer, R.A. and Brown, G.K. (1996) *Beck Depression Inventory ® II*. San Antonio, TX: Pearson.

Becker, H. (1993) How I learned what a crock was. *Journal of Contemporary Ethnography, 22*, 28-35.

Beech, M. (2002) The way forward? *Journal of Community Nursing, 16 (3)*, online edition. Available at http://www.jcn.co.uk/journal.asp?Year=2002&Month=03&ArticleID=441, accessed 4 August 2009. NB Registration is mandatory before you can access this article via www.jcn.co.uk.

Bennett, J., Done, J., Harrison-Read, P. and Hunt B. (1995) A side effect scale/checklist to assess the side effects of anti psychotics by community psychiatric nurses. In E. White and C. Brooker (eds) *Community Psychiatric Nursing. A Research Perspective*. London: Chapman and Hall, pp. 1-19.

Bennis, W. and Nanus, B. (1985) *Leaders: The Strategies for Taking Charge*. New York: Harper and Row.

Bland, M., Bridge, C., Cooper, M., Dixon, D., Hay, L. and Zerberto, A. (2002) Professional nursing. Procedural restraint in children's nursing: using clinical benchmarks. *Professional Nurse, 17*, 712-715.

Blumer, H. (1969) *Symbolic Interactionism: Perspective and Method*. Berkeley, CA: University of California Press.

Brent Teaching Primary Care Trust (2004) *District Nursing Service Guidelines*. Available at http://www.brenttpct.org/doxpixandgragix/DNGUIDELINES.pdf, accessed 4 August 2009.

British Heart Foundation (2004) *Coronary Heart Disease Statistics*. London: The British Heart Foundation. Available at http://www.heartstats.org/.

Brown, J.B. and Addington-Hall, J. (2008) How people with motor neurone disease talk about living with their illness: a narrative study. *Journal of Advanced Nursing, 62*, 200-208.

Brown, S.A., Harrist, R.B., Villagomez, E.T., Segura, M., Barton, S.A. and Hanis, C. L. (2000). Gender and treatment differences in knowledge, health beliefs, and metabolic control in Mexican Americans with type 2 diabetes. *Diabetes Education, 26 (3)*, 425-438.

Bryman, A. and Cramer, D. (1997) *Quantitative Data Analysis with SPSS for Windows. A Guide for Social Scientists*. London: Routledge.

Bysouth, D. (2007) "Jolly good nutter": a discursive psychological examination of bipolar disorder in psychotherapeutic interactions. PhD thesis, Murdoch University, Australia. Available at http://wwwlib.murdoch.edu.au/adt/pubfiles/adt-MU20071217.34447/02Whole.pdf, accessed 15 August 2009.

Carney, T.F. (1990) *Collaborative Inquiry Methodology*. Windsor, Ontario, Canada: University of Windsor, Division for Instructional Development.

Carr, W. and Kemmis, S. (1986) *Becoming Critical*. Lewes: Falmer Press.

Castonguay, G. (2008) Short-stretch or four-layer compression bandages: an overview of the literature. *Ostomy/Wound Management, 54 (3)*, 50-55.

Clabo, L.M.L. (2008) An ethnography of pain assessment and the role of social context on two postoperative units. *Journal of Advanced Nursing, 61*, 531-539.

Clegg, F. (1982) *Simple Statistics: A Course Book for the Social Sciences*. Cambridge: Cambridge University Press.

Cohen, J. (1988) *Statistical Power Analysis for the Behavioral Sciences*. New York: Academic Press.

Coubrough, A. (2008) Minister calls for London's views on care for older people. *Nursing Times*, 24 July. Available at http://www.nursingtimes.net/whats-new-in-nursing/minister-calls-for-londons-views-on-care-for-older-people/1744134.article, accessed 15 August 2009.

Cowan, J. (1998) *On Becoming an Innovative University Teacher*. Buckingham: SRHE and Open University Press.

Cox, J.L., Holden, J.M. and Sagovsky, R. (1987) Detection of postnatal depression: development of the 10-item Edinburgh Postnatal Depression Scale. *British Journal of Psychiatry, 150*, 782-786.

Crew, S. (2006) A qualitative study on effects of working unsocial hours. *Nursing Times, 102 (23)*, 30-33. Available at http://www.nursingtimes.net/ntclinical/a_qualitative_study_on_effects_of_working_unsocial_hours.html, accessed 15 August 2009.

Dartford and Gravesham NHS Trust (undated) *Bridging team*. Available at http://www.dvh.nhs.uk/page.asp?node=394&sec=Bridging_Team, accessed 4 August 2009.

Davies, C. (2003) Establishing referral criteria. *Journal of Community Nursing, 17 (7)*. Online edition available at http://www.jcn.co.uk/journal.asp?Year=2003&Month=07&ArticleID=597, accessed 4 August 2009. NB Registration is mandatory before you can access this article via www.jcn.co.uk.

Davies, C.A. (1999) *Reflexive Ethnography: A Guide to Researching Selves and Others*. Abingdon: Routledge.

Denzin, N. (1978) *Sociological Methods: A Sourcebook*, 2nd edn. New York: McGraw Hill.

Department of Health (2001) *The National Service Framework for Older People*. London: HMSO.

Dheensa, S. and Williams, G. (2008) *The Psycho-Social Effects of Living with Neurofibromatosis Type 1: An Interpretative Phenomenological Analysis*. Poster presented at Health Psychology Annual Conference, organised by Division of Health Psychology of The British Psychological Society and the European Health Psychology Society, Bath, 9-12 September, 2008.

Dheensa, S. and Williams, G. (2009) 'I have NF. NF does not have me': an interpretative phenomenological analysis of coping with Neurofibromatosis Type 1. *Health Psychology Update, 18 (1)*, 3-8.

Dickens, G., Stubbs, J. and Haw, C. (2007) Difficulties in administering medication to older mental health inpatients. *Nursing Times, 103 (15)*, 30-31.

Doll, R. and Hill, A.B. (1950) Smoking and carcinoma of the lung: preliminary report. *British Medical Journal, 2*, 739-748.

Donne, J. (undated) *Devotions Upon Emergent Occasions, Meditation XVII*. See the following for the full quotation: http://isu.indstate.edu/ilnprof/ENG451/ISLAND/index.html, accessed 4 August 2009.

Eller, L.S., Kleber, E. and Wang, S.L. (2003) Self-reported research knowledge, attitudes and practices of health professionals. *Nursing Outlook, 51*, 165-170.

Folkman, S. and Lazarus, R.S. (1978) If it changes, it must be a process: study of emotion and coping during three stages of a college examination. *Journal of Personality and Social Psychology, 48*, 150-170.

Foucault, M. (2003) *The Birth of the Clinic*. London: Routledge.

Gabrel, C. and Jones, A. (2000) The National Nursing Home Survey: 1995 summary. *Vital and Health Statistics, 146*, 1-83.

Gibbs, G. (1988) *Learning by Doing: A Guide to Teaching and Learning Methods*. London: Further Education Unit.

Glaser, B. (1978) *Theoretical Sensitivity: Advances in the Methodology of Grounded Theory*. Mill Valley, CA: Sociology Press.

Greenhalgh, T. (2001) *How to Read a Paper*, 2nd edn. London: BMJ Books.

Guba, I. and Lincoln, Y. (2001) Guidelines and checklist for constructivist (aka Fourth Generation) evaluation. Available at http://www.wmich.edu/evalctr/checklists/constructivisteval.pdf, accessed 22 September 2009.

Gustavsen, B. (2001) Theory and practice: the mediating discourse. In P. Reason and H. Bradbury (eds) *Handbook of Action Research*. London: Sage, pp. 17-26.

Hairon, N. (2007) NICE guidance on antenatal and postnatal mental health. *Nursing Times, 103 (13)*, 25-26. Available at http://www.nursingtimes.net/ntclinical/nice_guidance_on_antenatal_and_postnatal_mental_health.html, accessed 15 August 2009.

Hammersley, M. and Atkinson, P. (1995) *Ethnography: Principles in Practice*, 2nd edn. London: Tavistock.

Harper, N. (2006) Investigating the techniques adopted to socially readjust after the onset of epilepsy in adulthood. Unpublished B.Sc. (Hons) Psychology with Social Science dissertation, Nottingham Trent University, Nottingham.

Harrington, A. (ed.) (1997) *The Placebo Effect. An Interdisciplinary Exploration*. Cambridge, MA: Harvard University Press.

Hobgood, C., Villani, J. and Quattlebaum, R. (2005) Impact of *emergency department* volume on registered nurse time at the bedside. A*nnals of Emergency Medicine, 46*, 481-489.

Hodgkins, C., Rose, D. and Rose, J. (2005) A collaborative approach to reducing stress among staff. *Nursing Times, 101 (28)*, 35-37.

Hrobjartsson A. and Gotzsche, P. C. (2001) Is the placebo powerless? An analysis of clinical trials comparing placebo with no treatment. *New England Journal of Medicine, 344*, 1595-1602.

Imai, K. and Nakachi, K. (1995) Cross-sectional study of effects of drinking green tea on cardiovascular and liver diseases. *British Medical Journal, 310*, 693-696.

Jacobson, B.F., Munster, M., Smith, A. *et al.* (2008) The BEST study – a prospective study to compare business class versus economy class air travel as a cause of thrombosis. *South African Medical Journal, 93*, 522-528.

Janis, I. (1972). *Victims of Groupthink*. Boston, MA: Houghton Mifflin.

Johns Hopkins Medicine (undated) *Hospital at Home*. Available at http:// www.hospitalathome.org/DGM/, accessed 4 August 2009.

Jones, A. (2002) The National Nursing Home Survey: 1999 summary. *Vital and Health Statistics, 152*, 1-116.

Kanter, R.M. (1983) *The Change Masters: Innovation for Productivity in the American Corporation*. New York: Simon and Schuster.

Kipling, R. (2001) *Just So Stories*. Mineola, NY: Dover Publications.

Kolb, D.A. (1984) *Experiential Learning: Experience as the Source of Learning and Development*. Englewood Cliffs, NJ: Prentice-Hall.

Larkin, M., Watts, S. and Clifton, E. (2006) Giving voice and making sense in interpretative phenomenological analysis. *Qualitative Research in Psychology, 3*, 102-120.

Laungani, P. and Williams, G. A. (1997) Patient-focused care: effects of organisational change on the stress of community health professionals. *International Journal of the Institute of Health Education, 35 (4)*, 108-114.

Lazarus, R.S. and Folkman, S. (1984) *Stress, Appraisal and Coping*. New York: Springer.

Lewin, K. (1951) *Field Research in Social Sciences*. New York: Harper and Row.

Limb, M. (2004) An evaluation survey of self-concept issues in adult clients undergoing limb reconstruction procedures. *Journal of Orthopaedic Nursing, 8,* 34–40.

Luck, L., Jackson, D. and Usher, K. (2008) STAMP: components of observable behaviour that indicate potential for patient violence in emergency departments. *Journal of Advanced Nursing, 59 (1),* 11–19.

Maltby, J., Day, L. and Macaskill, A. (2010) *Personality, Individual Differences and Intelligence.* Harlow: Pearson Education.

Maltby, J., Day, L. and Williams, G. (2007) *Introduction to Statistics for Nurses.* Harlow: Pearson Education.

Maslach, C. and Jackson, S.E. (1986) *Maslach Burnout Inventory*, 2nd edn. Palo Alto, CA: Consulting Psychologists Press.

Mays, N. and Pope, C. (1996) *Qualitative Research in Health Care.* London: BMJ Publishing.

McGarry J. (2003) The essence of 'community' in community nursing: a district nursing perspective. *Health and Social Care in the Community, 11 (5),* 423–430.

McGarry, J. (2007a) *Defining Roles, Relationships, Boundaries and Participation between Older People and Nurses within the Home Setting: An Ethnographic Study.* Doctor of Health Science thesis, University of Nottingham.

McGarry J. (2007b) Nursing relationships in ethnographic research: what of rapport? *Nurse Researcher, 14 (3),* 7–14.

McGarry, J. (2009) Defining roles, relationships, boundaries and participation between older people and nurses within the home: an ethnographic study. *Health and Social Care in the Community, 17 (1),* 83–91.

McGarry J. and Arthur, A. (2001) Informal caring in late life: a qualitative study of the experiences of older carers. *Journal of Advanced Nursing, 33,* 180–187.

McGarry, J. and Thom, N. (2004) User and carer involvement in nurse education programmes: towards the development of a supportive and meaningful participant framework. *Nursing Times, 100 (18),* 36–39.

McKnight, M. (2006) The information seeking of on-duty critical care nurses: evidence from participant observation and in-context interviews. *Journal of the Medical Library Association, 94,* 145–151.

Mead, M. (1928) *Coming of Age in Samoa.* New York: William Morrow.

Mead, M. (1930) *Growing up in New Guinea.* New York: William Morrow.

Mead, M. (1935) *Sex and Temperament in Three Primitive Societies.* New York: William Morrow.

Miles, M. and Huberman, A. (1994) *Qualitative Data Analysis: An Expanded Sourcebook,* 2nd edn. London: Sage.

Modigh, C., Axelsson, G., Alavanja, M., Andersson, L. and Rylander, R. (1996) Pet birds and risk of lung cancer in Sweden: a case-control study. *British Medical Journal, 313,* 1236–1238.

Moseley, J.B., Jr., Wray, N.P., Kuykendall, D., Willis, K. and Landon, G. (1996) Arthroscopic treatment of osteoarthritis of the knee: a prospective, randomized placebo-control trial. *American Journal of Sports Medicine, 24*, 28-43.

Moseley, J.B., O'Malley, K., Petersen, N.J., Menke, T.J., Brody, B.A., Kuykendall, D.H., Hollingsworth, J.C., Ashton, C.M. and Wray, N.P. (2002) A controlled trial of arthroscopic surgery for osteoarthritis of the knee. *New England Journal of Medicine, 347 (2)*, 81-88.

Naerde, A. (2000) Symptoms of anxiety and depression among mothers of pre-school children: effect of chronic strain related to children and child care-taking. *Journal of Affective Disorders, 58 (3)*, 181-199.

National Cancer Institute (2008) National Cancer Institute: U.S. National Institutes of Health. Available at http://www.cancer.gov/, accessed 31 July 2009.

National Primary Care Research and Development Centre University of Manchester (2007) *Manual. General Practice Assessment Questionnaire (GPAQ) Version 2.1*. For further information on the GPAQ and also how to obtain a version for nurses, access the following website http://www.gpaq.info/, accessed 15 August 2009.

NMC (2008) *The Code. Standards of Conduct, Performance and Ethics for Nurses and Midwives*. London: Nursing and Midwifery Council.

(NRES) National Research Ethics Service (2007) *Guidance for Applicants to the National Research Ethics Service*. London: NRES/National Patient Safety Agency.

(NRES) National Research Ethics Service (2008) *Defining research. Issue 8*. London: NRES/National Patient Safety Agency.

Øvretveit, J. (1995) Team decision-making. *Journal of Inter-Professional Care, 9*, 41-51.

Papa, K.S. (2008) *Symbolic Interactionism: Re-examining the Environment*. Published 12 August 2008. Available online at http://community.advanceweb.com/blogs/ltc_5/archive/2008/08/12/symbolic-interactionism-re-examining-the-environment.aspx, accessed 5 August 2009.

Petticrew, M. and Roberts, H. (2003) Evidence, hierarchies, and typologies: horses for courses. *Journal of Epidemiology and Community Health, 57*, 527-529.

Pittet, D., Allegranzi, B., Sax, H., Chraiti, M.-N., Griffiths, W. and Richet, H. (2007) Double-blind, randomized, crossover trial of three hand rub formulations: fast-track evaluation of tolerability and acceptability. *Infection Control and Hospital Epidemiology, 28 (12)*, 1344-1351.

Population Reference Bureau (2004) *Country Profiles for Population and Reproductive Health: Policy Developments and Indicators*. Washington, DC: Population Reference Bureau. Available at http://www.prb.org/.

Powell, H., Murray, G. and McKenzie, K. (2004) Staff perceptions of community learning disability nurses' role. *Nursing Times, 100 (19)*, 40-42.

Quirk, A. and Lelliott, P. (2002) Acute wards: problems and solutions. A participant observation study of life on an acute psychiatric ward. *Psychiatric Bulletin, 26*, 344-345.

Reason, P. and Bradbury, H. (eds) (2007) *Handbook of Action Research*. London: Sage.

Ritchie, J. and Lewis, J. (2003) *Qualitative Research Practice: A Guide for Social Science Students and Researchers*. London: Sage.

Rolfe, G. (1998) The theory-practice gap in nursing: from research-based practice to practitioner-based research. *Journal of Advanced Nursing, 28 (3)*, 672–679.

Rosendahl, E., Lundin-Olsson, L., Kallin, K., Jensen, J., Gustafson, Y. and Nyberg, L. (2003) Prediction of falls among older people in residential care facilities by the Downton index. *Aging Clinical and Experimental Research, 15 (2)*, 142–147.

Rosenthal, R. (1991) *Meta-analytic Procedures for Social Research*, Rev. edn. Newbury Park, CA: Sage.

Royal College of Nursing (2003) *Developing Referral Criteria for District Nursing Services: Guidance for Nurses*. London: RCN.

Russell, C., Toussard, D. and Porter, M. (2002) What's rapport got to do with it? The practical accomplishment of fieldwork in relations between young female researchers and socially marginalised older men. *The Qualitative Report, 7 (1)*, 1–18.

Schoolfield, M. and Orduña, A. (1994) Understanding staff nurse responses to change: utilization of a grief-change framework to facilitate innovation. *Clinical Nurse Specialist, 8*, 57–62.

Scott, B.M. (2003) *Situational Positioning: A Grounded Theory of Registered Nurse Decision-making in Western Australian Nursing Homes*. PhD thesis, Curtin University of Technology, School of Nursing and Midwifery, Australia. Available at http://espace.library. curtin.edu.au:80/R?func=dbin_jump_full&object_id=13781, accessed 5 August 2009.

Silverman, D. (1987) *Communication and Medical Practice*. London: Sage.

Silverman, D. (2007) *A Very Short, Fairly Interesting and Reasonably Cheap Book about Qualitative Research*. London: Sage.

Skrabanek, P. and McCormick, J. (1994). *Follies and Fallacies in Medicine*, 4th edn. Whithorn: Tarragon Press.

Smith, J.A. (1996) Beyond the divide between cognition and discourse: using interpretative phenomenological analysis in health psychology. *Psychology and Health, 11*, 261–271.

Smith, M. (2005) Does encouragement boost visual acuity testing results? *Nursing Times, 101*, 35, 38–41.

Stotts, R.C., Roberson, P. K., Hanna, E. Y., Jones, S. K. and Smith, C. K. (2003) A randomised clinical trial of nicotine patches for treatment of spit tobacco addiction among adolescents. *Tobacco Control, 12(4)*, 11–15.

Strachan, D.P., Butland, B.K. and Anderson, H.R. (1996) Incidence and prognosis of asthma and wheezing illness from early childhood to age 33 in a national British cohort. *British Medical Journal, 312*, 1195–1199.

Strauss, A. and Corbin, J. (1998) *Basics of Qualitative Research Techniques and Procedures for Developing Grounded Theory*, 2nd edn. London: Sage.

Tavakol, M., Torabi, S. and Zeinaloo, A.A. (2006) Grounded theory in medical education research. *Medical Education Online, 11 (30)*, 1–6. Available at http://www.med-ed-online.org/ volume11.htm, accessed 5 August 2009.

The Healthcare Commission (2007) *Caring for Dignity: A National Report on Dignity in Care for Older People while in Hospital*. London: Healthcare Commission.

Thomas, P. (2006) General medical practitioners need to be aware of the theories on which our work depend. *Annals of Family Medicine, 4*, 450-454.

Ung, Y.C., Maziak, D.E., Vanderveen, J.A. *et al.* (2007) [18]Fluorodeoxyglucose positron emission tomography in the diagnosis and staging of lung cancer: a systematic review. *Journal of National Cancer Institute, 99*, 1753-1767.

Vallenga, D., Grypdonck, M.H.F., Tan, F.I.Y., Lendemeijer B.H.G.M. and Boon, P.A.J.M. (2008) Improving decision-making in caring for people with epilepsy and intellectual disability: an action research project. *Journal of Advanced Nursing, 61*, 261-272.

Wakefield, A.J., Harvey, P. and Linnell, J. (2004) MMR—responding to retraction. *The Lancet, 363, (9417)*, 1327-1328.

Ward, E., King, M., Lloyd, M. *et al.* (2000) Randomised controlled trial of non-directive counselling, cognitive-behaviour therapy, and usual general practitioner care for patients with depression. I: Clinical effectiveness. *British Medical Journal, 321*, 1383-1388.

Ware, J.E., Snow, K.K., Kosinski, M. and Gandek, B. (1993) *SF-36® Health Survey Manual and Interpretation Guide*. Boston, MA: New England Medical Center, The Health Institute. Further information available from http://www.sf-36.org/tools/sf36.shtml#LIT, accessed 15 August 2009.

Watts, S., O'Hara, L. and Trigg, R. (in press) Living with Type 1 diabetes: a by-person qualitative exploration. *Psychology and Health*, DOI: 10.1080/08870440802688588

Williams, G.A. (2002) Cross-cultural and sex differences in job stress, somatisation, and mental ill-health. In R. Roth and F. Farley (eds) *The Spiritual Side of Psychology at Century's End*. Lengerich: Pabst Publishers, pp. 269-279.

Williams, G.A. and Albery, I.P. (2003) *Neuroticism Biases Work Stressor-Strain Links and Should be Statistically Controlled*. Poster presented at 5th Annual Conference of European Academy of Occupational Health Psychology, Berlin, 20-21 November 2003.

Williams, G.A. and Laungani, P. (1999) Analysis of teamwork in an NHS Community Trust: an empirical study. *Journal of Inter-Professional Care, 13*, 19-28.

Willig, C. (2001) *Introducing Qualitative Research in Psychology. Adventures in Theory and Method*. Maidenhead: Open University Press.

Willis, B. and Wortley, P. (2007) Nurses; attitudes and beliefs about influenza and the influenza vaccine: a summary of focus groups in Alabama and Michigan. *American Journal of Infection Control, 35*, 20-24.

World Medical Association (2000) *Declaration of Helsinki Ethical Principles for Medical Research Involving Human Subjects*. Available at http://www.wma.net/e/ethicsunit/helsinki.htm, accessed 4 August 2009.

Worrall, K. and Williams, G.A. (2004) *Exploring the Relevance of 'Flow' in Explaining Paediatric Nurses' Satisfaction and Enjoyment at Work*. Paper presented at the British Psychological Society Annual Conference, Imperial College, London, 15-17 April 2004.

Xu, Y. and Kwak, C. (2007) Comparative trend analysis of characteristics of foreign and native nurses in the United States of America. *International Nursing Review, 54*, 78-84.

Index

Note: Boxes, Figures and Tables are indicated by *italic page numbers*, and Glossary terms by **emboldened numbers**